Intraoperative Flow Cytometry

Georgios Alexiou • Georgios Vartholomatos
Editors

Intraoperative Flow Cytometry

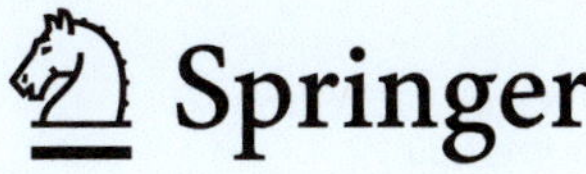 Springer

Editors
Georgios Alexiou (iD)
Dept. of Neurosurgery
University of Ioannina
Ioannina, Greece

Georgios Vartholomatos (iD)
Unit of Molecular Biology and
Translational Flow Cytometry
University Hospital of Ioannina
Ioannina, Greece

ISBN 978-3-031-33519-8   ISBN 978-3-031-33517-4   (eBook)
https://doi.org/10.1007/978-3-031-33517-4

This Springer imprint is published by the registered company Springer Nature Switzerland AG
The registered company address is: Gewerbestrasse 11, 6330 Cham, Switzerland

This book is dedicated to

*my wife Iocasti and my children Evrysthenis
and Alexandros.*

Georgios Vartholomatos

This book is dedicated to

my parents and grandparents.

Georgios Alexiou

Foreword

Current evolution of point-of-care diagnostics and precision medicine requires affordable and precise cell counting technologies. Since surgical removal is typically the first course of treatment of malignant tumors, definition of their resection margins requires such precision and accuracy. Achieving clear tumor resection margins is imperative to avoid re-intervention and to diminish the rates of cancer recurrency. Several approaches and technologies have been suggested to precisely characterize tumor margins in order to ensure complete removal.

Aneuploidy and high proliferative potential are distinct hallmarks of neoplastic cell frozen section analysis, which constitutes the standard intraoperative assessment for tumor margin evaluation and tumor resection. However, in recent years, the technique of flow cytometry represents the most applied method for measuring cellular DNA content in individual cells. Modern flow cytometers have evolved into more user-friendly versions, mainly through the use of intuitive digital interfaces and simplified operation protocols. Hence, intraoperative flow cytometry (iFC) has recently been proposed as a new approach to analyze DNA content/ploidy and cell cycle distribution during surgical resection of tumors to characterize cancer cells and to evaluate the status of resection margins.

Pioneers in this effort are the editors, authors, and coauthors of this book. The iFC approach was initially implemented in central nervous tumor surgeries using an innovative rapid cell cycle analysis protocol (the Ioannina protocol) they developed for the intraoperative identification of neoplastic cells. The utility of this protocol has been subsequently evaluated in several additional cancer types, including head and neck malignancies, breast cancer, pancreatic tumors, hepatocellular and other gastrointestinal malignancies. The results of this evaluation are presented in great detail in Parts III–VI of the book, with each part being prefaced by a review of currently used standard methods in the assessment of tumor surgical margins. It is concluded that, in most cases, iFC presents a high sensitivity and specificity, and an accuracy of over 90%. This diagnostic quality combined with an analysis time less than 10 min makes iFC a novel reliable tool in the surgical theater.

It is worthy to note that Parts I and II of the book are devoted to an informative description of the basic principles and the sample data analysis of both flow cytometry as a technic and specifically iFC; these sections are presented after a compelling presentation of the history of flow cytometry, very sentimental for the readers who recall those times.

It is without a doubt that large-scale studies are required to evaluate this very promising method. However, those interested in implementing novel approaches, especially oncologists and surgeons not familiar with the technology of flow cytometry, will find this book extremely useful. As the advent of iFC expands the horizons of use of flow cytometry in surgical oncology, this book can be a valuable introduction to those who wish to enter the field. In its last chapter, the perspectives of iFC are presented, including the development of novel protocols for other types of cancer-excision surgery, the addition of phenotypic markers to cell cycle analysis, the application of real-time iFC analyzers, and the correlation of iFC data with imaging findings.

Dear reader, welcome to the world of iFC! Whether you are familiar with the field or not, you will find real value in reading through this book cover to cover.

School of Medicine   Anastasios E. Germenis
University of Thessaly
Volos, Greece

Academy of Athens
Athens, Greece
agermen@med.uth.gr

Preface

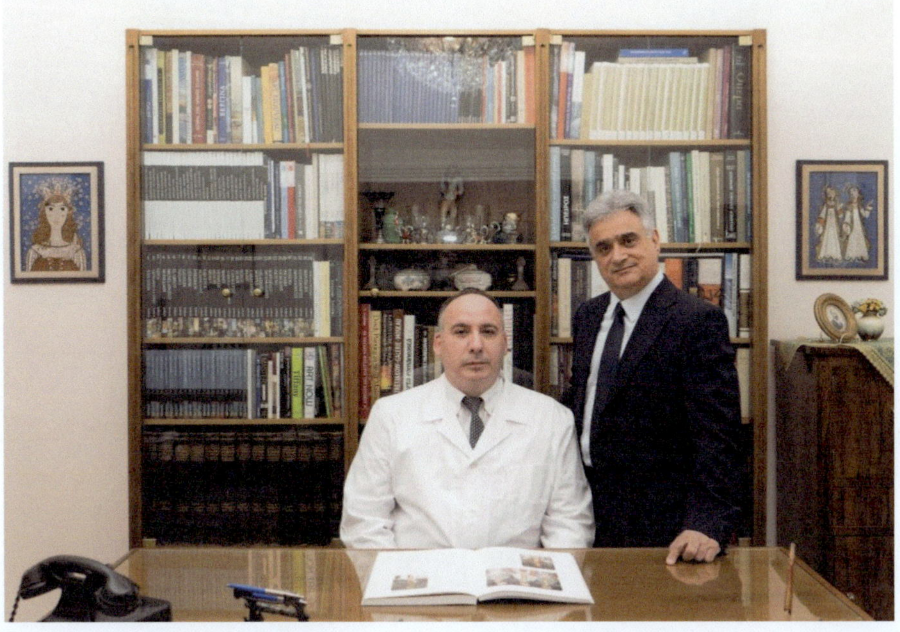

We are excited to present the first book on intraoperative flow cytometry. This book grew out of work conducted at the University Hospital of Ioannina, Greece. The book includes six parts: general topics, intraoperative flow cytometry, intraoperative flow cytometry in central nervous system malignancies, breast cancer, head and neck malignancies, gastrointestinal malignancies, and future perspectives. We aim to report current knowledge on this novel intraoperative technique for solid tumor surgery that comes from several disciplines that collaborated to refine this method. The book is intended as an introduction to the field of intraoperative flow cytometry for basic scientists, neurosurgeons, general surgeons, head and neck surgeons, and related disciplines such as radiologists, pathologists, and oncologists. As summarized in the final chapter, the future holds many additional promising applications. Certainly, as with any novel technique, excitement must be tempered by the knowledge obtained following ongoing studies and clinical experience. Finally, we would like to express our gratitude to all contributors for their effort, and we hope our readers will share our enthusiasm.

Ioannina, Greece   Georgios Alexiou
                                                                  Georgios Vartholomatos

Contents

Part I
General Topics

Chapter 1
History of Flow Cytometry

Katherina Psarra and Alexandra Fleva

1.1 Introduction

As the history of scientific discipline studies its evolution, this is what will be narrated in this chapter: the evolution of flow cytometry from its onset till today, or tomorrow (today is always a tomorrow for flow cytometry). It is worth recalling though that the Greek word istoria (history) is derived from istor (ιστωρ) meaning judge, appreciator, witness. This is the magic word for flow cytometry, witness. The people who write about the history of flow cytometry are real witnesses, they saw it from the beginning, they were there, they are still there, or some of them left very recently. Howard Shapiro left very recently, and he witnessed and wrote about "ancient history," "classical history," and "modern history" of flow cytometry in his classical book "Practical Flow cytometry."

An important and fascinating characteristic of flow cytometry related to the history is its multidisciplinary character. From the starting point until today (as this book will demonstrate) computer specialists, electronics experts, mathematicians, optical and fluidics engineers, and organic chemists worked together with biologists, physicians, and surgeons around the flow cytometer bench. All these people consider themselves lucky to have encountered flow cytometry and to collaborate with many scientists of different origins for the successful evolution of flow cytometry. All these researchers irrespectively of their scientific background consider themselves cytometrists and contribute with their intelligence and imagination in the spectacular and constant optimization of the machines and their applications.

K. Psarra (✉)
Immunology Histocompatibility Department, Evangelismos Hospital, Athens, Greece

A. Fleva
Department of Immunology – Histocompatibility, Flow Cytometry Laboratory, Papageorgiou General Hospital, Thessaloniki, Greece

© The Author(s), under exclusive license to Springer Nature Switzerland AG 2023
G. Alexiou, G. Vartholomatos (eds.), *Intraoperative Flow Cytometry*,
https://doi.org/10.1007/978-3-031-33517-4_1

1.1.1 History of the Machines

1.1.1.1 Microscopy

The history of the machines themselves, of flow cytometers, commences with the history of microscopy. Flow cytometers are considered automated fluorescent microscopes. Microscopes have been used, since the seventeenth century, to examine cells and tissue sections. After Leeuwenhoek, who visualized protozoa and bacteria by using a high-power magnifying lens, the first microscope was built in 1590. The first modern microscope was built by Carl Zeiss and his collaborators Ernst Abbe and the chemist Otto Schott in Jena Germany, at the end of the nineteenth century. In 1904 August Kohler of Zeiss observed fluorescent emission produced by ultraviolet light in an ultraviolet microscope. This technology was refined by many companies at the end of the World War I [1]. In the 1940s and 1950s, fluorescent stains incorporated into the nucleic acids of malignant cells and the cell suspension was placed on a glass slide and observed under a new device that included a lamp and filters. Fluorescence microscopy was emerged and added to the great inventions and helping tools for the flow cytometry's evolution.

1.1.1.2 The Coulter Principle

In the 1950s the Coulter brothers Wallace H. Coulter and Joseph R. Coulter Jr. founded an industry producing instruments to count cells automatically [2]. Andrew Moldavan had published a note in science in 1934 about a photoelectric technique for the counting of microscopic cells [3]. The Coulter principle was published on October 3, 1956, in Wallace's technical paper. "In the new counter, individual cells are directed to move through a small constricted electric current path suspended in fluid and detection is based upon differences in electrical conductivity between the cell and the suspending fluid" [4]. The Coulter principle applied for the measurement of the cell's or particle's volume has been embraced in the development of many sophisticated instruments, including flow cytometers. The Coulter counters incorporated many of the flow cytometers characteristics: single cells flow quickly through a flow cell, signals of these cells are detected electronically and analyzed automatically.

1.1.1.3 The Rise of Computers

At the end of the 1950s and the beginning of 1960s, computers made their appearance in several research institutions. From then on, discussions and collaborations began taking place, for the incorporation of mathematical models, computer diagnosis and computer use in several instruments and the automation of the results analysis.

Computers provided the possibility to document details of cells images and store them. Computers in the 1960s needed huge rooms with air-conditioning, required a lot of power and the cost was immense for a very small capacity in comparison to a nowadays laptops. But a few groups of analytical cytologists, among which the ones at the university of Chicago at the end of the decade of 1960 began using computers as they became smaller in size. The use of computers remained very expensive for all the first models of flow cytometers until the beginning of 1980s. Without computers the conception of gating (selecting a particular cells population) would not be possible. Once computers were connected to the early flow cytometers multiparametric flow cytometry became possible.

1.1.1.4   Hydrodynamic Focusing

In 1953 PJ Crosland-Taylor, working at the Middlesex Hospital in London, applied the principles of laminar flow to the design of a flow system. By injecting a suspension of red blood cells into the center of a faster flowing stream, the cells were aligned one after the other in a single line, introducing the principle of hydrodynamic focusing, which has been pivotal for the design of flow cytometers [5].

1.1.1.5   Flow Cytometers

In 1934 Andrew Moldavan in Montreal published a paper, proposing the counting of cells flowing in a capillary with the use of a photodetector attached to a microscope, but it was never documented that he actually built this machine. This flowing system along with the staining procedures developed over the next decade enabled the quantification of the flowing cell characteristics. In 1947 Gucker and his colleagues built an apparatus, where an air stream containing the sample was injected in the center of a larger air stream passing through the observation point of a microscope [6]. This apparatus is recognized as the first flow cytometer used for the evaluation of cells.

In 1965 Louis Kamentsky, after visiting Caspersson's laboratory in Stockholm to learn about micro-spectro-photometry, built a flow cytometer, based on microscopy. The machine used the scatter of blue light to estimate the size of the cells and UV absorption to estimate nucleic acid content. The rate of the cells flow was around 500 cells/second [7]. In 1967, an instrument was built to sort "unusual" from "normal" cells for a more detailed study and a computer was connected to the machine by Kamentsky and Melamed in 1969 [8].

Hemalog D produced by Technicon Corporation under the guidance of Ornstein is mentioned as the first commercial differential leukocyte counter by flow cytometry [9].

At the same time, Kamentsky and Melamed built their first sorter connected to the flow cytometer, using a syringe pump. In 1965, Mark Fulwyler in Stanford, Los

Alamos, built a sorter based on the recently developed ink jet printer technology, where droplets containing cells were produced and sorted [10].

In 1969, in Munster Germany, cellular DNA content of alcohol-fixed cells was determined by Dittrich and Göhde using ethidium bromide fluorescence, with a flow cytometer, later Partec Impuls cytophotometer (ICP) instrument, based on a microscope that included a flow chamber [11].

At the same year, the Los Alamos team led by Martin Van Dilla built an instrument where light illumination and collection axes were positioned at right angles to each other and to the direction of sample flow, incorporating hydrodynamic focusing also. In their publication on the detection of fluorescence from the Feulgen-DNA staining of Chinese hamster ovary cells and leukocytes, as well as of their Coulter volume, they anticipated further use of their device in the future [12].

At Stanford Leonard Herzenberg and his colleagues [13] built their instruments trying to sort living cells. Their first attempt using an arc lamp illumination was not very successful, but when they used fluorescently labeled antibodies and a water-cooled argon laser their attempt was a real success [14]. This led to the commercialization of the instrument with the name fluorescence—activated cells sorter (FACS) in 1974 by Becton—Dickinson (BD) now BD Biosciences (San Jose, CA, USA).

Mack Fulwyler directed Particle Technology a Coulter electronics subsidiary in Los Alamos (now Beckman Coulter). They built the TPS-1 (Two Parameter Sorter), which was the first flow cytometer produced and marketed by Coulter in 1975. It used an air-cooled 35-mW argon ion laser illumination and could measure forward scatter and fluorescence. Monoclonal antibodies invention and technology (César Milstein and Georges J. F. Köhler, Nobel Prize in physiology or medicine, in 1984.) led to the great impact of vast classification for internal and surface cellular components [15].

ISAC (the Society of Analytical Cytology, now the Society for Advancement of Cytometry) was founded in 1976. At that time BD, Coulter and Ortho were producing flow cytometers determining forward and side scatter and fluorescence of two different wavelengths. They were counting thousands of cells per second and were capable of sorting. DNA content analysis was considered very important as a risk factor especially concerning breast cancer and other tumors. A successful experiment by Loken, Parks, and Herzenbergin 1977 introduced fluorescence compensation [16].

1.1.1.6 Bench Top Flow Cytometers

A lot of instruments succeeded these first pioneer flow cytometers. We are all aware of the immense advances that have led to the modern flow cytometers, which form a part of clinical laboratories all over the world. All biosciences related research institutions and flow cytometrists will continually be a vital part of the evolution of flow cytometry since cell signals are always subject to artificial fluorescence and may not be what they appear to be as an electric signal. Therefore the human perceptive will never be replaced. A lot of applications will be presented in the following chapters and will prove the greatness of flow cytometry in the past, now, and in the future.

References

1. Clark G, Karsten FH. History of staining. 3rd ed. Baltimore: Williams and Wilkins; 1983, x + 304pp.
2. Marshal D. The Coulter principle: foundation of an industry. J Assoc Lab Autom. 2003;8(6):72–81.
3. Moldavan A. Photo-electric technique for the counting of microscopical cells. Science. 1934;80:188–9.
4. Coulter WH. High speed automatic blood cell counter and cell size analyzer. Proc Natl Electronics Conf. 1956;12:1034.
5. Crosland-Taylor PJ. A device for counting small particles suspended in a fluid through a tube. Nature. 1953;171:37–8.
6. Gucker FT Jr, O'Konski CT, Pickard HB, et al. A photoelectric counter for colloidal particles. J Am Chem Soc. 1947;69:2422–31.
7. Kamenstky LA, Melamed LA, Derman H. Spectrophotometer: new instrument for ultrarapid cell analysis. Science. 1965;150:630.
8. Kamenstky LA, Melamed LA. Spectrophotometric cell sorter. Science. 1967;156:1364.
9. Ornstein L, Ansley HR. Spectralmatching of classical cytochemistry and automated cytology. J Histochem Cytochem. 1974;22:453.
10. Fulwyler MJ. Electronic separation of biological cells by volume. Science. 1965;150:910.
11. Dittrich W, Göhde W. Impulsfluorometrie by einzelzellen in Suspensionen. Z Naturforsch. 1969;24b:360.
12. Van Dilla MA, Trujillo TT, Mullaney PF, et al. Cell microfluorimetry: a method for rapid fluorescence measurement. Science. 1969;163:1213.
13. Herzenberg LA, Sweet RG, Herzenberg LA. Fluorescence-activated cell sorting. Sci Am. 1976;234:108–15.
14. Bonner WA, Hulett HR, Sweet RG, et al. Fluorescence activated cell sorting. Rev Sci Instrum. 1972;43:404.
15. Köhler G, Milstein C. Continuous cultures of fused cells secreting antibody of predefined specificity. Nature. 1975;256:495–7.
16. Loken MR, Parks DR, Herzenberg LA. Two-color immunofluorescence using fluorescence-activated cell sorter. J Histochem Cytochem. 1977;25:899.

Chapter 2
Basic Principles of Flow Cytometry

Marianna Tzanoudaki and Evgenia Konsta

2.1 Introduction

Flow cytometry (FC) represents the technology which enables the multiparametric assessment of various particles such as eukaryotic cells, bacteria, plankton, LATEX beads or cell organelles, and other subcellular particles. The particles are in the form of cell suspension and flow in front on a light source at a rate of several thousand per second. The light that is generated by the interaction of the particles and the light beam is transferred through a complex configuration of filters and mirrors to multiple light detectors. The generated light is enriched with the use of fluorescent dyes, which can be selectively bound on cells, mainly using monoclonal antibodies. The collected light signals are then amplified, digitally converted, and eventually entered in a computer system. Results are based on the analysis of thus generated data, with the use of specialized software.

The above stand for classical flow cytometry which can be described as a successful combination of hematology analyzer and fluorescence microscope, applying the latest advances in microscopy, biochemical analysis, and computer evolution. Flow cytometers can be considered as automated immunofluorescence microscopes, which have the significant advantage over the latter that they can examine and measure cells individually, at a much higher rate, assessing many more parameters than those measured with microscopy (Fig. 2.1). This fact allows identification and study

M. Tzanoudaki (✉)
Department of Immunology & Histocompatibility, Specific Reference Centre for Primary Immunodeficiencies -Paediatric Immunology, "Aghia Sophia" Children's Hospital, Athens, Greece

E. Konsta
Laboratory of Microbiology, Department of Water Quality Control, EYDAP, Athens, Greece

G. Alexiou, G. Vartholomatos (eds.), *Intraoperative Flow Cytometry*, https://doi.org/10.1007/978-3-031-33517-4_2

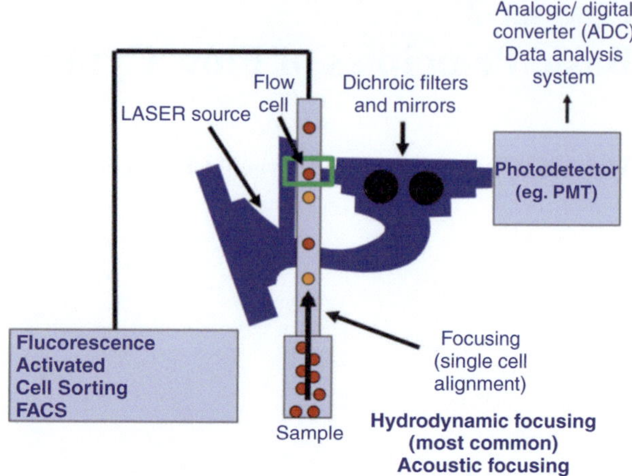

Fig. 2.1 Schematic comparison of a flow cytometer to a microscope

of very small cell populations and rare features, indicating that sensitivity of cytometry far exceeds than that of microscopic observation. Although flow cytometers are expensive, they are user friendly, highly specialized and with a high degree of automation [1–5].

Nowadays, FC constitutes a diagnostic tool in clinical laboratories but also an extremely useful technology in research laboratories. This technology can be used in fields as various as Hematology, Oncology, Immunology, Infectious Diseases, Transplantation, Microbiology, and even Marine Environment Biology.

Flow cytometry has been recently enriched by new technologies such as spectral flow cytometry, mass cytometry, and single cell sequencing, taking advantage of evolutions in computer science, mass spectrometry, and nucleic acid sequencing, respectively. An additional long-standing extension of flow cytometry is fluorescence activated cell sorting (FACS) in which any individual cell, can be selectively separated from the suspension, based on their characteristics [1–3, 6, 7]. As these technologies have not yet been applied on intraoperative DNA analysis, the next paragraphs are going to focus on the basic principles of classical flow cytometry.

2.2 The Flow Cytometer and How It Works

A flow cytometer consists of three systems (Fig. 2.2): (a) *hydrodynamic system*, which forces cells (or particles) to flow one after the other in front of a light beam where they interact with it, (b) *optical system*, which creates and collects the optical signals produced, and (c) *computer system*, which converts and processes signals and stores them, allowing re-evaluation and different analysis approaches [4, 8].

Fig. 2.2 Basic configuration of a classical single LASER Flow Cytometer. The addition of more LASER sources increases the number of fluorochromes that can be simultaneously detected

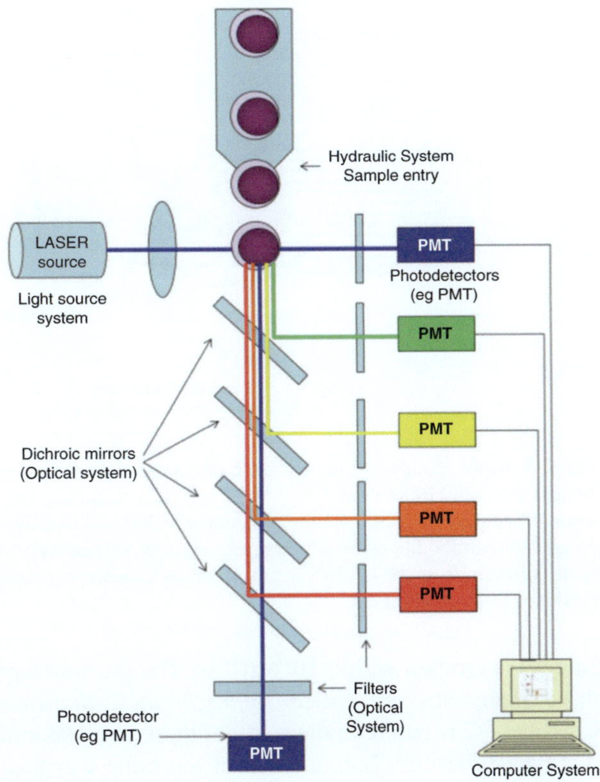

2.2.1 *The Hydrodynamic System: How Particles Are Aligned*

An essential condition of FC analysis is that the suspended cells are aligned in a narrow linear flux, which will lead them in front of the light source and allow uniform illumination of each cell separately. This is usually achieved by hydrodynamic focusing and the use of a fluid, called Sheath Fluid that exerts pressure on the cell suspension without mixing with it. Proper operation of the velocities and pressures of sheath fluid and cell suspension allows the alignment of the flow of cells without turbulence. Sheath fluid can be substituted by sound waves in Acoustic Flow Cytometers [1–4, 6–8].

2.2.2 *Interaction of Light with Particles: Light Scatter and Fluorescence*

When a light beam falls on a particle it may have two possible fates: It may either be absorbed or scattered (diffracted or reflected). If light is absorbed by molecules that are excited by its specific wavelength, light of longer wavelength (i.e., lower

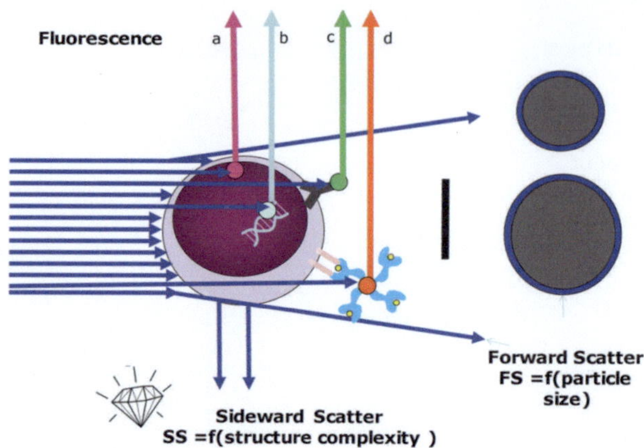

Fig. 2.3 Light scatter and fluorescence phenomena generated by the incidence of LASER light beams on a cell. Fluorescent dyes may be naturally occurring (**a**), may specifically bind on nucleic acids (**b**) or may be conjugated to molecules which specifically recognize cell structures, such as monoclonal antibodies or MCH tetramers (**c** and **d**, respectively). Note that scattered light is of the same wavelength as the LASER beam, whereas fluorescence radiation wavelengths depend on the existence of fluorescent dyes

energy) is emitted within 10^{-9}–10^{-6} s. The phenomenon is called fluorescence and these molecules are called *fluorochromes, fluorophores, or fluorescent dyes*. Classical FC is based on the study of these two phenomena (Fig. 2.3).

Light *diffraction* [i.e., a beam of the same wavelength shifted at a small angle (1–10°)] is called horizontal or forward scatter (FSC) and mainly depends on particle size. Light *reflection* (i.e., a change in the beam direction at an angle to the perpendicular to the particle's surface), when it is diffuse, is called vertical or side scatter (SSC) and depends on the particle's structural complexity (such as cell granulation).

Fluorescent molecules can be naturally found in cells (especially in dying or apoptotic cells). However, FC is mainly based on the specific binding of fluorescent dyes (Fluorochromes) on the particles of interest. This can be achieved either by using dyes which specifically bind on certain molecules, such as the nucleic acid dyes (ethidium bromide (EB) and propidium iodide (PI)) which are widely used in intraoperative flow cytometry and are discussed in Chap. 5. However, most FC applications use fluorochromes conjugated with molecules with specific binding properties as (first and foremost) monoclonal antibodies, but also MHC tetramers or mRNA probes.

In FC, fluorochromes fall into several groups including small organic molecules, phycobiliproteins, quantum dots (Qdots), polymer dyes, tandem dyes, fluorescent proteins, nucleic acid dyes, proliferation dyes, viability dyes, and calcium indicator dyes. The development of tandem dyes, containing two fluorochromes, the first exciting the second one, has increased the number of labeled proteins to be used. Selection of fluorochromes depends on the instrument's LASER wavelengths (excitation wavelength) and the fluorescent dye's emission spectra (which must be compatible with the instrument optical system and different from one another). Throughout the years, there has been an increasing demand for fluorochromes with different emission spectra so that cells could be simultaneously stained for many characteristics. The need for excitation light of different wavelengths has increased the number of LASERs in each instrument.

Fluorochromes should be ideally stimulated all by the same wavelength and have different emission spectra. Nevertheless, emission spectra of usual fluorochromes show partial overlap, generating false positive signals in the PMTs designated to other fluorochromes (Fig. 2.4). The false positive signals may be removed by using an additional electronic procedure, called *compensation of spectral overlap* [4, 6–8].

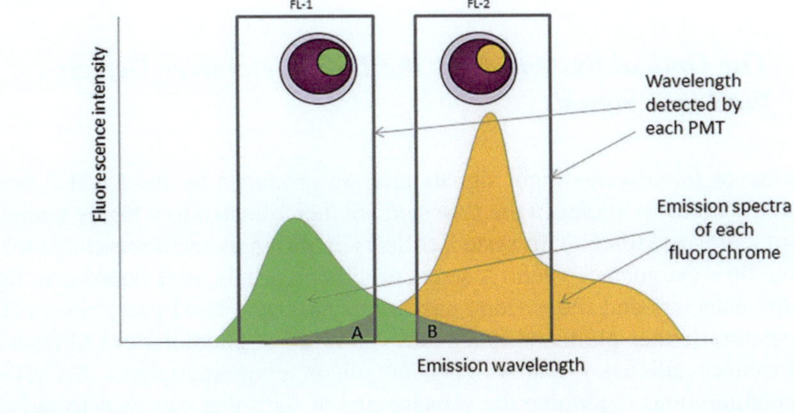

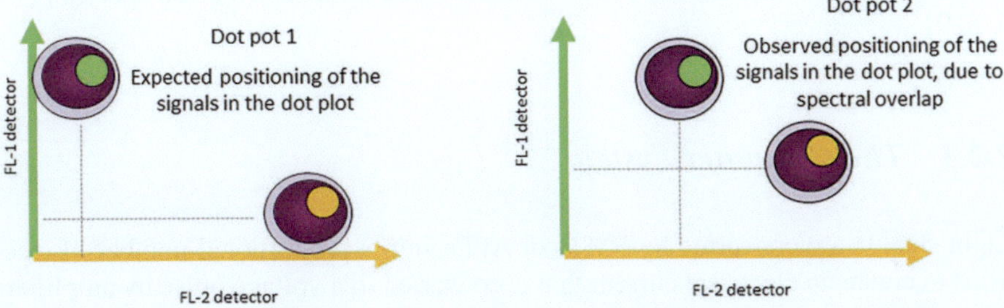

Fig. 2.4 Explanation of spectral overlap by using two imaginary fluorochromes green and orange. Green is measured in the FL-1 channel while orange in FL-2 channel. Grey parts A and B indicate false positive signals in neighboring channels due to spectral overlap

2.2.3   The LASER Beam

To draw safe and predictable conclusions from its incidence on particles, the light beam should be monochromatic (of a certain wavelength), coherent (all of the light waves in phase), directional (all rays parallel to each other), and bright. This is achieved by using LASER light. Flow cytometers are equipped with various categories of LASER sources: gas LASERs, solid state LASERs: crystals and most commonly LASER diodes (e.g., red, green or violet diode LASERs or near-UVdiode LASERs). Lenses are used to shape and focus LASER beam, as it must be carefully aligned to the particle suspension stream. The specific characteristics of the instrument's LASERs dictate the choice of fluorochromes. More LASERs of different wavelengths can exist in the same instrument, increasing the number of fluorochromes that can be used simultaneously and thus the number of studied parameters [1, 2, 4, 6, 8].

2.2.4   The Optical System: How the Flow Cytometer Detects the Light Signals

The scatter or fluorescence light signals that are produced by the LASER beam interaction with the particles in the *flow cell*, are then directed to a highly complex system of lenses and filters. This system collects light signals and directs them to the electronic flow cytometer system. A series of dichroic filters steer fluorescent light to specific detectors and filters (long pass, short pass, and band pass) towards the photodetectors [either photomultiplier tubes (PMTs) or photodiodes (APDs-with better quantum efficiency than PMTs), or silicon photomultipliers (SiPMTs)]. These configurations determine the wavelengths of light that can be detected and therefore the fluorochromes that can be used based on their emission spectra [1–4, 6, 8, 9].

2.2.5   The Computer System

Light signals are converted by PMTs or APDs into a proportional number of electrons to create an electrical current that is converted to a voltage pulse by amplifiers (pre- and main amplifiers). This amplification can be adjusted by the users by modifying photodetector Voltage or Gain. Voltage pulse is then digitized by an analog to digital converter (ADC). The reported digitized numbers can be used to describe three signal properties: integrated area (proportional to the intensity of the original light signal), height or width. Amplification may be linear (mostly for scatter signals and DNA analysis) or logarithmic (for fluorescence signals). Generally, developments in the past two to three decades have led to the replacement of analog circuitry with only linear amplification followed by fast high bit-depth digitization and purely digital signal processing. Binary signals fall into channels representative of different light intensities, whose number depends on the number of bits. The more the channels the better the signal resolution [1–4, 6–9].

2.2.6   Data Display and Analysis

Signals converted to digital data can be displayed as histograms or plots, using either linear, logarithmic or semi-logarithmic (logicle) axes. Frequency distribution histograms are single parameter plots, where the x-axis represents the intensity of the signal fluorescence and the y-axis shows the number of cells (events) per digital channel. Dot plots are 2-dimensional plots in which it is possible to simultaneously present and study two parameters: one on x-axis and one on y-axis (Fig. 2.5). Each dot represents a single event generated by the passage of a cell in front of the LASER beam. Dots may be given different colors, depending on the values of various other parameters, providing thus additional information on the studied cells. Two-dimensional plots also include the density (dot) plot, where two parameters are displayed as frequency distribution and the contour plot, where density of the events is displayed as contour lines (Fig. 2.6). Moreover, there are 3-D plots as well as radar plots combining multiple parameters. However, increase in the number of parameters and complexity in experiments is leading to the use of newer cluster data analysis algorithms such a PCA, SPADE, and t-SNE [10].

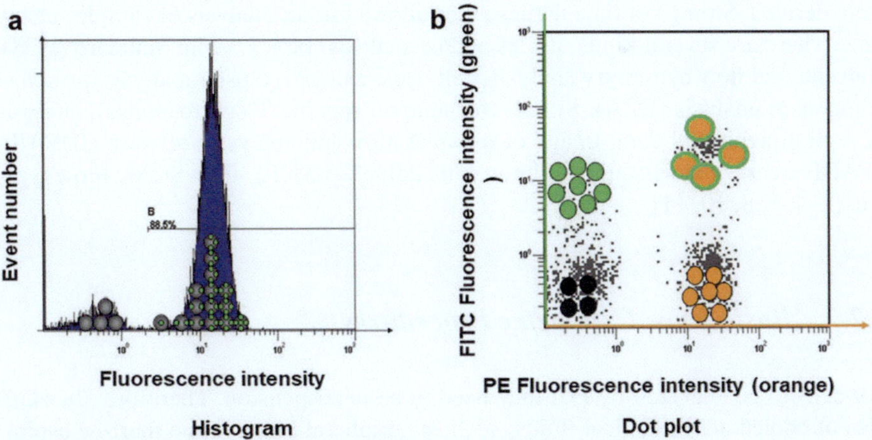

Fig. 2.5 (**a**) Typical monoparametric histogram, representative of the number of events (cells) designated to digital channels according to fluorescence intensity. (**b**) Typical dot plot, in which dots represent events (cells) placed according to fluorescence intensity of two different fluorochromes

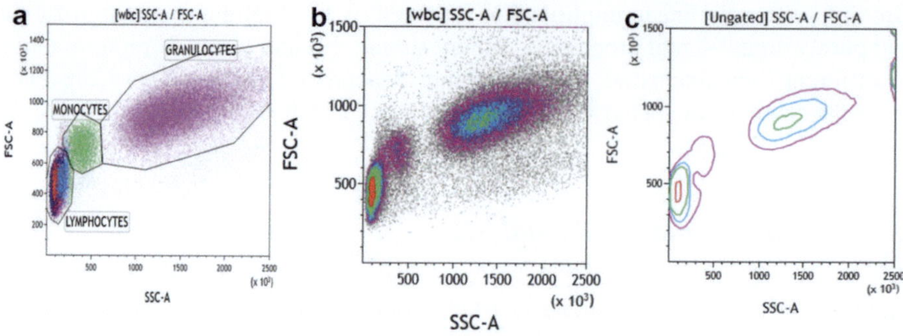

Fig. 2.6 The three basic types of 2-parametric plots: (**a**) Typical dot plot, (**b**) density plot, and (**c**) contour plot

Events in dot clusters or histogram peaks can be electronically selected with the use of *gates*. Gates can be drawn in various shapes (polygons, squares, rectangles, freehand, etc.) and enable statistics display on the cell subset of interest (event count, absolute count, percentages, mean/median fluorescence intensity, etc.). Moreover, the gated events can be used in many additional ways: new plots may be generated, including only the gated population with new gates drawn in them. This process multiply repeated is called *sequential gating* and is essential for the analysis of rare subsets (Fig. 2.7). Boolean logic rules may be additionally applied to enhance the acquired information. Deciding which gate to draw in which dot plot combinations is called *gating strategy*, is an essential part of the analysis and depends on the Flow Cytometrist's expertise and knowledge.

Finally, all analysis data can be collected and stored in files. In these files, all fluorescence and scatter measurements are combined with the cell from which they were derived. Storage of data in these files allows further analysis of samples at any time. There are several kinds of files and/or analysis: FCS 3.1 File Standard (FCS), conventional flow cytometry analysis, cell cycle analysis, cluster analysis, principal component analysis (PCA), SPICE (for antigen-specific T cell response), analysis of high dimensional data, image data exploration and analysis software (IDEAS), SPADE trees, "t-stochastic neighbor embedding" (t-SNE), FlowSOM, FlowType, etc. [2–4, 6, 8, 10, 11]

2.2.7 Basic Flow Cytometry Procedures

For cells to be analyzed by FC, they need to be in suspension. Therefore, the samples of choice are biological fluids, such as peripheral blood, bone marrow aspiration or cerebrospinal fluid. Samples prone to clotting, as peripheral blood or bone marrow, need to be collected in anticoagulant containing tubes (usually EDTA or heparin). In the case of solid tumors or any tissue sample, cells must be

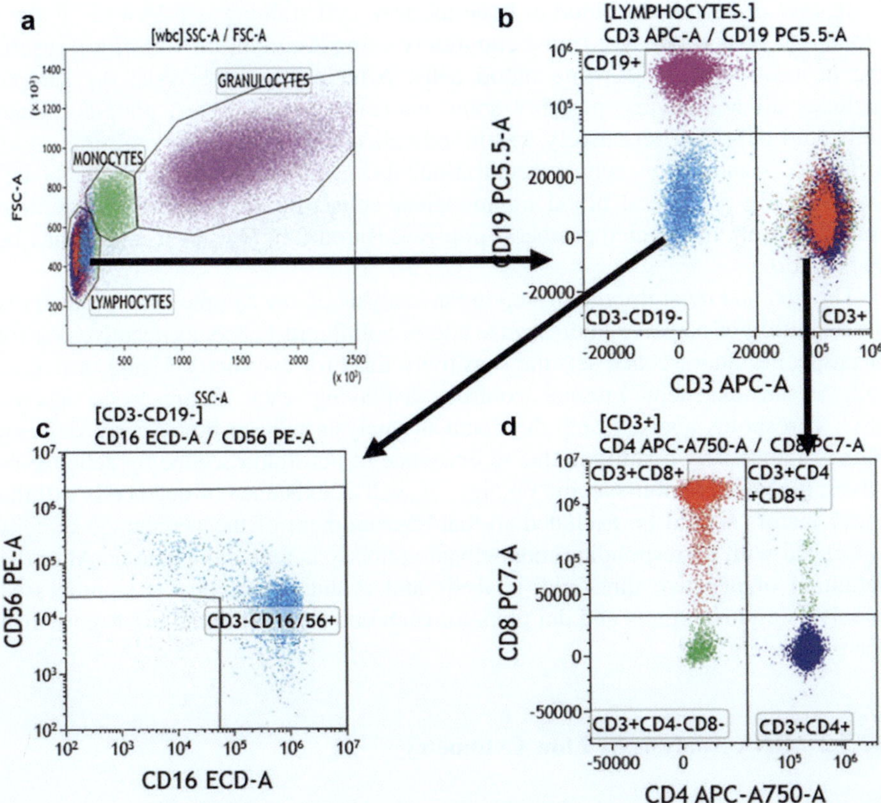

Fig. 2.7 A plot of forward versus side scatter for leukocytes from the peripheral blood (A) indicates that regions can be drawn around cells with different scatter characteristics, marking lymphocytes, monocytes, and neutrophils. These regions can be used to define gates. Plot B includes only those events of the lymphocyte gate (i.e., it is gated in lymphocytes). Plots C and D include events from specific quadrants of plot B. Plot C is gated on CD3-CD19 events and plot D is gated on CD3 + CD19 events. Using this kind of sequential gating one characterizes the basic lymphocyte subsets. (APC, ECD, PC5.5, PE PV7, and APC-A750 symbolize different fluorochromes.)

homogenized and released from the tissue with appropriate enzymes (pepsin, trypsin, etc.) or mechanical disintegration [2, 4, 6, 8, 12].

2.2.7.1 Classical Clinical Flow Cytometry

Generally, in FC, the treatment of cells with labeled monoclonal antibodies before analysis allows the identification of surface antigens, cytoplasmic antigens, and components of the cell nucleus, thus determining cellular origin, stage of differentiation, and function. Regarding the study of intracellular antigens, sample can be further processed to make the cell membrane permeable.

In case of peripheral blood or bone marrow, cell staining is followed by a red blood cell lysis procedure (most commonly using Ammonium Chloride), resulting in a suspension of white blood cells. After erythrocyte lysis, the sample includes all leukocytes, possibly some nucleated erythrocytes, platelets, dead cells, and debris. Alternatively, red blood cell lysis may precede staining, in an effort to standardize cell concentration, in a process called "bulk lysis." Occasionally peripheral blood mononuclear cells may be selected by gradient centrifugation. In selected protocols non-Red Blood Cell lysis procedures may be chosen too.

The first and most important step in the analysis of any sample in a cytometer is the definition of negative fluorescence and/or autofluorescence, as negative control or unspecific fluorescence sets the sensitivity limit for cytometry. Using unstained cells is an excellent internal control, displaying each fluorescence against SSC. Thresholds above which the result of analysis will be positive are defined. This is a necessary condition, due to existence of autofluorescence by cells themselves, the possible non-specific binding, as well as existence of dead cells. All the above factors should be excluded so that measurement of the percentage of cells associated with corresponding monoclonal antibody is real and accurate. After the definition of negative threshold, analysis and evaluation of results is processed mainly using histograms and dot plots for each one or a combination of more than one parameters [13].

2.2.7.2 DNA Analysis by Flow Cytometry

Flow Cytometric DNA analysis will be described in detail in Chap. 5.

2.2.8 Applications of Flow Cytometry

Flow cytometry is a modern, fast and reliable technique with multiple applications.

In hematology, it is used for the study of Leukemias, Lymphomas, Myelodysplastic Syndrome, and Multiple Myeloma, thus contributing to diagnosis, determination of the cell lineage, assessment of maturation stage, classification, detection of measurable residual disease (MRD) for treatment monitoring and, in some cases, prognosis and detection of PNH (paroxysmal nocturnal hemoglobinuria) clones [3, 6, 14].

In Immunology it contributes to the delineation of mechanisms underlying not only immune responses to pathogens and vaccines, but also autoimmunity or cancer immunology, with antigen-specific cell studies and cytokine profile evaluation. Most importantly, it is an essential clinical tool for the diagnosis and monitoring of primary and secondary immunodeficiencies (such as HIV infection). It may be combined with functional assays for Lymphocyte proliferation or function, intracellular Ca++ influx studies or kinase phosphorylation [2, 3, 6, 7, 15–17].

In the context of Hematopoietic Stem Cell Transplantation, it is essential for CD34+ enumeration and the assessment of immune reconstitution. In solid organ transplantation it is used for donor-recipient serological crossmatch [3, 7, 18].

DNA and cell cycle analysis has been among the first applications of FC and will be discussed in detail in the next chapters. Briefly, it determines the percentages of cells that are in various phases of cell cycle, ploidy, and DNA changes, which often accompany many malignancies [4, 6, 8, 19]. Measurement of apoptosis markers by rapid and quantitative measurement as well as measurement of cell proliferation based on a variety of markers [2, 7, 19].

In addition to the study of various cell populations, flow cytometry can identify other particles, such as organelles, chromosomes, nuclei, mitochondria, and extracellular vesicles or even microorganisms or beads [2, 3, 6, 7].

2.3 Quality Control in Flow Cytometry Experiments

Although Flow Cytometry is a very exciting method, it is also a tool that should be handled with caution! The path towards important discoveries is teeming with pitfalls that may lead to erroneous, misleading, or discrepant results. Therefore, whoever wants to venture in its world, should be aware of the factors that may influence result quality and of ways to monitor and control them. Knowledge of the above important facts will not only help scientists—preventing them from time and resource consuming mistakes, frustration, and rejected manuscripts—but also, and most importantly, will protect the patients who depend on them.

Moreover, the high variability of acquired signals and results among multiple centers had been hampering the introduction of flow cytometry in multicenter studies for years. Efforts for standardization of flow cytometry protocols have been increasingly adopted, paving the path for large scale clinical studies. This is also important for the implementation of the newest computational algorithms, whose basic and most important prerequisite for consistent results is the use of high-quality data, derived from standardized protocols [10, 20–23].

2.3.1 How Is Quality Is Assessed in Flow Cytometry?

To answer this key question, we should first recall some basic parameters which characterize a flow cytometry experiment. These are the Fluorescence Intensity (FI) of the signals, the Median or Median Fluorescence Intensity (MFI) of a cluster of signals and net results. These parameters are used to calculate a series of statistical indexes, whose description is beyond the scope of this book. Of those, the one that is the probably most useful for monitoring Quality Control in everyday practice is the Coefficient of Variation (CV = Standard Deviation × 100/mean)).

What should be kept in mind by every ambitious Cytometrist is that CV mirrors measurement precision and is strongly related to method resolution. It can be applied either within a certain experiment by using the Fluorescence intensity generated by theoretically identical particles or among different experiments, by using the MFI and the result values. Ideally, all identical particles should fall in the same intensity channel and CV of their FIs should be zero. Similarly, all identical experiments, either performed in the same instrument or performed in centers situated in different continents, should produce exactly the same result and the CV of MFI and the results should be zero too. As we do not live in a perfect world, we just aim to achieve the lowest possible CV. Just like in the case of high-quality focusing lens on a telescope, a low CV will permit us to detect even subtle differences among various cell subsets, which could otherwise be blurred. It the case of DNA and cell cycle analysis, this is of utmost importance. Whoever disregards the importance of maintaining the lowest possible CV, will just miss any subtle aneuploidies [20–22].

An additional value that describes the quality of a FC experiment is the signal-to-noise ratio or stain index (SI). The SI describes the difference of fluorescent intensity between positive and negative signals. The goal of an optimally designed protocol is not only to achieve bright signals of the positive populations, but also to keep the signals of negative subsets (i.e., the "noise") as dim as possible. Maintaining the highest possible SI will improve the discrimination of different populations and enhance the sensitivity of the method [4, 8].

One must keep in mind that continuous quality control is required for generating consistent and reproducible results. This encompasses method validation, daily checks of instrument performance, use of internal controls as well as participation in external quality control schemes [24–26].

2.3.2 Factors that Influence Result Quality and Recommended Corrective Actions

Result quality is influenced by a variety of factors which depend on the specific Flow cytometric method used. Since classical flow cytometry (as compared to spectral cytometry, mass cytometry, and single cell sequencing) is mostly used in DNA analysis for clinical purposes, the factors described below mostly concern this method. They can roughly be classified into (1) Instrument related, (2) Preanalytical, (3) Analytical, and (4) Data analysis related (Table 2.1) [21, 23, 25, 27, 28].

Table 2.1 Major factors influencing result quality in flow cytometry

Factor	Consequences of poor performance	Corrective actions
Instrument related		
Poorly maintained instrument fluidics	Turbulent flow causing elevated measurement CVP	Clean instrument daily and before rare event analysis experiments
	Increase of noise	
	"Carry over" phenomenon	
Light beam and flow stream alignment	Elevated CV in signal intensity measurement	Check signal intensity CV daily with calibration beads
		Keep instrument on a stable surface
		Keep a steady room temperature
Photodetector and LASER source instability	Non-standardized dot plot images	Check signal intensity stability, and adjust photodetector gain with calibration beads
	Unreliable quantitational measurements (DNA analysis included)	Use TIME parameter to detect any instability within a certain run
Preanalytical		
Poorly designed antibody combination (panel)	Excess spillover among channels, resulting in non-specific signals, low discriminatory capacity, and low specificity and sensitivity	Carefully design antibody panel adhering to multicolor panel rules
		Use freely available panel builder software
		Consult published protocols and optimized multicolor immunofluorescence panels (OMIPs)
		Test selected panels before their final implementation
Poor sample quality	Excess noise, suboptimal staining	Use fresh samples
		Use cell preservative if applicable
		Discard clotted samples

(continued)

Table 2.1 (continued)

Factor	Consequences of poor performance	Corrective actions
Poorly titrated reagents	Suboptimal signal to noise ratio, leading to poor discriminatory capacity especially of weak signals	Always titrate reagent quantity in relation to cell concentration
		Consider titration when opening a new lot of "research only" reagents
		Keep cell concentration within a narrow range
Variable incubation time and temperature	Non-standardized dot plot images	Define standard operating procedures and stick to them
Pipetting errors	Erroneous results	Apply a system for organizing reagents according to panels
		Always check pipetted reagent volume in the tip
		Ensure the tip is empty after pipetting
		Drop reagents on the bottom of the tube and NOT its walls
		Use premixed antibody combinations if available
		Use cell subsets with known immunophenotype as internal controls, for checking correct pipetting
Reagent instability	Erroneous results	Maintain optimal storage conditions
		Protect from light
		Double check in-house cocktails
		Use tandem dyes for high turn-over markers, to reduce their shelf life
Analytical factors		
Too elevated flow rate	Turbulent flow causing elevated measurement CV	Maintain the lowest flow rate possible, especially when increased precision is required (DNA analysis)
	Increase in percentage of doublets	
Suboptimal or not fixed photodetector voltage/gain settings	Suboptimal signal to noise ratio, leading to poor discriminatory capacity	Perform "gaintration" experiments
	Problematic compensation of spectral overlap	Use target settings if available
		Do not interfere with voltage/gain settings once compensation is completed

Table 2.1   (continued)

Factor	Consequences of poor performance	Corrective actions
Poor compensation of spectral overlap	False positive or false negative results	Perform compensation experiments every 2–4 weeks
		Perform compensation experiments on the cell subset of choice
		Perform compensation experiments using each specific panel reagent
		Do not import compensation settings from other panels
		Avoid weakening (manual adjustment of compensation)
Low number of acquired events	Low sensitivity	Calculate minimum total event count based on the target population percentage and on maximum permitted CV
	Low target cell subset count causing elevated measurement CV	
Data analysis		
Failure to remove confounding signals	Poor discriminatory capacity	Use FS/SS plots to exclude debris
	Low sensitivity	Use FS-H/FS-A plots to exclude doublets
		Use TIME parameter to exclude events generated by air bubbles or during clogging of the instrument
		If possible, use viability dyes to remove dead/apoptotic cells
Poorly designed gating strategy	Inconsistent results	Consult published protocols and optimized multicolor immunofluorescence panels (OMIPs)
		Ask for experienced operator assistance
Failure to adhere to a specific gating strategy	Inconsistent results	Use the same gating strategy for all samples
	Non-reproducible results	Reanalyze all samples in case of alterations in gating strategy
Poor training	Erroneous/non-reproducible results	Do not perform FC without proper training
		Experiment with data before
		Ask for experienced operator assistance
Overall performance		
		Continuously validate you methods
		Participate in external quality schemes

2.3.2.1 Instrument Related Factors

Proper instrument maintenance is of utmost importance, as a poorly performing Flow Cytometer may be an important source of errors [20, 21, 26–28].

Firstly, instrument fluidics must be kept in a perfect condition. Any accumulated debris will cause turbulence which will increase signal variability and result in increased CV. Moreover, debris may generate signals which will increase unwanted noise. Most importantly, cells from a previous experiment may remain in the tubing system and generate signals that will be erroneously added to the following run, resulting in a "carry-over" effect. It is therefore important to thoroughly clean the instrument, not only when switching it on and off, but also before any measurements requiring high sensitivity, like DNA analysis. Additionally, the use of the TIME parameter may be helpful for gating out, any "carry-over" signals.

Alignment of the flow stream to the LASER beam needs to be carefully adjusted, as a poor alignment may contribute to an increased CV in Signal Intensity. Fortunately, the alighnment of most contemporary instruments is kept relatively stable over time. However, it may be easily distorted by mechanical factors (such as moving the instrument or placing it on vibrating surface) or by extreme temperature fluctuations. Therefore, keeping a stable position and environmental temperature are crucial for instrument performance. Alignment should be checked daily, by monitoring the CV of the signals generated by commercially available beads. Any CV increase that is not corrected after thoroughly cleaning the instrument, warrants technical support.

Instability of photodetector sensitivity and LASER beam intensity used to be important issues in the past. Although modern Flow Cytometers have significantly been improved regarding the above issues, Photodetector sensitivity may still deteriorate over time and needs to be regularly assessed. Especially in experiments that heavily rely on signal intensity measurements, (just like those of DNA and cell cycle analysis), it is important to calibrate the instrument to minor sensitivity fluctuations and keep a low CV of MFI in between experiments and throughout the years. Moreover, any attempts of multicenter instrument harmonization may be hampered if this instability is not circumvented. This is achieved by the use if yet another kind of commercially available calibration beads with strictly defined fluorescence intensity. In most modern instruments, once the beads do not generate their target MFI values, signal amplification is automatically adjusted to correct MFI as needed.

2.3.2.2 Preanalytical Factors

Introducing high-quality samples in the flow cytometer is crucial for producing consistent and reliable results. Preparation steps (i.e., panel design, reagent selection, sample collection, and staining procedure) all involve procedures that are prone to errors [7, 23, 27, 28].

Panel design is a major step during the implementation of new protocols. Increasing availability of antibody clones and fluorochrome conjugates inflates the number of possible combinations, making the problem even more perplexing. Rules that may help successful panel design either rely on fluorescence intensity (dictating the use of bright fluorochromes for detecting dimly expressed markers and vice versa) or on fluorochrome spectral overlap and spillover (proposing that fluorochromes which a high spillover percentage should be conjugated with mutually exclusive markers, i.e., markers that are not expected to be co-expressed). However, the optimal antibody clone often depends on the study question and the cell type of interest. Moreover, and frustratingly enough, even the most meticulous design may yield disappointing results. This is the reason why multiple candidate combinations should be tested before reaching the final decision [29]. To save time and money, one could refer to already published panels and especially those issued by large study groups or belonging to the OMIP (Optimized Multicolor Immunofluorescence Panels) group of protocols. The latter can be found in

https://onlinelibrary.wiley.com/doi/toc/10.1002/(ISSN)1552-4930. OMIPscollection

Sample quality constitutes yet another factor which may be accounted for highly variable or discrepant results. Anticoagulant used (was it EDTA or heparin?), sampling method and conditions (risk of hemodilution bone marrow samples), time from sampling, cellularity, any use of freezing and thawing methods, any prior stimulation should be carefully documented. Apart from certain self-evident facts (e.g., the older the sample gets the poorer the result quality), there is not always a golden rule as to the best sample parameters, which, however, should be harmonized among different experiments or various centers.

Staining protocol is also a major determinant of result quality. Most importantly, the optimal final concentration of the staining reagents must be carefully determined in titration experiments. Less than optimal concentration will result in dim staining of the positive events, whereas too much reagent will increase unspecific fluorescence signals (noise). Both of the above result in a low signal-to-noise ratio and poor discrimination of the positive population. Notably, reagent titration depends on cell concentration, especially in extremely concentrated or diluted samples. It is also important to consider that the addition of multiple reagents in the cell suspension changes its final volume, influencing the final concentration of each single reagent. This means that the reagent volume to be pipetted is usually different than the one used in single stain titration experiments. Failure to properly titrate the reagents may produce mistakes that cannot be compensated in later stages. Titration may be warranted for every new lot of reagents, especially if there is an elevated risk of lot-to-lot variability, as in the case of "research only" products [27, 28, 30].

Apart from reagent concentration, staining conditions, such as incubation time and temperature, strongly influence the results. Many protocols propose incubation on ice, to minimize non-specific staining, but require prolonged incubation time. In addition to staining reagents, choice of red blood cell lysis solution or any fixation or permeabilization solution, as well as centrifugation and washing steps all have an impact on the results. Again, there is no golden rule on the optimal protocol, other than the need for establishing predetermined Standard Operating Procedures (SOPs), which should be followed in every experiment.

Technical issues during the staining procedure may also constitute a source of variability. Pipetting errors (mis pipetting the wrong reagent, forgetting to pipet reagents or pipetting the reagents on the walls of the tube, rather than to its bottom) can occur even in the most experienced laboratories. Although, premixed antibody combinations may reduce the risk of mispipetting, there are stability issues, especially in the case of in-house cocktails. Hence, validated commercially available ones may be a useful alternative. Stability issues may arise regarding single reagents too, especially those containing tandem dyes (i.e., dyes consisting of two different fluorochromes, with one parent fluorochrome exciting the other). Breaking down of tandem dyes will give false positive signals in the wavelength of the parent fluorochrome and yield erroneous results. Therefore, maintaining optimal storage conditions (mainly recommended temperature and protection from exposure to light) may prevent future failures [27, 30].

2.3.2.3 Analytical Factors

The final image that is generated during the analysis of a properly stained sample in a classic Flow Cytometer depends heavily on the acquisition and compensation settings of the instrument. Acquisition settings should always be determined before the analysis, whereas compensation settings can be modified in later stages as well [20, 21, 23, 27, 28].

Acquisition settings mainly include the flow rate, the photodetector voltage/gain, and threshold determination. As an increased flow rate (i.e., the velocity of the cell suspension) may cause turbulence and increase the CV of signal intensity, it is important to maintain the lowest flow rate possible in experiments requiring low CVs, like DNA analysis. This is in contrast with rare event analysis experiments, in which the need for acquisition of as many events as possible in a reasonable amount of time, occasionally permits an increase in the flow rate, in the expense of the CV [31].

Setting the photodetector voltage and gain, determines the intensity of the electric signal that is generated by each light signal, which will in turn determine how far away from the "0" point on the plot axes the population of interest (and the noise too!) will be situated. Optimal settings may be calculated in "gaintration" experiments, based on the signal-to-noise ratio. However, in multicenter studies, target settings are given, which can be achieved with the use of multiple peak beads. Gain and voltage settings are adjusted so that the MFI of each peak falls within predetermined limits. In cannot be overemphasized that it is extremely important not to interfere with fluorescence voltage and gain settings once they are determined for a set of experiments, especially in DNA analysis [4, 8].

Apart from voltage gains, it is usually possible to set a lowest threshold, below which photodetector signals are not recorded. This usually concerns the Forward Scatter Photodetector and helps preventing the inclusion of debris signals in the analysis. However, if a threshold is too high, important signals may be discarded too, this being a commonly made mistake.

The number of acquired events may also influence the results, especially in the case of rare event analysis. The optimal number of events is mainly determined by the number of cells of interest (target events) that should be acquired, as this directly influences the measurement's CV. Acquiring too few events may reduce the sensitivity of a method. Moreover, differences in the number of acquired events may be a source of discrepant results between runs [31–33].

Compensation of fluorochrome spectral overlap is also a crucial step towards generating high-quality results. It is extremely important that compensation is carefully adjusted and that is specific to the reagents used. Undercompensating may give false positive results, whereas over-compensating may hide cell subsets. In short, both distort dot plot images and constitute a serious source of errors (Fig. 2.8). Spillover compensation is automatically calculated in modern Flow Cytometers once the proper single tube experiment has been concluded. This experiment involves staining cells (or commercially available compensation beads) with a single marker in every tube. In this way percentage of interference with other fluorescence channels can be calculated and reduced from the respective signals. It is of utmost importance that the reagents used are the ones of the experiment. Importing compensation settings from other experiments, even if they contain the same fluorochromes, may be too risky. Moreover, calculations should be specific for the cell type of interest, as different cell types (i.e., lymphocytes, monocytes, mesenchymal cells, cancer cells) exhibit various levels of autofluorescence and signal intensities. Finally, in most instruments, whose photodetectors have logarithmic properties, compensation settings are specific for the photodetector voltage/gain settings that have been chosen. Any interference with the voltage settings will need calculation of new compensation settings. This is not the case in instruments with linearly behaving photodetectors, in which compensation settings may be adjusted to any gain alterations. What is important to remember (and relieving to most cytometrists)

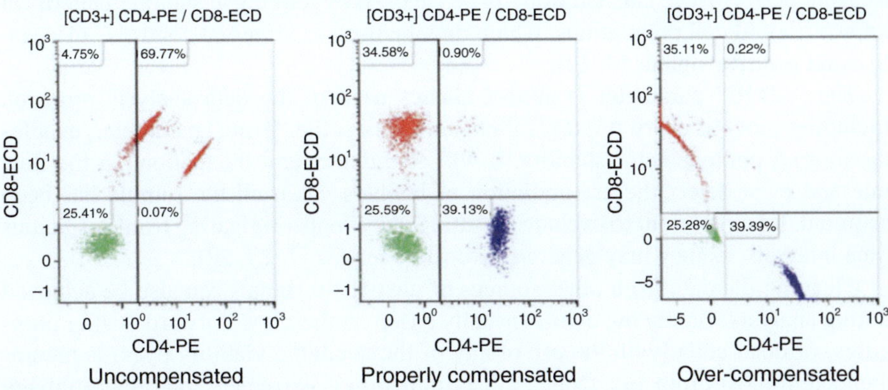

Fig. 2.8 Dot plots of the classical CD4+ vs. CD8+ combination, showing how suboptimal compensation settings may distort dot plot images and, hence, results. Note the semi-logarithmic (logicle) scale on the axes, which is particularly useful for detecting over-compensation issues (right)

is that spillover compensation can be adjusted after acquisition too, during data analysis. However, it is useful to have compensated data during acquisition, as this will permit the detection of mistakes that may be corrected before it is too late [4, 8, 27, 28, 34].

2.3.2.4 Data Analysis Related Factors

Data analysis, it yet another challenging or (according to many cytometrists) the most challenging part of a flow cytometry experiment [4, 27, 35]. There are numerous gating strategies published in books and journals, some of them being part of consensus guidelines and widely implemented. They are totally experiment dependent and, once again, there are no golden rules as to the optimal data analysis strategy. Modern software, using machine learning algorithms, have changed the way flow cytometrists look at data and have revolutionized flow cytometry analysis. However, in view of all this tremendous amount of information, there are some basic rules that, if followed, help improve result quality.

To start with, it is important that exactly the same gating strategy is used, when comparing experiments. One major source of mistakes is comparing results generated by different gating strategies. It is commonly the case that the definition of cell subsets differs among various data analysis protocols. Fortunately, one of the advantages of flow cytometry is that it gives the opportunity of re-analyzing the data and harmonize the way results are generated between runs or among different laboratories.

Most analysis protocols, though, include some common steps that help improve experiment quality. Drawing ungated dot plots of all markers versus Sideward or Forward Scatter is always recommended. Not only does it give information on the proper performance of the reagents, but also it may detect any pipetting errors. Reagent performance can additionally be checked by looking at staining patterns of known normal cell populations, which may be used as "internal controls" of negative and positive signals [4, 13].

The "TIME" parameter is almost always used in the data analysis protocol. Including plots of every fluorescent channel versus the "Time" parameter, enables monitoring photodetector stability. It will also detect any fluctuations in the flow rate and even detect the accumulation of bubbles when all the sample has been acquired. It is important to exclude by gating any events originating from suspicious time intervals, as they may generate erroneous results [7, 27, 28].

Cleaning the data from other sources of unspecific signals can also be achieved during analysis. Gating out debris (usually based on their low Forward Scatter properties) or dead cells (with the use of any of the available viability dyes) is recommended in most protocols. Doublet discrimination is extremely important in many experiments that detect aberrant co-expressions (as two aggregated cells will generate one signal expressing both their markers) and in DNA analysis (as two aggregated cells may falsely generate a signal of an aneuploid cell). Doublets are excluded based on the differences of the pulse generated by them from the one generated by normal single cells. The ratio of pulse area/pulse height is commonly used, as well

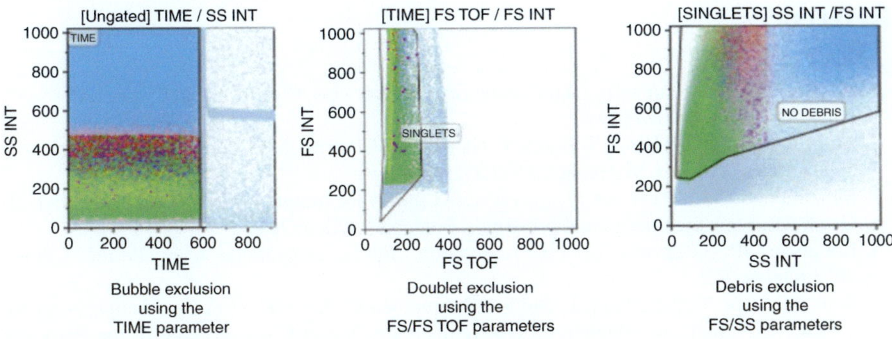

Fig. 2.9 Basic tools for "cleaning" FC data, to facilitate their further analysis

as the "time-of-flight" parameter (which is increased in doublets) [7, 27, 28] (Fig. 2.9).

An obstacle than always needs to be overcome is subjectivity in cytometric data analysis. Gating strategies cannot always describe the exact positioning of the gates nor the exact ways to discriminate cell populations, negative from positive or bright from dim expression. Many decisions rely on the use of controls, be it isotypic (anti-mouse antibody of the same isotype and conjugated with the same fluorochrome as the one in use), fluorescence minus one (eliminating one antibody from the combination to check for false positive signals in the respective channel), unstimulated or normal control. Still, to avoid discrepant or inconsistent results, extensive training is required and interlaboratory collaborations are set, in an effort to harmonize the way results are generated. As a compromise, it may even be agreed that speaking the same language is more important than conquering the absolute truth. New computational tools are struggling to overcome this limitation, but there is still a long way until we reach a level in which any cell subset discrimination is unanimous and undisputable [10, 11, 27, 35].

2.4   Concluding Remarks

Flow cytometry is an exciting, versatile, and continuously evolving method for fast multiparametric cell analysis. Although bioinformatics has started to change the way data are analyzed, most clinical applications rely on manual gating and subjective interpretation. Therefore, complying with the rules that have been established for generation of quality results is of utmost importance for interlaboratory collaborations for the patients' profit. It cannot be overemphasized that a successful Cytometrist knows the basic principles and the possible pitfalls, is well trained by experienced colleagues, creates collaborations with other laboratories and is always ready to doubt his own practices. For timidity in view of the grandeur of biological, physical, and chemical phenomena, is the only way to adapt to an evolving and demanding field, such as flow cytometry.

References

1. Büscher M. Flow Cytometry Instrumentation – an overview. Curr Protoc in Cytom. 2018; e52. https://doi.org/10.1002/cpcy.52.
2. Adan A, Alizada G, Kiraz Y, Baran Y, Nalbant A. Citometría de flujo: principios básicos y aplicaciones. Crit Rev Biotechnol. 2017;37:163–76.
3. McKinnon KM. Flow cytometry: an overview. Curr Protoc Immunol. 2018;120(1):5.1.1–5.1.11.
4. Givan AL. Flow cytometry: first principles. Somerset: Wiley; 2013.
5. Robinson JP. Overview of flow cytometry and microbiology. Curr Protoc Cytom. 2018;84(1):e37.
6. Béné M, Nebe T, Bettelheim P, Buldini B, Bumbea H, Kern W, et al. Immunophenotyping of acute leukemia and lymphoproliferative disorders: a consensus proposal of the European LeukemiaNet Work Package 10. Leukemia. 2011;25(4):567–74.
7. Cossarizza A, Chang HD, Radbruch A, Acs A, Adam D, Adam-Klages S, et al. Guidelines for the use of flow cytometry and cell sorting in immunological studies. Eur J Immunol. 2019;49(10):1457–973.
8. Shapiro HM. Practical flow cytometry. New York: Wiley; 2005.
9. Henderson LO, Marti GE, Gaigalas A, Hannon WH, Vogt RF Jr. Terminology and nomenclature for standardization in quantitative fluorescence cytometry. Cytometry. 1998;33(2):97–105.
10. Saeys Y, Van Gassen S, Lambrecht BN. Computational flow cytometry: helping to make sense of high-dimensional immunology data. Nat Rev Immunol. 2016;16(7):449–62.
11. Lugli E, Roederer M, Cossarizza A. Data analysis in flow cytometry: the future just started. Cytometry A. 2010;77(7):705–13.
12. Scheffold A, Kern F. Recent developments in flow cytometry. J Clin Immunol. 2000;20(6):400–7.
13. Hulspas R, O'Gorman MRG, Wood BL, Gratama JW, Sutherland DR. Considerations for the control of background fluorescence in clinical flow cytometry. Cytometry B Clin Cytom. 2009;76B(6):355–64.
14. Porwit A, Béné MC. Multiparameter flow cytometry in the diagnosis of hematologic malignancies. Cambridge University Press; 2018.
15. Del Zotto G, Antonini F, Pesce S, Moretta F, Moretta L, Marcenaro E. Comprehensive phenotyping of human PB NK cells by flow cytometry. Cytometry A. 2020;97(9):891–9.
16. Telford WG. Multiparametric analysis of apoptosis by flow cytometry. In: Hawley TS, Hawley RG, editors. Flow cytometry protocols. New York: Springer; 2018. p. 167–202.
17. Yin Y, Mitson-Salazar A, Prussin C. Detection of intracellular cytokines by flow cytometry. Curr Protoc Immunol. 2015;110(1):6.24.1–6.24.18.
18. Gratama JW, Sutherland DR, Keeney M, editors. Flow cytometric enumeration and immunophenotyping of hematopoietic stem and progenitor cells. Seminars in hematology. Elsevier; 2001.
19. Darzynkiewicz Z, Bedner E, Smolewski P, editors. Flow cytometry in analysis of cell cycle and apoptosis. Seminars in hematology. Elsevier; 2001.
20. Glier H, Heijnen I, Hauwel M, Dirks J, Quarroz S, Lehmann T, et al. Standardization of 8-color flow cytometry across different flow cytometer instruments: a feasibility study in clinical laboratories in Switzerland. J Immunol Methods. 2019;475:112348.
21. Jamin C, Le Lann L, Alvarez-Errico D, Barbarroja N, Cantaert T, Ducreux J, et al. Multi-center harmonization of flow cytometers in the context of the European "PRECISESADS" project. Autoimmun Rev. 2016;15(11):1038–45.
22. Kalina T, Flores-Montero J, Lecrevisse Q, Pedreira CE, van der Velden VHJ, Novakova M, et al. Quality assessment program for EuroFlow protocols: summary results of four-year (2010–2013) quality assurance rounds. Cytometry A. 2015;87(2):145–56.
23. Le Lann L, Jouve P-E, Alarcón-Riquelme M, Jamin C, Pers J-O. Standardization procedure for flow cytometry data harmonization in prospective multicenter studies. Sci Rep. 2020;10(1):1–8.

24. Kalina T, Flores-Montero J, Van Der Velden V, Martin-Ayuso M, Böttcher S, Ritgen M, et al. EuroFlow standardization of flow cytometer instrument settings and immunophenotyping protocols. Leukemia. 2012;26(9):1986–2010.
25. Lambert C, Yanikkaya Demirel G, Keller T, Preijers F, Psarra K, Schiemann M, et al. Flow cytometric analyses of lymphocyte markers in immune oncology: a comprehensive guidance for validation practice according to laws and standards. Front Immunol. 2020;11:2169.
26. Novakova M, Glier H, Brdičková N, Vlková M, Santos AH, Lima M, et al. How to make usage of the standardized EuroFlow 8-color protocols possible for instruments of different manufacturers. J Immunol Methods. 2019;475:112388.
27. Cherian S, Hedley BD, Keeney M. Common flow cytometry pitfalls in diagnostic hematopathology. Cytometry B Clin Cytom. 2019;96(6):449–63.
28. Tettero JM, Freeman S, Buecklein V, Venditti A, Maurillo L, Kern W, et al. Technical aspects of flow cytometry-based measurable residual disease quantification in acute myeloid leukemia: experience of the European LeukemiaNet MRD working party. HemaSphere. 2022;6(1):e676.
29. Flores-Montero J, Kalina T, Corral-Mateos A, Sanoja-Flores L, Perez-Andres M, Martin-Ayuso M, et al. Fluorochrome choices for multi-color flow cytometry. J Immunol Methods. 2019;475:112618.
30. Illingworth AJ, Marinov I, Sutherland DR. Sensitive and accurate identification of PNH clones based on ICCS/ESCCA PNH consensus guidelines—a summary. Int J Lab Hematol. 2019;41:73–81.
31. Roederer M. How many events is enough? Are you positive? Cytometry A. 2008;73(5):384–5.
32. Donnenberg AD, Donnenberg VS. Rare-event analysis in flow cytometry. Clin Lab Med. 2007;27(3):627–52.
33. Hedley B, Keeney M. Technical issues: flow cytometry and rare event analysis. Int J Lab Hematol. 2013;35(3):344–50.
34. Roederer M. Spectral compensation for flow cytometry: visualization artifacts, limitations, and caveats. Cytometry. 2001;45(3):194–205.
35. Maurer-Granofszky M, Schumich A, Buldini B, Gaipa G, Kappelmayer J, Mejstrikova E, et al. An extensive quality control and quality assurance (QC/QA) program significantly improves inter-laboratory concordance rates of flow-cytometric minimal residual disease assessment in acute lymphoblastic leukemia: an I-BFM-FLOW-network report. Cancers. 2021;13(23):6148.

Chapter 3
Sample-Data Analysis

Georgios S. Markopoulos

3.1   Introduction

Flow cytometry is among the methods of choice for quantifying cellular phenotype. The main requirement is to obtain cells into a homogeneous liquid mixture. This mixture is commonly prepared in a preanalytical step, in which cells (or subcellular structures) are incubated by fluorochrome-bound antibodies, or other fluorescent dyes, such as dyes that specifically bind nucleic acids, lipids, etc. When the sample is ready for analysis, it will pass through the cytometer to examine the presence of fluorochromes in each cell and infer the existence of specific proteins, the quantity of DNA, etc.

A typical flow cytometer contains three main interconnected systems: a hydraulics system, an optical system, and an electronics system (Fig. 3.1). First, cell mixture is passed through the hydraulics system in which cells are hydrodynamically focused in order to be sequentially analyzed as single events. Next, they pass through an interrogation point, as part of an optical system that contains laser(s) for excitation of bound fluorophores and filters for the detection of scatter and fluorescence emission signals. Lastly, through the electronics system, optical signals are digitized and stored into a unified format. Data analysis is also performed by the electronics system by using an appropriate software [1].

In this chapter, we will provide a primer on sample-data analysis, from data acquisition to knowledge production.

G. S. Markopoulos (✉)
Faculty of Medicine, Neurosurgical Institute, School of Health Sciences, University of Ioannina, Ioannina, Greece

Haematology Laboratory, Unit of Molecular Biology and Translational Flow Cytometry, University Hospital of Ioannina, Ioannina, Greece

G. Alexiou, G. Vartholomatos (eds.), *Intraoperative Flow Cytometry*,
https://doi.org/10.1007/978-3-031-33517-4_3

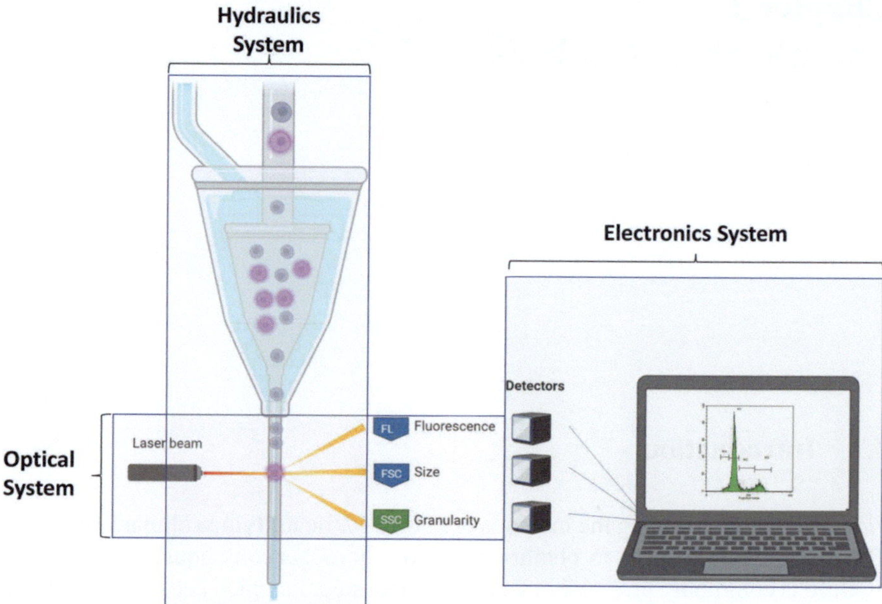

Fig. 3.1 The interconnected systems of a flow cytometer. A flow cytometer is composed of three interconnected systems. A hydraulics system manages the hydrodynamic focusing of the sample, in order to achieve passing individual cells/events through an interrogation point, where they "meet" beam(s) from laser(s) source(s). Interrogation point is also part of the optical system in which cells are excited by the laser and emit fluorescence. Forward and side scatter of fluorescence is detected, as well as individual channels from the emitted fluorescence of each cell. Specific detectors from the electronic system convert emitted photons to electrical signals, which are digitized and stored in a flow cytometry standard. Sample analysis also occurs in the electronics system, by specific software

3.1.1 Data Acquisition in the Electronics System

In a typical flow cytometer, the electronics system picks the fluorescence signals of individual cells by specific detectors, also called photomultipliers. Once in a detector, the signal, which is composed of emitted photons, is converted into electronic current that is composed of electrons, creating an electric pulse. Within the electronics system the signal is amplified and converted from analog to digital, passing through distinct amplifiers and analog-to-digital signal converters, respectively. For each event analyzed (for example a cell or a subcellular structure) the electronics system creates a digital signal for every parameter, such as forward scatter (FSC), side scatter (SSC), and individual fluorescence channels, dependent on the cytometer settings [1].

Several advancements in the field have made it possible to analyze signals beyond fluorescence or to detect and analyze the whole spectrum of fluorescence. Mass cytometry is an advancement of cytometry in which individual events are passed through a mass spectrometer, instead of analyzing fluorescence [2]. The main advantage of using a mass cytometer is the ability to quantify more parameters than conventional flow cytometry, providing a potency of analyzing 40–100 parameters per event. Mass cytometry also comes with some disadvantages, such as the much higher cost for equipment and sample labeling, as well as the challenge to accurately acquire biological knowledge from complex data.

In imaging flow cytometry, a camera is added to the conventional signal detectors to also provide data on a cell's morphology [3]. In that way, the user has a supplementary source of information to validate fluorescence data and to provide more accurate characterization on cell populations.

A promising advance of flow cytometry is spectral flow cytometry, offering the detection of the whole emission spectrum per event, a feat that makes possible to analyze more than 30 parameters with high sensitivity and resolution, by minimizing the need of compensation due to spectral overlap of different fluorochromes [4].

Beyond instrumentation, advances in the field of informatics lead to the development of powerful analysis protocols and software, which offer advanced functionality, such as visualization of multiple parameters, separation of population based-on morphological and phenotypic features, unsupervised analysis, support of high-throughput pipelines, and integration of deep-learning algorithms [5, 6].

3.1.2   Storage Standard for Cytometry Files

The data acquired by the electronic system are stored in a flow cytometry standard (FCS) format that was first adopted in 1984. The file extension standard for most flow cytometry files is FCS, in order to be recognized and opened by different data analysis software. The first established standard (FCS version 1.0) was revised in 1990 (as FCS 2.0) and 1997 (as FCS 3.0), in accordance with the developments in the field. The current established standard is that of FCS 3.1, a minor revision of the last version [7]. An FCS 3.1 file is a text file composed of data organized into at least three and sometimes four segments: HEADER, TEXT, DATA, and ANALYSIS. The HEADER is utilized as a "map" to the other segments of the file. The TEXT contains general information and descriptions of the dataset. DATA segment contains raw data values that have been acquired by the electronics system. ANALYSIS segment is optional, it can be added by an operator to an FCS file and contains results following data processing (cell cycle analysis, cell sub-population, etc.) [7].

The structured and organized storage of flow cytometry experiments facilitated by the FCS standard offers a transparent means of data sharing and analysis by different software and operators throughout the world. In addition, the presence of optional segment of ANALYSIS enables, except from experimental data sharing, the opportunity to distribute the analysis strategies that support the development of standards based on the work done by experts in field.

3.2 Presentation of Current Techniques for Sample Analysis

Sample analysis is an essential part in knowledge production from acquired flow cytometric data. Modern flow cytometers come with powerful software capable of both acquisition and analysis. In the analysis part, a common flow cytometry analysis software can perform at least the following: (I) Finding and selecting/"gating" a population of interest, based on standard scatter and fluorescence properties, (II) analyzing one parameter of interest, (II) performing a comparative analysis of two (or more) parameters. Following the impressive flourishing in the production of next-generation flow cytometers during the last years, modern software for analysis have also been developed. Today, the characterization of common or novel cell populations can be performed by simultaneous analysis of several parameters and in some cases with the assistance of artificial intelligence and machine learning algorithms [6, 8, 9].

Flow cytometrists, apart from the FCS file, have established a standard for sample analysis, the Minimum Information about a Flow Cytometry Experiment (MIFlowCyt) standard [10]. MIFloCyt has been developed in 2008 by a cross-disciplinary international collaborative group that included inter-alia bioinformaticians, software developers, instrument manufacturers, and research scientists. This international consortium has worked under the consultation by the International Society for Advancement of Cytometry (ISAC) Data Standards Task Force (DSTF). The information that are included in a MIFlowCyt compliant experiment are: Experiment Overview (stating the purpose, variables, conclusions, and quality control); Flow Sample (stating material, source, treatment, and reagents/analytes used); Data Analysis (including list-mode data, compensation and gating information, descriptive statistics); Instrument Details (including instrument identification, fluidics configuration, optical configuration, and electronic configuration). Together, MIFloCyt is a list of recommendations stating that the minimum information required to report flow cytometry (FCM) experiments in order to facilitate data clarity, availability, third-party understanding and reuse from the international community of cytometrists.

3.2.1 A Primer on Flow-Cytometry Software

Flow cytometry data analysis software represents the "heart" of the electronics system. From the development of commercial flow cytometers till today, the available packages of software can be part of a flow cytometry instrument and dedicated to assist both acquisition and analysis. In addition, there are several software that offer functionality on conventional flow cytometry analysis, while they also offer next-generation capabilities for multiparameter data. Table 3.1 provides a list on popular flow cytometry software packages and their main functionalities.

Table 3.1 Popular Contemporary Flow Cytometry Analysis Software

Name (Developer)	Functionality (based on developer data)	Lisence
FCS Express (De novo Software)	Conventional flow cytometry analysis (FCS files visualization, population gating, proliferation analysis, cell cycle analysis), high dimensional data reduction, image cytometry, spectral flow cytometry, pipelines	Proprietary
FlowJo (Treestar)	Conventional flow cytometry analysis, archival cytometry standard, high dimensional data reduction, R-tools, analysis platforms, plugins	Proprietary
Cyflogic (Cyflo Ltd)	Conventional flow cytometry analysis	Free
WinList (Verity Software)	Conventional flow cytometry analysis, mass cytometry, spectral flow cytometry	Proprietary
ModFit LT (Verity Software)	Advanced DNA content and cell cycle analysis	Proprietary
GemStone (Verity Software)	High dimensional flow cytometry analysis, mass cytometry, spectral flow cytometry	Proprietary
BD FACSCanto, BD FACSuite BD FACSChorus BD FACSDiva (BD Biosciences)	Instrument software for acquisition and analysis of flow cytometry data Conventional flow cytometry analysis BD FACSCanto and BD FACSuite: Clinical applications BD FACSChorus and BD FACSDiv: Research applications	Proprietary
Kaluza Series (Beckman Coulter)	Conventional flow cytometry analysis High dimensional flow cytometry analysis Instrument software for acquisition	Proprietary
Cytobank (Beckman Coulter)	Conventional flow cytometry analysis, mass cytometry, spectral flow cytometry High dimensional flow cytometry analysis and dimensionality reduction (viSNE, SPADE, FlowSOM, CITRUS, or sunburst packages) Machine learning assisted analysis Cloud-based analysis	Proprietary (free community version)
Infinicyt (Cytognos)	Conventional flow cytometry analysis, mass cytometry, spectral flow cytometry High dimensional flow cytometry analysis and dimensionality reduction Principal component analysis Supervised automated analysis Unsupervised automated analysis	Proprietary
R and Bioconductor (several developers, open access license)	Conventional flow cytometry analysis, mass cytometry, spectral flow cytometry Package-related functionality and ability to create personalized workflows (based on R programing language)	Free (open access)

Most modern software packages provide capabilities for conventional flow cytometry analysis that covers the majority of common clinical and research applications. However, based on the individual software, additional functionalities may be available. For example, while the majority of flow cytometry software offer cell cycle and DNA content analysis, Modfit LT is a tool dedicated to more advanced DNA content quantification capabilities. Other tools, such as Cytobank, offer innovative functionality towards data sharing and online collaboration between cytometrists [11].

3.2.2 Gating a Population of Interest

Flow cytometry is commonly used for the quantification of cell populations in order to assess physiology and/or pathology in a given sample. Among the most successful applications of flow cytometry are the ones in hematology [12] and immunology [13]. The quantification of individual sub-populations in peripheral blood or other body fluids offers an accurate diagnosis of several diseases, such as hematologic malignancies and autoimmune syndromes. In addition, it can offer prognostic insights and monitor the patient for recurrence of cancer cells using a clinical protocol for measurable (or minimal) residual disease (MRD) [14].

A first step in conventional flow cytometry analysis is the optical depiction and separation of populations of interest based on scatter and/or fluorescence features. A well-established example is presented here, which is the separation of lymphocyte sub-populations in a sample from peripheral blood (Fig. 3.2). To present the analyzed populations we can use a two-dimensional plot, such as a dot-plot, to represent side scatter (that quantifies internal complexity of cells) and CD45 marker expression, also known as lymphocyte common antigen, which a cluster of differentiation/CD marker expressed in different levels in cell populations present in peripheral blood [12].

A population of cells can be separated and tagged by drawing a region or "gate" around it. This strategy is called gating. The events that are present in a specific gate can be further analyzed for other parameters within the given sample, by applying that region gating in subsequent plots. The analysis of this gated population can also be applied to other samples, to quantify several markers within a common feature that is represented in the isolated gate region.

In our example, based on lymphocyte structure and phenotype we can apply gate 1 (Region R1 in Fig. 3.2), based on the knowledge that we expect lymphocytes to have a lower internal complexity and thus a lower side scatter than other white blood cells. In comparison, a more complex structure can be seen in monocytes (recognized in a gate in region R2) and the highest complexity in polymorphonuclear cells (gated in region R3). Logical gating is then applied to the other analyzed parameters. The presented analysis is three color and two different samples are used with the applied gating in lymphocytes to discern different sub-population. In sample one CD3/CD19 discrimination is done and in the second sample a CD4/CD8 is performed. The principles of logical gating can be applied to several more parameters. Logical gating has been the basis of several conventional flow cytometry

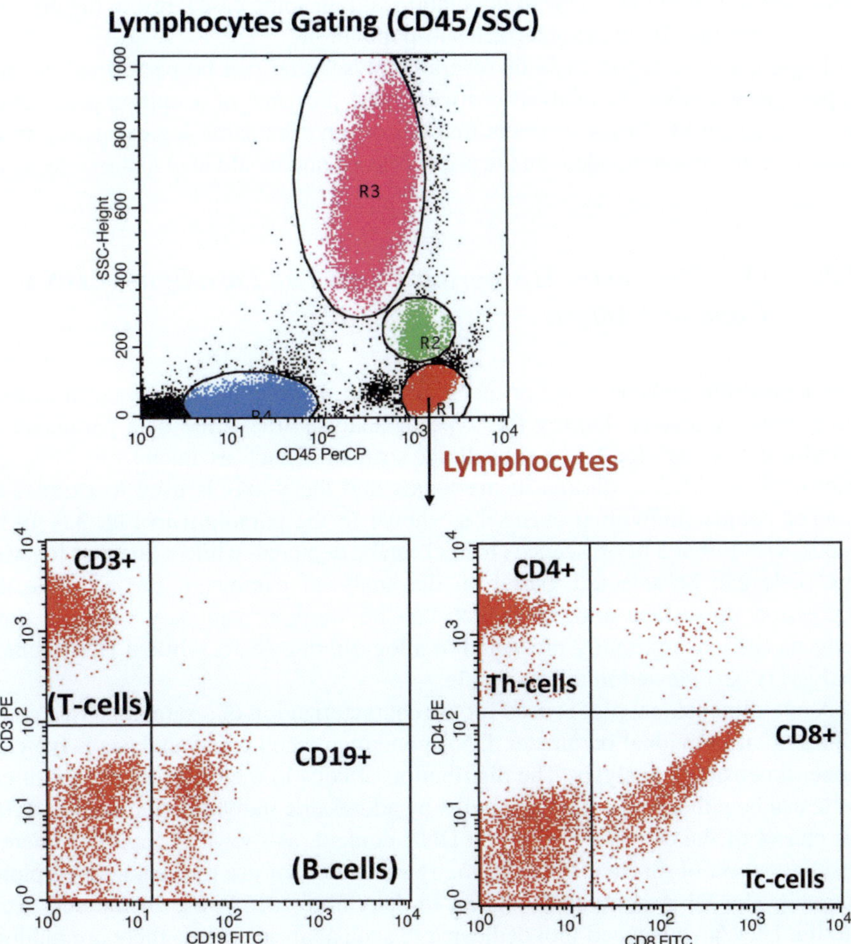

Fig. 3.2 An example of analysis using gating strategy in a sample from peripheral blood. White blood cells were stained with fluorescent dye-bound antibodies that recognize the markers: lymphocyte common antigen CD45 (CD45-perCP), T-lymphocyte marker CD3 (CD3-PE), B-lymphocyte marker CD19 (CD19-FITC), helper T-cells marker CD4 (CD4-PE), and cytotoxic T-cells marker CD8 (CD8-FITC). In a first step, CD45 expression and side scatter is used to recognize lymphocytes by designing a gate in region R1 around side scatter low (low complexity) and CD45-high population. Next, by applying that gate to CD3/CD19 dot-plot we can discriminate between T- and B-cells. Finally, CD4/CD8 plot data can be used to quantify helper and cytotoxic T-lymphocyte sub-populations. In both cases, a "cross" is drawn to separate the plot into four quadrants, in order to discriminate low and high-expressing populations for each parameter in X- and Y-axes, respectively. [The image is a courtesy of Georgios Vartholomatos]

analyses, including clinical and research applications. However, in a panel of multiparameter, next-generation flow cytometry data, two-parameter plots are often not the preferable way of analysis and the presence of new analysis software may add functionalities into the analyzed population and, in some cases, reveal the presence of novel, previously uncharacterized sub-populations.

Logical gating is the basis of several analyses that can be performed on most popular flow cytometry analysis software. The presence of a unified protocol for data storage in FCS files warrants that performing the same logical gating in the same FCS file is independent on the used program and would lead to the same result.

3.2.3 One Parameter Histogram Plots: The Paradigm of DNA Content Analysis

One parameter analysis is the primer evaluation that can be performed in conventional flow cytometry. During this type of analysis, the value of a parameter on individual "events" (cells, or subcellular structures such as nuclei mitochondria, microvesicles, etc.) is plotted in the x-axis and the y-axis is used to express the number counts (individual events), as shown in the paradigm in Fig. 3.3. In the x-axis, a scatter or a fluorescence channel can be depicted, while a linear or logarithmic scale can be selected, based on the analyzed parameter. For example, the expression of surface antigen (which can be weak or can vary multiple times between cells) is optimally presented in a logarithmic scale, while a DNA content analysis is best viewed in a linear scale.

A one-dimensional plot is used for the characterization of a sample, based on the values of an individual parameter. DNA content and cell cycle analysis is typically a one-dimensional analysis. The distribution of cells in the different phases of cell cycle can be either performed manually, by addressing individual markers to different phases of the cell cycle based on DNA content, as shown in Fig. 3.3. There is also the option of discrete flow cytometry software that use to the so-called ploidy modeling the DNA content histogram to determine each phase of the cell cycle. ModFit LT is an advanced tool dedicated to such analyses, while there are modules in most modern flow cytometry software to model DNA content histograms (Table 3.1).

Practically, the separation of cell cycle phases by a one-dimensional analysis is possible based on the differential DNA content in each cell cycle phase [15]. The main event in a cell cycle that makes this possible is DNA replication that takes place in S (synthesis) phase. An active cell cycle, accompanied by a high proliferative potential is also a hallmark of cancer [16, 17], making the conventional DNA content analysis by flow cytometry an irreplaceable tool in the cancer research [15].

Intraoperative flow cytometry (iFC) is the use of flow cytometry to define tumor biology and assess tumor margins during surgery. The rationale of iFC is based on the accurate detection of DNA content that reflect the unique biology of cancer cells [17]. The distinct features of cancer cells in comparison to their normal counterparts allowed the successful analysis by iFC in several types of malignancy, including central nervous system, head and neck, breast, liver, pancreatic, and colorectal

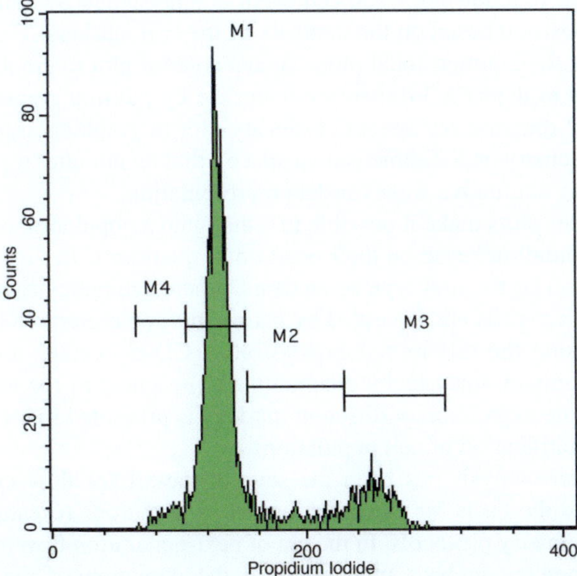

Fig. 3.3 A paradigm of one parameter analysis. The analyzed parameter is the quantity of DNA, based on propidium iodide fluorescence. The preanalytical step requires stain with propidium iodide, to bind nucleic acids. The presented histogram is separated using four different areas, by the respective markers M1, M2, M3, and M4, that correspond, based on the mean fluorescence, to cells in G1, S, G2/M phases and subG1 cells, respectively. Cells in G2/M are characterized by a dual mean fluorescence intensity than cells in G1, due to the completion of DNA replication. Cells in S phase (undergoing DNA replication) are characterized by a mean fluorescence intensity between cells in G1 and G2/M phases. SubG1 cells correspond to cells that undergo cell death and the quantity of nuclear DNA is less than cells in G1, due to a nuclear breakdown. (The image is a courtesy of Georgios Vartholomatos.)

malignancies. The analytical performance of flow cytometry for accurate DNA content analysis, along with the ease and speed of the method has distinguished iFC as an accurate diagnostic tool among the next-generation margin evaluation techniques [18–24]. The details of intraoperative flow cytometry analysis are presented in Chaps. 4 and 5.

3.2.4 Two Parameter Analysis: Dot Plots and Alternative Visualization Methods

The comparative expression of two markers or the expression of a marker in conjunction to scatter properties can be performed using a two-parameter plot. Paradigms of two parameter analysis have been elucidated in Fig. 3.2, in which two-parameter dot plots made it possible to separate lymphocyte sub-populations in peripheral blood. In a dot-plot, each cell/event is represented by a distinct dot that hold a unique position based on the intensity of the two markers. There are several other depictions for 2-dimensional plots, such a contour plot (a graphical representation technique to depict a 3-dimensional surface by plotting z-axis slices, called contours, on a 2-dimensional space) or density plot (a graphical representation of 3-dimensional density on a 2-dimensional space), that do not alter the final result of analysis but offer alternative ways for data representation.

Two-parameter plots make it possible to either gate a population of interest or to characterize population based on their position in quadrants. In Fig. 3.2, top panel shows a paradigm of the first type of analysis, where lymphocyte, monocyte, and polymorphonuclear cells are separated by gating in three regions (R1, R2, and R3, respectively), using the differential expression of CD45 (x-axis) and side scatter (y-axis). Paradigms of analyses by quadrants are presented in the lower panels of Fig. 3.2, where the expression of different markers is presented in each axis, allowing accurate quantification of cell populations.

Two-parameter analysis has been the state-of-the-art for flow cytometry data visualization and the basis for the development of numerous research studies and clinical flow cytometry protocols. In the era of next-generation flow cytometry protocols, two-parameter analysis may assist in the depiction of the relationships between specific parameters. However, in a modern protocol of multiple parameters, a new generation of analysis tools is necessary for data representation and accurate analysis [25].

3.2.5 Next Generation Data Analysis of High Dimensional Data

The recent advances in technology have surfaced the need for analysis of high dimensional data of cell populations that contain 20 or more parameters per event. For example, spectral flow cytometry has the ability of analyzing at least 40 parameters in a single sample [26], while mass cytometry has a proved the ability of analyzing at least 50 parameters [27]. The visualization methods of one- and two-parameter data, as well as sequential gating, used in conventional flow cytometry make it hard, if not impossible to draw meaningful conclusions from such complex samples. Therefore, several analytical methods for data visualization and analysis have been developed.

The first "obstacle" in multiparameter data analysis is a visualization method, since hundreds of plots would be needed to visualize each parameter. The main solution is algorithms that enable the so-called dimension reduction, in which viewing and analysis of high dimensional data is possible in two- or three-dimensional plots. Popular examples of such algorithms are principal component analysis (PCA) [28], t-distributed stochastic neighbor embedding (tSNE) [29], and spanning-tree progression analysis of density-normalized events (SPADE) [30]. The next step in multiparameter data analysis is data classification and knowledge production. Several methodologies have been developed to assist in the classification of populations in a sample, in determination of the status of a sample as a physiological or pathological, as well as the determination of novel cellular populations. Artificial intelligence and machine learning has been recently implemented in modern software to assist both supervised and unsupervised data classification and characterization [31–33]. Algorithms for dimension reduction and complex data classification are embedded in most modern flow cytometry analysis packages (see Table 3.1 for details).

3.3 Future Perspectives

Flow cytometry, since its development in the late twentieth century, has been evolved as the science of quantification of cellular phenotype and into a powerful tool assisting both research and diagnosis purposes. Data analysis is in the core of flow cytometry and has been progressed in parallel to the recent technical innovations in the field. The new generation of flow cytometrists should be aware of the data analysis tools of conventional flow cytometry, such as one- and two-dimension plots and sequential gating, as an integral part of their training, as a step-by-step process towards understanding biological processes that involve single cell dynamics. This type of training will prove valuable before entering the exciting avenues of multiparameter flow cytometry and data tools that support it.

References

1. Shapiro HM. Practical flow cytometry. New York: Wiley; 2005.
2. Spitzer MH, Nolan GP. Mass cytometry: single cells, many features. Cell. 2016;165:780–91.
3. Manohar SM, Shah P, Nair A. Flow cytometry: principles, applications and recent advances. Bioanalysis. 2021;13:181–98. https://doi.org/10.4155/bio-2020-0267.
4. Nolan JP. The evolution of spectral flow cytometry. Cytometry A. 101:812. https://doi.org/10.1002/cyto.a.24566.
5. Cheung M, Campbell JJ, Whitby L, Thomas RJ, Braybrook J, Petzing J. Current trends in flow cytometry automated data analysis software. Cytometry A. 2021;99:1007–21.
6. Pedreira C, da Costa ES, Lecrevise Q, Grigore G, Fluxá R, Verde J, Hernandez J, van Dongen J, Orfao A. From big flow cytometry datasets to smart diagnostic strategies: the EuroFlow approach. J Immunol Methods. 2019;475:112631.
7. Spidlen J, Moore W, Parks D, Goldberg M, Bray C, Bierre P, Gorombey P, Hyun B, Hubbard M, Lange S, et al. Data file standard for flow cytometry, version FCS 3.1. Cytometry A. 2010;77:97–100. https://doi.org/10.1002/cyto.a.20825.
8. Cualing HD. Automated analysis in flow cytometry. Cytometry. 2000;42:110–3.

9. Salama ME, Otteson GE, Camp JJ, Seheult JN, Jevremovic D, Holmes DR III, Olteanu H, Shi M. Artificial intelligence enhances diagnostic flow cytometry workflow in the detection of minimal residual disease of chronic lymphocytic leukemia. Cancers (Basel). 2022;14:2537.

10. Lee JA, Spidlen J, Boyce K, Cai J, Crosbie N, Dalphin M, Furlong J, Gasparetto M, Goldberg M, Goralczyk EM. MIFlowCyt: the minimum information about a flow cytometry experiment. Cytometry A. 2008;73:926–30.

11. Chen TJ, Kotecha N. Cytobank: providing an analytics platform for community cytometry data analysis and collaboration. Curr Top Microbiol Immunol. 2014;377:127–57.

12. Ortolani C. Flow cytometry of hematological malignancies. Hoboken, NJ: Wiley; 2021.

13. Cossarizza A, Chang HD, Radbruch A, Acs A, Adam D, Adam-Klages S, Agace WW, Aghaeepour N, Akdis M, Allez M. Guidelines for the use of flow cytometry and cell sorting in immunological studies. Eur J Immunol. 2019;49:1457–973.

14. Dix C, Lo T-H, Clark G, Abadir E. Measurable residual disease in acute myeloid leukemia using flow cytometry: a review of where we are and where we are going. J Clin Med. 2020;9:1714.

15. Pozarowski P, Darzynkiewicz Z. Analysis of cell cycle by flow cytometry. Methods Mol Biol. 2004;281:301–11.

16. Kastan MB, Bartek J. Cell-cycle checkpoints and cancer. Nature. 2004;432:316–23.

17. Hanahan D, Weinberg RA. Hallmarks of cancer: the next generation. Cell. 2011;144:646–74.

18. Vartholomatos E, Vartholomatos G, Alexiou GA, Markopoulos GS. The past, present and future of flow cytometry in central nervous system malignancies. Methods Protoc. 2021;4:11.

19. Alexiou G, Vartholomatos G, Stefanaki K, Markopoulos G, Kyritsis A. Intraoperative flow cytometry for diagnosis of central nervous system lesions. J Cytol. 2019;36:134–5.

20. Vartholomatos G, Harissis H, Andreou M, Tatsi V, Pappa L, Kamina S, Batistatou A, Markopoulos GS, Alexiou GA. Rapid assessment of resection margins during breast conserving surgery using intraoperative flow cytometry. Clin Breast Cancer. 2021;21:e602–10.

21. Markopoulos GS, Glantzounis GK, Goussia AC, Lianos GD, Karampa A, Alexiou GA, Vartholomatos G. Touch imprint intraoperative flow cytometry as a complementary tool for detailed assessment of resection margins and tumor biology in liver surgery for primary and metastatic liver neoplasms. Methods Protoc. 2021;4:66.

22. Markopoulos GS, Goussia A, Bali CD, Messinis T, Alexiou GA, Vartholomatos G. Resection margins assessment by intraoperative flow cytometry in pancreatic cancer. Ann Surg Oncol. 2022:1–3.

23. Georvasili VK, Markopoulos GS, Batistatou A, Mitsis M, Messinis T, Lianos GD, Alexiou G, Vartholomatos G, Bali CD. Detection of cancer cells and tumor margins during colorectal cancer surgery by intraoperative flow cytometry. Int J Surg. 2022;104:106717.

24. Vartholomatos G, Alexiou GA, Tatsi V, Harissis H, Markopoulos GS. Next-generation margin evaluation techniques in breast conserving surgery: a memorandum on intraoperative flow cytometry. Eur J Surg Oncol. 2022;49:675.

25. Montante S, Brinkman RR. Flow cytometry data analysis: recent tools and algorithms. Int J Lab Hematol. 2019;41:56–62.

26. Bonilla DL, Reinin G, Chua E. Full spectrum flow cytometry as a powerful technology for cancer immunotherapy research. Front Mol Biosci. 2021;7:612801. https://doi.org/10.3389/fmolb.2020.612801.

27. Olsen LR, Leipold MD, Pedersen CB, Maecker HT. The anatomy of single cell mass cytometry data. Cytometry A. 2019;95:156–72.

28. Lugli E, Pinti M, Nasi M, Troiano L, Ferraresi R, Mussi C, Salvioli G, Patsekin V, Robinson JP, Durante C. Subject classification obtained by cluster analysis and principal component analysis applied to flow cytometric data. Cytometry A. 2007;71:334–44.

29. Van der Maaten L, Hinton G. Visualizing data using t-SNE. J Mach Learn Res. 2008:9.

30. Zaki MJ. SPADE: an efficient algorithm for mining frequent sequences. Mach Learn. 2001;42:31–60.

31. Béné MC, Lacombe F, Porwit A. Unsupervised flow cytometry analysis in hematological malignancies: a new paradigm. Int J Lab Hematol. 2021;43:54–64.
32. Luo S, Shi Y, Chin LK, Hutchinson PE, Zhang Y, Chierchia G, Talbot H, Jiang X, Bourouina T, Liu A-Q. Machine-learning-assisted intelligent imaging flow cytometry: a review. Advanced Intelligent Systems. 2021;3:2100073.
33. Monaghan SA, Li J-L, Liu Y-C, Ko M-Y, Boyiadzis M, Chang T-Y, Wang Y-F, Lee C-C, Swerdlow SH, Ko B-S. A machine learning approach to the classification of acute leukemias and distinction from nonneoplastic cytopenias using flow cytometry data. Am J Clin Pathol. 2022;157:546–53.

Part II
Intraoperative Flow Cytometry

Chapter 4
Basic Principles

Georgios Vartholomatos and Georgios Alexiou

4.1   Introduction

During carcinogenesis normal cells are transformed into neoplastic cells that create a tumor, through the gradual accumulation of genetic mutations and an epigenetic reprogramming. Cancer is the second leading cause of mortality, with an estimation of 19.3 million new cases and a toll of 10.0 million deaths in the year 2022. The estimation for the next 20 years remain dismal, accounting for at least 16 million deaths worldwide [1].

For at least 150 years the surgical removal of solid neoplasms is based on histopathological examination and pathoanatomical diagnosis following surgery. This whole process usually lasts from 2 to 4 weeks, which delays the final diagnosis and early treatment. In cases of stereotactic biopsy in the brain, a large percentage of biopsies come out non-diagnostic or of a lower degree of malignancy than the actual [2]. Intraoperatively, the surgeon to this day (through a frozen section biopsy) may have an estimate of the degree and type of malignancy of brain neoplasms as well as tumor margins. However, rapid biopsy has many drawbacks, since the time from sample collection to answer can reach 20–30 min, the incisions are usually of low quality, the technique is based on the experience of the pathologist, while sometimes the final diagnosis may differ from that of the final conclusion of the biopsy [3–5].

FC, since its conception, has been evolved from an analytical technique into the science of quantitative cell biology, including the analysis of cellular phenotype, as well as several cellular processes including proliferation and cell death [6]. The

G. Vartholomatos (✉)
Unit of Molecular Biology and Translational Flow Cytometry, University Hospital of Ioannina, Ioannina, Greece

G. Alexiou
Department of Neurosurgery, University of Ioannina, Ioannina, Greece
e-mail: galexiou@uoi.gr

G. Alexiou, G. Vartholomatos (eds.), *Intraoperative Flow Cytometry*,
https://doi.org/10.1007/978-3-031-33517-4_4

main requirement for performing flow cytometry is to obtain cells in a uniform liquid mixture. A major advantage of FC over similar methods, such as microscopy, is the quantitative nature of the results, since a large number of cells/events can be analyzed in very short period of time.

A very early application of FC is that of DNA content analysis [7]. DNA content analysis by FC would soon prove to be useful on the characterization of human tumor cells. As regards brain tumors, early studies showed that malignant lesions can contain hyperploid DNA content [8] and that loss-of-heterozygosity is analogous to the CNSM stage [9]. In addition DNA content analysis in benign lesions (such as meningiomas, neuroblastomas, and low-grade astrocytomas) revealed mainly diploid cells with low proliferation index, while most malignant tumors (mainly gliomas and glioblastomas) had aneuploid populations and/or a significantly higher proliferation index [10]. Another early study revealed that FC analysis could be also useful apart from solid brain tissue, for the analysis of cerebrospinal fluid to study the possibility of infiltrating cancer cells [11]. The results of the aforementioned studies are paradigms of the utility of DNA content analysis in the characterization of brain tumor cells and the possibility of being utilized as a diagnostic tool.

In the current chapter we will discuss how these ideas were used and developed to form into shape the concept of intraoperative flow cytometry, which is the use of DNA content analysis for the diagnosis of malignant lesions during a surgical operation.

4.2 Basic Discussion on Intraoperative Flow Cytometry History and Applications

Flow cytometric analysis of DNA content, even though is probably the first established application of flow cytometry and exhibited a promising potential to differentiate between cancer and normal cells, has never been systematically used in the past as a diagnostic or a prognostic tool for brain malignancies.

However, the revolution of molecular biology techniques has stalled the establishment of FC DNA analysis as a diagnostic tool in the clinic or the operating theater [12]. Fortunately, flow cytometric DNA content analysis entered the clinic during the last decade, when a novel concept was developed, which was the analysis of DNA content distribution, during the surgical excision of brain cancer. This led to intraoperative flow cytometry (iFC), which is the analysis of excised tissue for characterization of cancer cells and the evaluation of tumor margins.

The conceptual basis of an intraoperative flow cytometric method was first recognized in a retrospective study in which a series of tumor samples taken from 56 patients were analyzed for DNA content by flow cytometry. A cell cycle distribution analysis was proved useful in discriminating between grade I meningiomas to grade

II/III and between low-grade gliomas to higher grade gliomas and glioblastomas. Importantly, in patients with glioma, the results of DNA content analysis were in concordance with clinical results over a 5-year period, offering a potential of prognostic significance [13].

The logic behind iFC is the cytometric analysis in a rapid manner, which offers the opportunity for intraoperative diagnosis, as an adjunct or alternative to the pathology evaluation during surgery. A rapid protocol that offers cell cycle analysis of central nervous system lesions and their surgical margins in 6 min per sample was developed by our team in the University Hospital of Ioannina (Ioannina Protocol) [14].

The study has analyzed the utility of iFC in a group including 31 patients. Following iFC analysis of DNA content, a significant increase in S and G2/M fractions (their sum is referred as Tumor Index) in cell cycle phases has been found between low-grade and high-grade tumors. In patients with glioblastoma, the most aggressive primary brain tumor, the significant differences found between cancer and tumor margins G0/G1 phase fractions and in tumor index, suggested that there is a potential in delineating tumor margins by iFC [14].

In parallel to the ioannina protocol, a team of researchers based in Women's Medical University, in Tokyo, Japan has developed a similar protocol of iFC, achieving an analysis time of 10–12 min per sample. Based on their results from 328 specimens from patients with glioma, they calculated an optimal malignancy index (percentage of cells with abnormal DNA content) of 6.8%, resulting in 88% sensitivity and 88% diagnostic specificity [15].

Both research groups have highlighted in a joint publication the significance of iFC on tumor surgery of intracranial neoplasms. Briefly, iFC has exhibited the ability to aid in the identification of tumor margins in glioma and in the diagnosis of a tumor's grade, the capacity to diagnose intracranial lymphomas and to prognose the clinical outcome in glioma [16]. In a prognosis point of view, iFC may aid intraoperative diagnosis by calculating tumor or malignancy index, which can be evaluated as a novel prognostic factor if it is calculated following chemotherapy with temozolomide and radiotherapy [17].

The verified impact of iFC in tumors of the central nervous system has led to the development of specialized iFC protocols in order to aid the diagnosis in tumor surgeries of head and neck, breast, liver, pancreatic, and colorectal malignancies [18–23]. The iFC protocols are characterized for their accuracy in DNA content analysis, the rapid and easy implementation and their low cost. Due to that, iFC has been distinguished as a precise diagnostic method among next-generation margin evaluation techniques [24]. It has been suggested as adjunct or alternative to several novel margin evaluation techniques, the use of the fluorescent dye 5-Aminolevulinic Acid (5′ALA) and intraoperative magnetic resonance imaging analysis [25–27], the analysis of tumor metabolites using mass spectrometry [28, 29], intraoperative squash smear cytology [30, 31], and cavity shaving technique [32], among others.

4.3 Basic Principles on Sample Size Requirements

The accuracy of flow cytometry in quantifying cellular phenotype is partly based on the potential to rapidly analyze a large number of cells/events for several parameters. This potential, as well as parameters as precision and variability in the end result is largely impacted by the number of cells per analyzed sample. In different analyses it has been calculated that a different number of cells may be appropriate to have an acceptable result. An extreme paradigm to this notion is measurable/minimal residual disease (MRD) in hematological malignancies, where cytometric analysis should denote the presence of leukemic cells at a frequency that is below routine morphology by morphology or that of cytogenetics, to reach sensitivity down to at least 1 cell per 10^4–10^6 leukocytes [33]. Such sensitivity requires the analysis of 500,000–1 million cells to obtain an analytical power of 0.1%, that is an agreed cut-off value for an MRD-positive sample [34].

In iFC, sample size requirement has been also evaluated and a consensus has been reached. In brain cancer, a number of 5000–10,000 cells is optimal for an accurate DNA content analysis [13]. The same is true for head and neck lesions [35] and colon cancer [23], while in liver and hepatocellular carcinoma 5000 cells were adequate for analysis [21, 22]. In all the above cases a high accuracy has been reached, processing the aforementioned number of cells. Notably, in breast cancer, iFC analysis involved a number of 2000 cells, which has been sufficient for cancer cell characterization and margin evaluation with an accuracy of 92.5% [20, 24, 32]. The sample size of 5000 cells is considered optimal in the manner that it may reach the detection of the presence of pathological cells in a fraction of roughly 1% in a margin sample, an assumption that can be made by using the golden standard approach of pathological assessment as a reference. Further analysis with the next-generation molecular techniques, such as deep sequencing [36], may assist in the establishment of this notion and also in a more thorough evaluation of the accuracy of iFC as well as a more systematic assessment of sample size requirements, towards negative margin surgical interventions.

4.4 Sample Acquisition, Storage, and Use

During the development of different "variants" of iFC in the assessment of tumor biology and margin status in surgical interventions from several tissues, it has been made clear that a special approach should be considered. This conclusion has been the result of recuring discussions between cytometrists and surgeons, with respect to the special environment of each tissue/organ and the individualized conditions and requirements in each surgical intervention. Having that in mind, the sample collection has been essential in the development of accurate intraoperative flow cytometry methodologies. The different techniques for cell collection in different tissues are summarized in Table 4.1.

Table 4.1 Methods for sample collection in different variations of intraoperative flow cytometry

Tissue/ cancer type	Cell collection and separation method	Ref.
Brain	Cancer cells and cells in tumor margins: collection and mince of the tissue (Medimachine System, BD Bioscience) Filtration (consult no. 10, Medicons, BD Bioscience) and resuspension in PBS	[13, 14]
Breast	Cancer cells: collection by using fine needle aspiration (FNA) methodology Cells in tumor margins: collection of cells from the surface of each margin by using a Cytobrush (Cooper Surgical, Trumball, CT) Tumor and margin samples were filtered using CellTrics filters (Sysmex Europe, Norderstedt, Germany) to obtain single cell suspensions in PBS	[20]
Head and neck	Cancer cells and cells in tumor margins: collection and mince of the tissue (Medimachine System, BD Bioscience) Filtration (consult no. 10, Medicons, BD Bioscience) and resuspension in PBS	[35]
Liver	Cancer cells: collection by using fine needle aspiration (FNA) methodology Cells in tumor margins: the resected area of the liver is imprinted into the membrane of a sterilized pouch (Wipak Medical) and rinsed in PBS filtration using CellTrics filters (Sysmex Europe, Norderstedt, Germany) and resuspension in PBS	[21]
Pancreas	Cancer cells: collection by using fine needle aspiration (FNA) methodology Cells in tumor margins: the resected area of the liver is imprinted into the membrane of a sterilized pouch (Wipak Medical) and rinsed in PBS Filtration using CellTrics filters (Sysmex Europe, Norderstedt, Germany) and resuspension in PBS	[22]
Colon and rectum	Tumor and normal tissue samples: excision of tissue and raking, to obtain homogeneous cell solution Filtration using CellTrics filters (Sysmex Flow Cytometry Europe), in order to obtain single cell suspension in PBS	[23]

Briefly, directly following tumor excision, samples from cancerous tissue can be collected either as excised solid tissue or as fine needle aspirates. Margin samples have been collected either as solid tissue, as brushed tissue or as touch imprints. Medimachine or raking has been used as a means to detach cells in solid tissues. In all cases, filtration is necessary to obtain single cell homogenates, devoid of aggregates that would clog a flow cytometer and influence the end result of analysis. All the obtained cells should be rinsed in phosphate-buffered saline (PBS) or a similar isotonic solution before analysis. Staining with propidium iodide (125 mM final concentration) for a minimum of 3 min, according to Ioannina protocol, is the last preanalytical step before flow cytometric analysis of DNA content. This procedure has been originally utilized for the analysis of DNA content in central nervous system tumors [14] and has been adopted in the context of several other procedures. It should be noted that in parallel, corresponding samples are being sent for pathology examination, according to the reference diagnostic protocols for each tumor type, to evaluation tumor type and histopathological grade according to the proposed grading systems.

4.5   Conclusions

Intraoperative flow cytometry has emerged as a direct application of DNA content analysis to first analyze tumor biology and evaluate margin status in intracranial malignancies. The success of iFC led to be proposed as a reliable next-generation margin evaluation methodology and the development of several other iFC variations of tumor excision surgeries for additional types [37], with candidates such as head and neck malignancies [35, 38] and breast cancer [39], as well as liver cancer [21], pancreatic cancer [22] and colorectal cancer [23]. In all these cases, iFC has emerged as a consistent, accurate diagnostic tool with both high sensitivity and specificity, that is above 90% in most cases. A next step is to further diminish the time between sample acquisition and cytometric analysis from 6 min per sample, into seconds, a that would ultimately lead to near real-time a feat that may be possible in the near future [40, 41]. Flow cytometry is currently being revolutionized by the development of new acquisition techniques, such as spectral flow cytometry [42] and mass cytometry [43], while analysis is being assisted by powerful algorithms that are based on machine learning [44]. Such developments may be incorporated in next-generation iFC protocols that would further improve their diagnostic accuracy. A critical factor in all these developments is the training of the new generation of scientists involved in surgical oncology to apply iFC protocols as part of their surgical routines. We hope that this book would assist towards this direction and would act as a roadmap for new scientists to learn about and apply iFC protocols.

References

1. Sung H, Ferlay J, Siegel RL, Laversanne M, Soerjomataram I, Jemal A, Bray F. Global cancer statistics 2020: GLOBOCAN estimates of incidence and mortality worldwide for 36 cancers in 185 countries. CA Cancer J Clin. 2021;71:209.
2. Jackson RJ, Fuller GN, Abi-Said D, Lang FF, Gokaslan ZL, Shi WM, Wildrick DM, Sawaya R. Limitations of stereotactic biopsy in the initial management of gliomas. Neuro Oncol. 2001;3:193–200.
3. Jaafar H. Intra-operative frozen section consultation: concepts, applications and limitations. Malays J Med Sci. 2006;13:4–12.
4. Novis DA, Zarbo RJ. Interinstitutional comparison of frozen section turnaround time. Arch Pathol Lab Med. 1997;121:559.
5. Plesec TP, Prayson RA. Frozen section discrepancy in the evaluation of central nervous system tumors. Arch Pathol Lab Med. 2007;131:1532–40.
6. Shapiro HM. Practical flow cytometry. New York: Wiley; 2005.
7. Horan PK, Wheeless LL. Quantitative single cell analysis and sorting. Science. 1977;198:149–57.
8. Frederiksen P, Reske-Nielsen E, Bichel P. Flow cytometry in tumours of the brain. Acta Neuropathol. 1978;41:179–83. https://doi.org/10.1007/BF00690432.
9. Kawamoto K, Herz F, Wolley R, Hirano A, Kajikawa H, Koss L. Flow cytometric analysis of the DNA distribution in human brain tumors. Acta Neuropathol. 1979;46:39–44.
10. Hoshino T, Nomura K, Wilson CB, Knebel KD, Gray JW. The distribution of nuclear DNA from human brain-tumor cells: flow cytometric studies. J Neurosurg. 1978;49:13–21.

11. Helson L, Traganos F, Allen JC. Brain tumor cells; flow cytofluorometric analyses in cerebrospinal fluid. N Y State J Med. 1982;82:1255–9.
12. Danielsen HE, Pradhan M, Novelli M. Revisiting tumour aneuploidy—the place of ploidy assessment in the molecular era. Nat Rev Clin Oncol. 2016;13:291–304.
13. Alexiou GA, Vartholomatos E, Goussia A, Dova L, Karamoutsios A, Fotakopoulos G, Kyritsis AP, Voulgaris S. DNA content is associated with malignancy of intracranial neoplasms. Clin Neurol Neurosurg. 2013;115:1784–7. https://doi.org/10.1016/j.clineuro.2013.04.015.
14. Alexiou GA, Vartholomatos G, Goussia A, Batistatou A, Tsamis K, Voulgaris S, Kyritsis AP. Fast cell cycle analysis for intraoperative characterization of brain tumor margins and malignancy. J Clin Neurosci. 2015;22:129–32.
15. Shioyama T, Muragaki Y, Maruyama T, Komori T, Iseki H. Intraoperative flow cytometry analysis of glioma tissue for rapid determination of tumor presence and its histopathological grade. J Neurosurg. 2013;118:1232–8.
16. Alexiou GA, Vartholomatos G, Kobayashi T, Voulgaris S, Kyritsis AP. The emerging role of intraoperative flow cytometry in intracranial tumor surgery. Clin Neurol Neurosurg. 2020;192:105742.
17. Saito T, Muragaki Y, Shioyama T, Komori T, Maruyama T, Nitta M, Yasuda T, Hosono J, Okamoto S, Kawamata T. Malignancy index using intraoperative flow cytometry is a valuable prognostic factor for glioblastoma treated with radiotherapy and concomitant temozolomide. Neurosurgery. 2019;84:662–72.
18. Vartholomatos E, Vartholomatos G, Alexiou GA, Markopoulos GS. The past, present and future of flow cytometry in central nervous system malignancies. Methods Protoc. 2021;4:11.
19. Alexiou G, Vartholomatos G, Stefanaki K, Markopoulos G, Kyritsis A. Intraoperative flow cytometry for diagnosis of central nervous system lesions. J Cytol. 2019;36:134–5.
20. Vartholomatos G, Harissis H, Andreou M, Tatsi V, Pappa L, Kamina S, Batistatou A, Markopoulos GS, Alexiou GA. Rapid assessment of resection margins during breast conserving surgery using intraoperative flow cytometry. Clin Breast Cancer. 2021;21:e602–10.
21. Markopoulos GS, Glantzounis GK, Goussia AC, Lianos GD, Karampa A, Alexiou GA, Vartholomatos G. Touch imprint intraoperative flow cytometry as a complementary tool for detailed assessment of resection margins and tumor biology in liver surgery for primary and metastatic liver neoplasms. Methods Protoc. 2021;4:66.
22. Markopoulos GS, Goussia A, Bali CD, Messinis T, Alexiou GA, Vartholomatos G. Resection margins assessment by intraoperative flow cytometry in pancreatic cancer. Ann Surg Oncol. 2022:1–3.
23. Georvasili VK, Markopoulos GS, Batistatou A, Mitsis M, Messinis T, Lianos GD, Alexiou G, Vartholomatos G, Bali CD. Detection of cancer cells and tumor margins during colorectal cancer surgery by intraoperative flow cytometry. Int J Surg. 2022;104:106717.
24. Vartholomatos G, Alexiou GA, Tatsi V, Harissis H, Markopoulos GS. Next-generation margin evaluation techniques in breast conserving surgery: a memorandum on intraoperative flow cytometry. Eur J Surg Oncol. 2022;49:675.
25. Alexiou GA, Vartholomatos G, Voulgaris S, Kyritsis AP. Letter: glioblastoma resection guided by flow cytometry. Neurosurgery. 2016;78:E761. https://doi.org/10.1227/NEU.0000000000001218.
26. Hauser SB, Kockro RA, Actor B, Sarnthein J, Bernays RL. Combining 5-Aminolevulinic acid fluorescence and intraoperative magnetic resonance imaging in glioblastoma surgery: a histology-based evaluation. Neurosurgery. 2016;78:475–83. https://doi.org/10.1227/NEU.0000000000001035.
27. Kockro RA, Hauser SB, Bernays RL. In reply: glioblastoma resection guided by flow cytometry. Neurosurgery. 2016;78:E761–2. https://doi.org/10.1227/NEU.0000000000001219.
28. Vartholomatos G, Alexiou G, Batistatou A, Kyritsis AP. Intraoperative cell-cycle analysis to guide brain tumor removal. Proc Natl Acad Sci U S A. 2014;111:E3755. https://doi.org/10.1073/pnas.1413155111.

29. Santagata S, Eberlin LS, Norton I, Calligaris D, Feldman DR, Ide JL, Liu X, Wiley JS, Vestal ML, Ramkissoon SH, et al. Intraoperative mass spectrometry mapping of an onco-metabolite to guide brain tumor surgery. Proc Natl Acad Sci U S A. 2014;111:11121–6. https://doi.org/10.1073/pnas.1404724111.

30. Alexiou GA, Vartholomatos G, Stefanaki K, Markopoulos GS, Kyritsis AP. Intraoperative flow cytometry for diagnosis of central nervous system lesions. J Cytol. 2019;36:134–5. https://doi.org/10.4103/JOC.JOC_45_18.

31. Jindal A, Kaur K, Mathur K, Kumari V, Diwan H. Intraoperative squash smear cytology in CNS lesions: a study of 150 pediatric cases. J Cytol. 2017;34:217–20. https://doi.org/10.4103/JOC.JOC_196_15.

32. Markopoulos GS, Harissis H, Andreou M, Alexiou G, Vartholomatos G. Intraoperative flow cytometry for invasive breast cancer conserving surgery: a new alternative or adjunct to cavity shaving technique? Surg Oncol. 2022;42:101712. https://doi.org/10.1016/j.suronc.2022.101712.

33. Dix C, Lo T-H, Clark G, Abadir E. Measurable residual disease in acute myeloid leukemia using flow cytometry: a review of where we are and where we are going. J Clin Med. 2020;9:1714.

34. Schuurhuis GJ, Heuser M, Freeman S, Béné M-C, Buccisano F, Cloos J, Grimwade D, Haferlach T, Hills RK, Hourigan CS. Minimal/measurable residual disease in AML: a consensus document from the European LeukemiaNet MRD working party. Blood. 2018;131:1275–91.

35. Vartholomatos G, Basiari L, Exarchakos G, Kastanioudakis I, Komnos I, Michali M, Markopoulos GS, Batistatou A, Papoudou-Bai A, Alexiou GA. Intraoperative flow cytometry for head and neck lesions. Assessment of malignancy and tumour-free resection margins. Oral Oncol. 2019;99:104344. https://doi.org/10.1016/j.oraloncology.2019.06.025.

36. Weinstein JN, Collisson EA, Mills GB, Shaw KR, Ozenberger BA, Ellrott K, Shmulevich I, Sander C, Stuart JM. The cancer genome atlas pan-cancer analysis project. Nat Genet. 2013;45:1113–20.

37. Vartholomatos G, Alexiou GA, Lianos GD, Harissis H, Voulgaris S, Kyritsis AP. Intraoperative cell cycle analysis for tumor margins evaluation: the future is now? Int J Surg. 2018;53:380–1. https://doi.org/10.1016/j.ijsu.2018.03.046.

38. Vartholomatos G, Basiari L, Kastanioudakis I, Psichogios G, Alexiou GA. The role of intraoperative flow cytometry in surgical margins of head and neck malignancies. Ear Nose Throat J. 2020;100:989S. https://doi.org/10.1177/0145561320931989.

39. Andreou M, Vartholomatos E, Harissis H, Markopoulos GS, Alexiou GA. Past, present and future of flow cytometry in breast cancer - a systematic review. EJIFCC. 2019;30:423–37.

40. Vartholomatos G, Alexiou GA, Batistatou A, Lykoudis E, Voulgaris S, Kyritsis AP. GV/GA Sarissa-lancet: a proposed real-time flow cytometer for intraoperative identification of glioma margins. Surg Innov. 2016;23:104–5. https://doi.org/10.1177/1553350615589860.

41. Vartholomatos G, Alexiou GA, Lianos GD, Kyritsis AP. From bench to operating theater: has the time come for a molecular scalpel? Future Oncol. 2017;13:121–3. https://doi.org/10.2217/fon-2016-0413.

42. Nolan JP. The evolution of spectral flow cytometry. Cytometry A. 101:812. https://doi.org/10.1002/cyto.a.24566.

43. Spitzer MH, Nolan GP. Mass cytometry: single cells, many features. Cell. 2016;165:780–91.

44. Luo S, Shi Y, Chin LK, Hutchinson PE, Zhang Y, Chierchia G, Talbot H, Jiang X, Bourouina T, Liu A-Q. Machine-learning-assisted intelligent imaging flow cytometry: a review. Adv Intelligent Syst. 2021;3:2100073.

Chapter 5
Sample: Data Analysis

Georgios Vartholomatos and Evrysthenis Vartholomatos

5.1 Introduction

Histopathologic assessment through microscopic examination of tissue has been the de facto method to evaluate the degree of malignancy as well as the status of surgical margins, making it the only available tool for surgical oncology that can guide the surgeon on the extent of resection. This information can be obtained by a "fast biopsy" by examination frozen tissue sections, for a period of at least 10–15 min per tissue sample.

Flow cytometry (FC) is an automated method of analyzing the physicochemical characteristics of cells and subcellular particles, based on the quantification of scatter and fluorescence provided that the sample under investigation is in the form of a homogeneous suspension. The analysis of DNA content and the quantification of cell cycle phases is the first established application of flow cytometry, where for a long time it has been abandoned as a diagnostic tool, overshadowed by the revolution of molecular biology and new molecular techniques [1]. Quantitative measurements of cellular DNA have shown that changes in the amount of DNA very often accompany malignancy [2].

A typical/conventional flow cytometer contains three systems that interact and make possible to analyze a sample: First a hydraulics system, in which cells in suspension can pass and hydrodynamically focused and move sequentially as individual events. Second, an optical system, in which cells and their bound fluorophores are excited by laser(s) irradiation and emit fluorescence that is detected by

G. Vartholomatos (✉)
Unit of Molecular Biology and Translational Flow Cytometry, University Hospital of Ioannina, Ioannina, Greece

E. Vartholomatos
Faculty of Medicine, School of Health Sciences, Neurosurgical Institute, University of Ioannina, Ioannina, Greece

© The Author(s), under exclusive license to Springer Nature Switzerland AG 2023
G. Alexiou, G. Vartholomatos (eds.), *Intraoperative Flow Cytometry*,
https://doi.org/10.1007/978-3-031-33517-4_5

individual filters, specialized either for the detection of scatter or fluorescence signals. Third, an electronics system, in which the quantified scatter and fluorescence signals are stored into a unified digital format for each sample and these files can be further analyzed by specialized software [3].

Flow cytometry can determine the total amount of DNA of a cell population as well as the percentage of cells located in each phase of the cell cycle. In recent studies it has been made clear that cell cycle analysis can help distinguish the grade of malignancy of brain tumors [4]. Until recently, the analysis of the cell cycle required for its determination, a time of at least 30 min and thus excluded any intraoperative application. Recently, our team has developed a rapid protocol that enables the analysis of the cell cycle within 6 min (which has the acceptance of the international scientific community under the name "Ioannina Protocol") [2]. This fact allows intraoperative analysis of the cell cycle in a surgical sample. Thus, it became possible to reliably intraoperatively classify intracranial tumors that came from both adults and pediatrics into low and high malignancy, and most importantly to determine whether the surgical limits of resection are beyond the tumor margins [5, 6].

The pioneering advantages of cytometry over other techniques (patho-anatomical and cytological assessment) lie in its great sensitivity and specificity for the identification of cancer cells, the reproducibility of the results, and the lower overall cost. Flow Cytometry allows for the analysis of multiple samples taken by the surgeon from various tumor locations during resection within a 6-minute timeframe. The samples are in the order of 2–5 mm³ and can be analyzed at the same time. Therefore, the immediate information of the surgeon about the type of malignancy and most importantly about whether he has disease-free limits is of strategic importance. Similarly, a Japanese research team that applies the trans-operative cytometry is in full alignment with our results, with the significant difference in response time which is twice as high (up to ~12 min) [7, 8]. Therefore, the surgeon is notified that a complete tumor exclusion has been made possible and the occlusion of the surgical wound could begin.

In the current chapter, we will discuss how sample-data analysis is performed in a typical iFC experiment and the things taken under consideration to assess malignancy.

5.2 Presentation of Current Techniques for Intraoperative Sample Analysis

5.2.1 A Brief Summary on Sample Preparation

During surgical assessment of a sample, a tissue can be either excised, extracted using a fine needle aspirate (FNA) or cells can be brushed or imprinted into a membrane and transferred into a solution. Solid tissues should be minced or homogenized into mixtures. Next, a PBS wash and filtration is necessary to exclude parts of tissue that have not been homogenized, in order to obtain homogeneous mixture of singular cells. This is the starting material for an intraoperative flow cytometry. The details on different variants of the method are based on the analyzed tissue and are presented in detail in the previous chapter.

5.2.2 Pre-analytical Considerations

It should be noted that before analysis, a number of tasks should be performed. First, independently of the assay, the instrument's performance should be evaluated in order to obtain results with the least variance. The correct alignment of the cytometer should be also validated before every experiment. In our case, the instrument performance in DNA content analysis has been performed using DNA QC particles (BD Biosciences), following the step-by-step instructions from the manufacturer manual.

Second, an internal control is necessary to determine the normal DNA content of non-dividing control cells. In our case we use ficoll-separated peripheral blood mononuclear cells (PBMCs) from healthy donors. Ficoll-separated PBMCs can be stained for 3 min with Ioannina Protocol staining solution containing a final concentration of 125 mM of PI. It is critical to use freshly prepared ficoll-separated PBMCs as a standard before every experiment in order to determine their DNA content, since long-term storage may lead to DNA degradation and a non-optimal peak of G0/G1 DNA content. Following analysis, we expect a single peak of mostly non-dividing cells in G0/G1 (in most cases >98% of total cells). This peak is the basis for analysis of cancer and margin samples and for the calculation of two indices that help determine malignancy, tumor index, and DNA index, as will be discussed in the next steps. A DNA content distribution of PBMCs is presented in Fig. 5.1.

Third, it should be noted that the type of analysis we perform is also based on the properties on the instrument used. For our intraoperative flow cytometry analyses, Ioannina protocol is based on propidium iodide and has been successfully used in several different cancer types [2, 9–17]. However, based on the excitation and emission properties of PI, analysis should be performed in a flow cytometer with specific optical system: 488 nm blue laser for excitation and a 617 nm (or near, compatible) emission channel. In our case, we used a compatible with PI BD FACSCalibur cytometer (BD Biosciences) with a 488 nm excitation laser and a 585/42 (FL2) emission filter. However, it should be noted that in case a cytometrist chooses another dye for DNA content quantification, a cytometer with compatible excitation and emission channels to the fluorescence properties to the chosen dye should be selected.

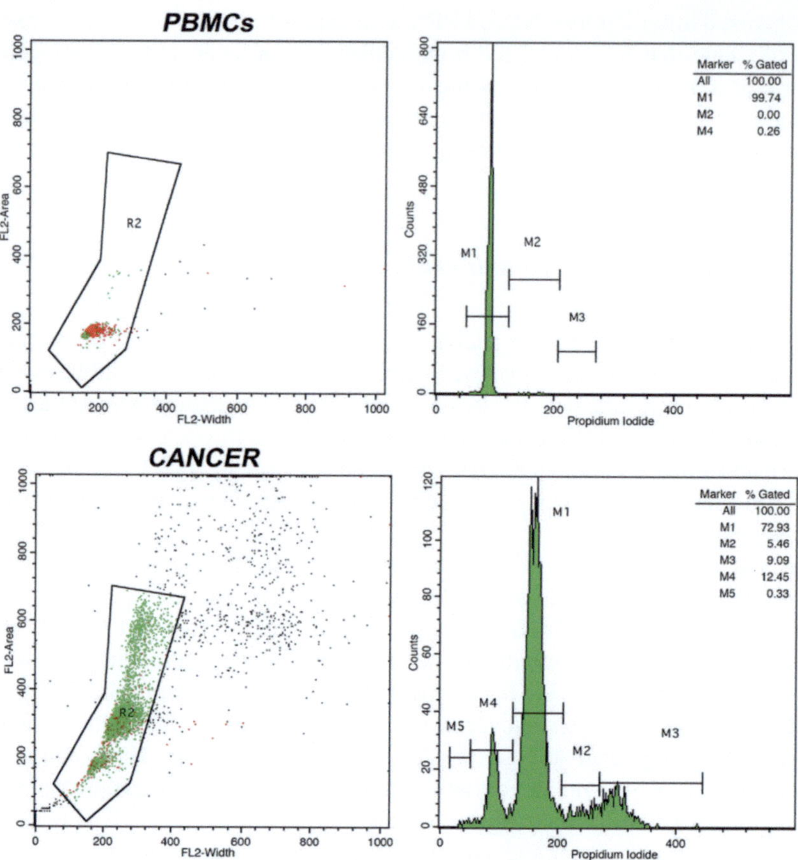

Fig. 5.1 A paradigm of intraoperative analysis of DNA content, based on propidium iodide fluorescence. Upper panel: analysis of DNA content in peripheral blood mononuclear cells (PBMCs); Lower panel: analysis of DNA content in a sample derived from a tumor tissue. In a preanalytical step, we obtain cells in solution which are stained with propidium iodide, a dye that is incorporated into nucleic acids. First, a two-dimensional analysis is performed (two dot-plots in the left), using FL2-width and FL2-area fluorescence, the fluorescence channel that represents emission of PI-fluorescence. A gating strategy (R2 region) is necessary to separate between real events that represent stained nuclei and non-specific events that are either cellular debris (lower left) or doublets (mostly events with a higher ratio of FL2-width to FL2-area). The gating strategy is executed initially to a PBMCs sample and is repeated for each other sample, including cancer and margin samples. Second, a histogram representing PI-fluorescence is each sample is used to quantify DNA content and cell cycle distributions. The presented histograms in the right are separated using different areas, by respective markers. In PBMCs markers M1, M2, M3 correspond, based on mean fluorescence intensity, to cells in G1, S, G2/M cell cycle phases, respectively. In cancer sample the DNA content distribution is separated by 5 markers. M1, M2, and M3 correspond to, as previously to cancer cells. G1, S, G2/M cell cycle phases, respectively. M4 corresponds to normal diploid DNA distribution, as determined by PBMCs analysis. In this case, this additional marker is necessary, since cancer cells exhibit hyperploidy. M5 corresponds to cell death, since represent nuclei that have lost a significant amount of their DNA (apoptotic cells, etc.). The percentage of cells in each phase (presented in the upper right in each histogram) is used to quantify markers that are used to determine malignancy and evaluate margin status

5.2.3   *Flow Cytometric DNA Content Analysis*

The foundations of iFC require an accurate DNA content analysis. The concept behind this is based on the fact that among the hallmarks of cancer is genomic instability and mutation, evading growth suppressors and sustaining proliferative signaling [18, 19]. Genomic instability is associated with significant chromosomal abnormalities [1, 20] that can be quantified by iFC as cells with aneuploidic chromosomal number. Sustaining proliferative signaling [21] as well as evading growth suppressors [22] leads to a large percentage of cells in S and G2/M cell cycle phases. The potential of iFC to accurate cell cycle phase determination matches these characteristics that distinguish cancer from normal cells.

A representative analysis of iFC in cancer, including an internal control is presented in Fig. 5.1. In the depicted analysis, fluorescence from propidium iodide is directly analogous to the DNA content of individual cells. A gating strategy is performed to separate cells from debris and aggregates. Next, follows the separation of cell subpopulation by markers in order to separate cells in different cell cycle phases. This is possible because cells in G2/M are characterized by a dual mean fluorescence intensity than that of cells in G1 phase, since DNA replication has been completed in these phases. Cells in S phase (synthesis phase in which cells undergo replication of their DNA) can be characterized by a mean fluorescence intensity between cells in G1 and G2/M phases, dependent on the proportion of replicated DNA. An additional fraction of SubG1 cells are the ones which the nuclear DNA quantity is less than that of cells in G1 phase, meaning chromosome loss (apoptotic cells, fractured nuclei, nuclear debri, etc.).

In our analysis, both cell determination and gating, as well as DNA content analysis are performed manually by the cytometrist. Conventional intraoperative flow cytometry analysis is a typical one-dimension analysis that can be performed in all modern software packages. In some cases, the selection of the appropriate analysis software may be based on the available cytometer. In our case, we have used CellQuest V3.1 (BD Biosciences), since it is the default software for acquisition and analysis for a FACSCalibul (BD Biosciences) flow cytometer. However, the files on a modern cytometer are saved in a unified standard, the FCS standard, that makes it possible to transfer and reanalyze a file with other analysis software programs that can offer DNA content analysis. There are several modern tools, such as Modfit LT, that can offer more advanced DNA content quantification capacity, including a more automated cell cycle peak evaluation. Modfit and other distinct flow cytometry software for DNA analysis regularly use ploidy modeling on a DNA content histogram in order to evaluate the subpopulations in each phase of the cell cycle. In addition, online tools such as Cytobank may offer near real time evaluation by cytometrists throughout the world [23].

5.2.4   Evaluation of Results

The use of a flow cytometry analysis software makes possible the determination of percentage of cells in G0/G1, based on the geometric mean of PBMCs fluorescence peak. Next, markers can define corresponding subpopulations that represent proliferating cells in S phase or the G2/M cell cycle phases. In addition, altered DNA content of G0/G1 peak can be detected, corresponding to aneuploidic cancer cells. During analysis of iFC findings, a number of indices have been developed to assist the interpretation of results and to lead to a more unified and robust analysis. Based on Ioannina Protocol, two indices have developed, while an additional index has been developed by the team in Tokyo, Japan.

An index for quantifying tumor aneuploidy is DNA index. DNA index is calculated as a fraction of the geometric mean of G1 peak of cancer cells divided to the geometric mean of G1 peak of normal PBMC cells. In that way DNA index is indicative of the presence aneuploidy. A DNA index of ~1 means that cancer cells are devoid of aneuploidic DNA and are diploid (Fig. 5.2). A DNA index more than 1.05 means hyperploidy (higher number of chromosomes or chromosomes with altered acquired quantity of DNA (Fig. 5.3). On the contrary a DNA index less than 0.95 is considered as hypoploid, meaning that cancer cells have lost chromosomes or chromosome parts (Fig. 5.4). In all cases, a DNA index $\neq$ 1 is indicative of cancer.

An index of cancer proliferation is that of Tumor-index which is considered as the total sum of the percentage of cancer cells in S and G2/M cell cycle phases. The tumor index can be informative of the resultant proliferative potential following

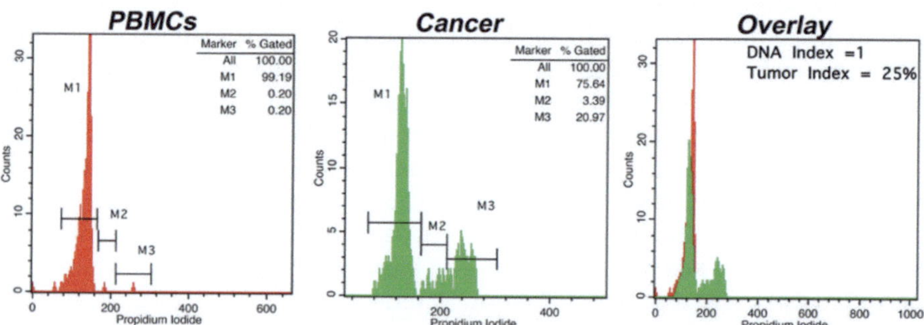

Fig. 5.2 A representative case of a diploid tumor. The DNA content distribution of PBMCs, cancer cells, and an overlay of both histograms is presented. DNA index has been calculated as 1 (the peak of G0/G1 of PBMCs) and the presence of cancer cells is based on the high tumor index of 25%

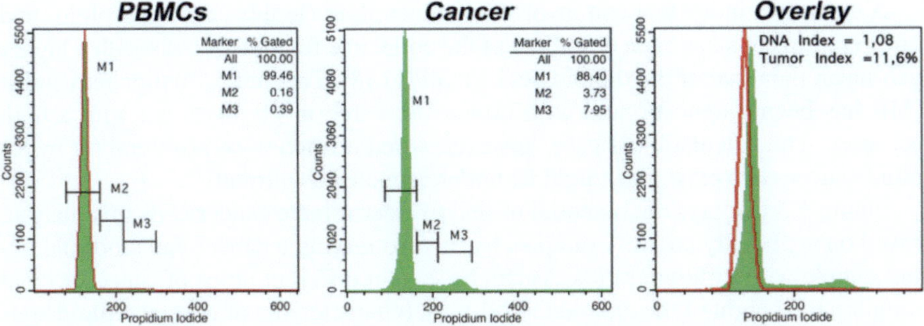

Fig. 5.3 A representative case of a hyperploid tumor. The DNA content distribution of PBMCs, Cancer cells and an overlay of both histograms are presented. DNA index has been calculated as 1.08, indicating hyperploidy (the peak of G0/G1 of PBMCs). Cancer cells are characterized by both hyperploidy and a high tumor index of 11.6%

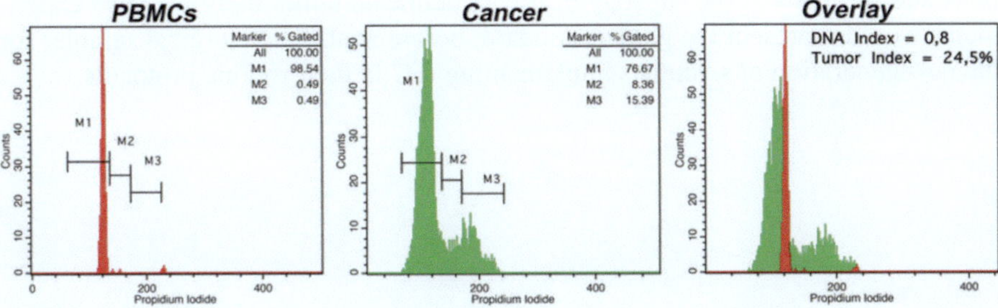

Fig. 5.4 A representative case of a hypoploid tumor. The DNA content distribution of PBMCs, cancer cells, and an overlay of both histograms is presented. DNA index has been calculated as 0.8, indicating hypoploidy (the peak of G0/G1 of PBMCs). Cancer cells are characterized by both hypoploidy and a high tumor index of 24.5%

carcinogenesis, since it is the collective fraction of cells that have an active cell cycle and circulate in the S and G2/M phases. A high tumor index can be predictive of cancer cells, in the absence of a DNA index $\neq$ 1, while the cut-off value can be anywhere between 5% and 10.5%, a feat that is dependent on the cancer site and the proliferative potential of normal cells, leading to very high sensitivity, specificity, and accuracy [2, 9–17]. Figure 5.2 shows a typical paradigm of a diploid tumor with high tumor index (~25%). Aneuploidic tumors shown in Figs. 5.3 and 5.4 are also characterized by tumor index, which is characteristic for malignancy, up to 24.5%.

A collective index that can involve both aneuploid (in this case hyperploid) and proliferating cells has been described as the collective fraction of cells with a higher geo-mean than that of the diploid peak in G0/G1 [8]. This index, malignancy index (MI) has been diagnostic and with prognostic value in glioblastoma with a high accuracy. The calculation is easy, however, when a fraction of proliferating hypoploid cancer cells exist, this might be underestimated as normal.

Figure 5.5 displays the potential of iFC to discriminate cancer cells in a margin, based on artificially creating samples by in vitro mixing a cancer and a normal tissue sample with different ratios. As can be seen in different ratios of cancer/normal samples, the height of the diploid G0/G1 peak (characteristic of normal diploid nondividing cells, present on the left corner of the histogram) is inversely proportional to the population of malignant cells (co-localized with the DNA content distribution of cancer cells). In the last histogram (100% normal), the absence of malignant cells is prominent and may represent a negative margin during iFC assessment during surgery. This kind of analysis is of paramount importance for the training of cytometrists and surgeons of the capacity of iFC to delineate tumor margins. Such experiments would represent the golden standard, before analysis of surgical samples for the new generation of scientists implementing iFC in their routine protocols.

Fig. 5.5 Demonstration of the sensitivity of iFC in discriminating cancer cells by mixing in-vitro cancer and normal cells with different ratios. (**a**) DNA content analysis as individual histograms. A hyperploid cancer (DNA index = 1.7), with high proliferative potential (tumor index = 17%) is presented. Markers M1, M2, and M3 correspond to, G1, S, G2/M cell cycle phases, respectively. M4 corresponds to normal diploid DNA distribution. The percentage of cells in each marker is presented in each individual histogram. The analysis of cancer, normal and the results of in vitro mixing cancer cells (C) and normal cells (N) with different ratios and following analysis of DNA content is presented. (**b**) Overlay distributions. DNA content distribution of cancer cells is presented in solid green distribution. Overlays of in vitro mixing cancer cells (C) and normal cells (N) with different ratios (the respective ratios that are presented in panel A) is shown in red line overlay to achieve an optical comparison to the distribution of cancer cells

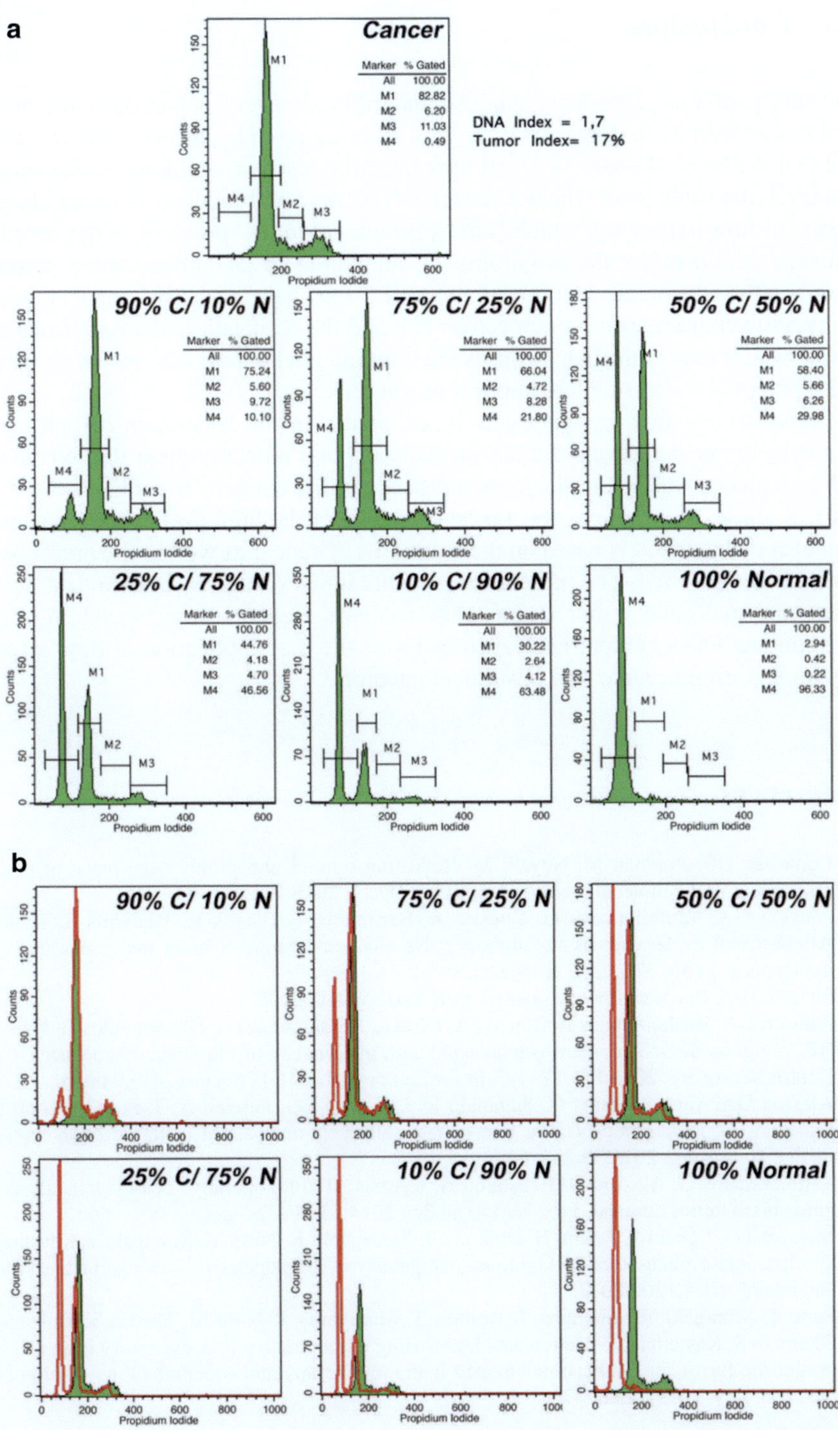

a
Cancer
Marker   % Gated
All   100.00
M1   82.82
M2   6.20
M3   11.03
M4   0.49
DNA Index = 1,7
Tumor Index= 17%

90% C/ 10% N
Marker   % Gated
All   100.00
M1   75.24
M2   5.60
M3   9.72
M4   10.10

75% C/ 25% N
Marker   % Gated
All   100.00
M1   66.04
M2   4.72
M3   8.28
M4   21.80

50% C/ 50% N
Marker   % Gated
All   100.00
M1   58.40
M2   5.66
M3   6.26
M4   29.98

25% C/ 75% N
Marker   % Gated
All   100.00
M1   44.76
M2   4.18
M3   4.70
M4   46.56

10% C/ 90% N
Marker   % Gated
All   100.00
M1   30.22
M2   2.64
M3   4.12
M4   63.48

100% Normal
Marker   % Gated
All   100.00
M1   2.94
M2   0.42
M3   0.22
M4   96.33

b
90% C/ 10% N
75% C/ 25% N
50% C/ 50% N
25% C/ 75% N
10% C/ 90% N
100% Normal

5.3 Conclusions

The utility of flow cytometry analysis has offered several advantages for tumor analysis as well as in diagnosis of several pathologies. This utility is based on the fact that the level of analysis is cell based, exhibit a sensitivity down to the single-cell level, the same level where a cancer cell occurs and functions. Another characteristic of flow cytometry, which is most prominent in iFC protocol, is the speed of analysis, which offers the possibility of adaptation in an intraoperative manner. Based on the advantages mentioned above, iFC may have a positive impact towards the specific characterization of a cancer cell and the delineation of a tumor margin. In that way it may contribute towards the ultimate goal of surgical oncology, which is the potential for a complete tumor removal.

Intraoperative flow cytometry is based partly on the separation of cell cycle phases by the so-called one-dimension analysis [24]. What separates the cells in the different phases is DNA replication, a procedure that happens in proliferating cells in the S phase. The logic of iFC takes advantage of the high proliferative potential of cancer cells, which is based on the hallmarks of cancer as well as the presence of aneuploidies [18, 25]. The presence of specific indices, such as DNA index, tumor index, and malignancy index, assists the analysis. Hence, a rapid variation of the conventional DNA content analysis transforms the first application of flow cytometry into an irreplaceable tool in surgical oncology.

References

1. Danielsen HE, Pradhan M, Novelli M. Revisiting tumour aneuploidy—the place of ploidy assessment in the molecular era. Nat Rev Clin Oncol. 2016;13:291–304.
2. Alexiou GA, Vartholomatos G, Goussia A, Batistatou A, Tsamis K, Voulgaris S, Kyritsis AP. Fast cell cycle analysis for intraoperative characterization of brain tumor margins and malignancy. J Clin Neurosci. 2015;22:129–32.
3. Shapiro HM. Practical flow cytometry. New York: Wiley; 2005.
4. Alexiou GA, Vartholomatos E, Goussia A, Dova L, Karamoutsios A, Fotakopoulos G, Kyritsis AP, Voulgaris S. DNA content is associated with malignancy of intracranial neoplasms. Clin Neurol Neurosurg. 2013;115:1784–7. https://doi.org/10.1016/j.clineuro.2013.04.015.
5. Alexiou GA, Vartholomatos G, Stefanaki K, Lykoudis EG, Patereli A, Tseka G, Tzoufi M, Sfakianos G, Prodromou N. The role of fast cell cycle analysis in pediatric brain tumors. Pediatr Neurosurg. 2015;50:257–63.
6. Vartholomatos G, Alexiou G, Batistatou A, Kyritsis AP. Intraoperative cell-cycle analysis to guide brain tumor removal. Proc Natl Acad Sci. 2014;111:E3755–5.
7. Matsuoka G, Eguchi S, Anami H, Ishikawa T, Yamaguchi K, Nitta M, Muragaki Y, Kawamata T. Ultrarapid evaluation of meningioma malignancy by intraoperative flow cytometry. World Neurosurg. 2018;120:320–7.
8. Saito T, Muragaki Y, Shioyama T, Komori T, Maruyama T, Nitta M, Yasuda T, Hosono J, Okamoto S, Kawamata T. Malignancy index using intraoperative flow cytometry is a valuable prognostic factor for glioblastoma treated with radiotherapy and concomitant temozolomide. Neurosurgery. 2019;84:662–72.

 9. Alexiou G, Vartholomatos G, Stefanaki K, Markopoulos G, Kyritsis A. Intraoperative flow cytometry for diagnosis of central nervous system lesions. J Cytol. 2019;36:134–5.
10. Vartholomatos G, Basiari L, Exarchakos G, Kastanioudakis I, Komnos I, Michali M, Markopoulos GS, Batistatou A, Papoudou-Bai A, Alexiou GA. Intraoperative flow cytometry for head and neck lesions. Assessment of malignancy and tumour-free resection margins. Oral Oncol. 2019;99:104344. https://doi.org/10.1016/j.oraloncology.2019.06.025.
11. Markopoulos GS, Glantzounis GK, Goussia AC, Lianos GD, Karampa A, Alexiou GA, Vartholomatos G. Touch imprint intraoperative flow cytometry as a complementary tool for detailed assessment of resection margins and tumor biology in liver surgery for primary and metastatic liver neoplasms. Methods Protoc. 2021;4:66.
12. Vartholomatos E, Vartholomatos G, Alexiou GA, Markopoulos GS. The past, present and future of flow cytometry in central nervous system malignancies. Methods Protoc. 2021;4:11.
13. Vartholomatos G, Harissis H, Andreou M, Tatsi V, Pappa L, Kamina S, Batistatou A, Markopoulos GS, Alexiou GA. Rapid assessment of resection margins during breast conserving surgery using intraoperative flow cytometry. Clin Breast Cancer. 2021;21:e602–10.
14. Georvasili VK, Markopoulos GS, Batistatou A, Mitsis M, Messinis T, Lianos GD, Alexiou G, Vartholomatos G, Bali CD. Detection of cancer cells and tumor margins during colorectal cancer surgery by intraoperative flow cytometry. Int J Surg. 2022;104:106717.
15. Markopoulos GS, Goussia A, Bali CD, Messinis T, Alexiou GA, Vartholomatos G. Resection margins assessment by intraoperative flow cytometry in pancreatic cancer. Ann Surg Oncol. 2022:1–3.
16. Markopoulos GS, Harissis H, Andreou M, Alexiou G, Vartholomatos G. Intraoperative flow cytometry for invasive breast cancer conserving surgery: a new alternative or adjunct to cavity shaving technique? Surg Oncol. 2022;42:101712. https://doi.org/10.1016/j.suronc.2022.101712.
17. Vartholomatos G, Alexiou GA, Tatsi V, Harissis H, Markopoulos GS. Next-generation margin evaluation techniques in breast conserving surgery: a memorandum on intraoperative flow cytometry. Eur J Surg Oncol. 2022;49:675.
18. Hanahan D, Weinberg RA. Hallmarks of cancer: the next generation. Cell. 2011;144:646–74.
19. Hanahan D. Hallmarks of cancer: new dimensions. Cancer Discov. 2022;12:31–46.
20. Fröhling S, Döhner H. Chromosomal abnormalities in cancer. N Engl J Med. 2008;359:722–34.
21. DeBerardinis RJ, Lum JJ, Hatzivassiliou G, Thompson CB. The biology of cancer: metabolic reprogramming fuels cell growth and proliferation. Cell Metab. 2008;7:11–20.
22. Amin AR, Karpowicz PA, Carey TE, Arbiser J, Nahta R, Chen ZG, Dong J-T, Kucuk O, Khan GN, Huang GS. Evasion of anti-growth signaling: a key step in tumorigenesis and potential target for treatment and prophylaxis by natural compounds. Semin Cancer Biol. 2015;35 Suppl:S55–77.
23. Chen TJ, Kotecha N. Cytobank: providing an analytics platform for community cytometry data analysis and collaboration. Curr Top Microbiol Immunol. 2014;377:127–57.
24. Pozarowski P, Darzynkiewicz Z. Analysis of cell cycle by flow cytometry. Checkpoint controls and cancer. Springer; 2004. p. 301–11.
25. Kastan MB, Bartek J. Cell-cycle checkpoints and cancer. Nature. 2004;432:316–23.

Part III
Intraoperative Flow Cytometry in CNS Malignancies

Chapter 6
Pathology of the Tumors of the Central Nervous System

Redi Bumci, Ioannis Parthymos, Constantinos Zamboglou,
and Anna C. Goussia

6.1 Introduction

Recent advances in cancer genomics and epigenomics have improved our knowledge of the molecular alterations underlying biology of the Central Nervous System (CNS) tumors. According to the recommendations of the cIMPACT-NOW consortium, the fifth edition of the WHO CNS classification published in 2021 (WHO CNS5 2021) advances the role of molecular markers in tumor definition, grading, and classification emphasizing the importance of integrated diagnoses and layered reports [1–10]. Now, for many CNS tumors the histological findings must be combined with knowledge on the presence or absence of particular molecular characteristics before pathologists arrive at an integrated diagnosis (Table 6.1).

The discovery of several molecular abnormalities and altered signaling pathways such as *IDH1/IDH2* (isocitrate dehydrogenase 1 and 2) gene mutations, deletions of chromosomes 1 and 19 (1p/19q codeletion), alterations of p53 (tumor suppressor gene *p53*), Rb (retinoblastoma susceptibility gene), WNT (Wingless), and other pathways have contributed significantly to our understanding of tumors' biology [1–13]. The emergence of therapies targeting specific molecular events emphasizes the value for the inclusion of molecular alterations in disease diagnostic approach.

R. Bumci · I. Parthymos
Department of Pathology, University Hospital of Ioannina, Ioannina, Greece

C. Zamboglou
Department of Radiotherapy, German Oncology Center, Limassol, Cyprus
e-mail: constantinos.zamboglou@goc.com.cy

A. C. Goussia (✉)
Department of Pathology, University Hospital of Ioannina, Ioannina, Greece

Department of Pathology, German Oncology Center, Limassol, Cyprus
e-mail: agoussia@uoi.gr; anna.gousia@goc.com.cy

© The Author(s), under exclusive license to Springer Nature
Switzerland AG 2023
G. Alexiou, G. Vartholomatos (eds.), *Intraoperative Flow Cytometry*,
https://doi.org/10.1007/978-3-031-33517-4_6

Table 6.1 An example of four-layered report structure[a]

Cerebrum	
Integrated diagnosis	Diffuse astrocytoma, IDH-mutated (CNS WHO grade 2)
Histological diagnosis	Diffuse infiltrating astrocytoma, mitotic activity is not detected, microvascular proliferation and/or necrosis are absent
WHO grade	2
Molecular information	*IDH1*- or *IDH2*-mutant, *ATRX*-mutant, *p53*-mutant, 1p/19q not co-deleted, H3-wildtype, *TERT* promoter-wildtype, *CDKN2A/B* non-deleted, *EGFR*-non amplified, +7/−10 chromosome copy number changes-negative

[a]A tumor in an adult patient
Abbreviations: *IDH* isocitrate dehydrogenase, *IDH1* isocitrate dehydrogenase 1, *IDH2* isocitrate dehydrogenase 2, *ATRX* alpha thalassemia/mental retardation syndrome X-linked, *p53* tumor suppressor gene p53, *H3* histone 3 gene, *TERT* telomerase reverse transcriptase, *CDKN2A/B* cyclin-dependent kinase inhibitors 2A/B, *EGFR* epidermal growth factor receptor

A wide variety of laboratory technologies has been used for CNS tumor diagnosis and classification, as evidenced in WHO CNS5 classification. Immunohistochemistry (IHC) is a simple and robust methodology for detecting protein expression indicative of the origin and the underlying molecular (e.g., mutational) status [11, 12, 14–16]. With respect to gliomas, antibodies directed towards molecules such as GFAP (glial fibrillary acidic protein), IDH1 p.R132H, ATRX (alpha thalassemia/mental retardation syndrome X-linked), p53 (tumor suppressor gene *p53)*, H3 K27M (histone 3), EGFR (epidermal growth factor receptor), and others are the routine standards for diagnostic, prognostic, and classification purposes. However, this technique has several limitations and over the last decade novel methodologies such as DNA and RNA sequencing, fluorescence in situ hybridization (FISH) or genome-wide SNP arrays have dramatically contributed to tumor diagnosis and classification [5, 17]. Very recently, DNA methylation profiling has emerged as a powerful tool for diagnostic and prognostic purposes, especially when used along with morphology and standard technologies. Importantly, in the WHO CNS5 Classification for some tumor entities the methylation profile is included into the Essential and Desirable Diagnostic Criteria [5, 18–20].

In this chapter, we review the updates in histopathology and molecular biology for the most common primary CNS tumors in adults and children-particularly gliomas, embryonal tumors, and meningiomas-highlighting important molecular features that are used to make an integrated diagnosis and provide robust prognostic information for a more tailored and effective therapeutic approach.

6.2 Gliomas

Gliomas are the most common primary brain tumors and comprise a broad category of neoplasms represented approximately 24.5% of all primary brain and other CNS tumors and 80.9% of malignant tumors according to the Central Brain Tumor

Registry of the United States (CBTRUS) [21]. Most gliomas occur in supratentorial sites (frontal, temporal, parietal, occipital lobes, combined; 61.6%) and only a small proportion of tumors occur in areas of the CNS other than the brain [21]. Gliomas affect all ages, and the incidence rate is higher in males than in females.

The 2021 CNS5 WHO classification divides gliomas into categories based on histopathological features, mutational profile, and copy number alterations (Table 6.2). According to this classification, diffuse gliomas are classified into adult-type and pediatric-type diffuse gliomas. This distinction is important to separate tumors with distinct molecular biology and different prognosis, even they may share overlapping histology. In addition, gliomas with circumscribed growth pattern are grouped separately from gliomas with diffuse and infiltrating growth pattern because the latter tend to have a more aggressive clinical behavior [5].

6.2.1 Adult-Type Diffuse Gliomas

In the group of adult-type diffuse gliomas, three main tumor entities are included: astrocytoma, IDH-mutant; oligodendroglioma, IDH-mutant, and 1p/19q-codeleted and glioblastoma, IDH-wildtype [5].

Table 6.2 2021 CNS5 WHO Classification of Gliomas [5]

Adult-type diffuse gliomas
• Astrocytoma, IDH-mutant
• Oligodendroglioma, IDH-mutant, and 1p/19q-codeleted
• Glioblastoma, IDH-wildtype
Pediatric-type diffuse low-grade gliomas
• Diffuse astrocytoma, MYB or MYBL1-altered
• Angiocentric glioma
• Polymorphous low-grade neuroepithelial tumor of the young
• Diffuse low-grade glioma, MAPK pathway-altered
Pediatric-type diffuse high-grade gliomas
• Diffuse midline glioma, H3 K27-altered
• Diffuse hemispheric glioma, H3 G34-mutant
• Diffuse pediatric-type high-grade glioma, H3-wildtype, and IDH-wildtype
• Infant-type hemispheric glioma
Circumscribed astrocytic gliomas
• Pilocytic astrocytoma
• High-grade astrocytoma with piloid features
• Pleomorphic xanthoastrocytoma
• Subependymal giant cell astrocytoma
• Chordoid glioma
• Astroblastoma, MN1-altered

6.2.1.1 Astrocytoma, IDH-Mutant

Astrocytoma, IDH-mutant is defined as a diffusely infiltrating glioma with *IDH1* or *IDH2* gene mutations, frequent *ATRX* or/and *p53* mutations and with the absence of 1p/19q codeletion.

The reported incidence rate is 0.44 per 100,000 population and the median age of diagnosis is 36 years; however, some cases can occur in older ages [22] Most tumors affect males than females. IDH-mutant astrocytomas can arise in any site of the CNS, develop sporadically and rarely in association with genetic syndromes (e.g., Li-Fraumeni syndrome) [23] In young adults and children, astrocytomas are characterized by germline mutations in mismatch repair genes [24].

Histopathology-Molecular Pathology

The histologic appearance varies depending on tumor grade (CNS WHO grades 2,3 or 4) [5, 25, 26]. Low-grade tumors consist of well differentiated glial cells with mild nuclear atypia and absent or very low mitotic activity, embedded in a loose microcystic matrix (Fig. 6.1). Higher grade tumors exhibit signs of anaplasia, increased mitotic activity, microvascular proliferation, and necrosis.

IDH-mutant astrocytomas harbor *IDH* (isocitrate dehydrogenase) gene mutations, commonly *IDH1* and less frequently *IDH2* [27]. *IDH* gene mutations lead to changes in cell metabolism and to accumulation of the oncometabolite 2-hydroxyglutarase, which promotes tumorigenesis [28, 29]. *IDH1* mutations are usually located at the codon 132 and the most frequent is the IDH1: c.395G > A p.R132. The rare *IDH2* mutations are found at codon 172 with the p.R172K mutation being the most frequent. In the majority of IDH-mutant astrocytomas (~90%), the presence of *IDH* mutations is associated with mutations of the *ATRX* gene, which is responsible for the alternative lengthening of telomeres [30–32]. Concurrent mutations include mutations of the *p53* gene [31]. All the above molecular

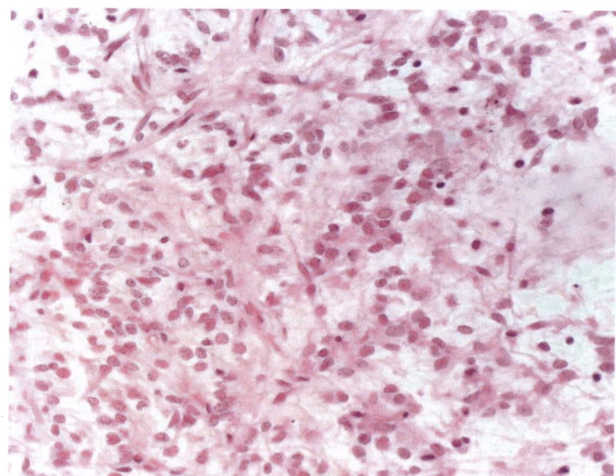

Fig. 6.1 Astrocytoma, IDH-mutant, CNS WHO grade 2. An infiltrating glioma showing features of a low-grade tumor with mild nuclear atypia and absence of mitoses (Hematoxylin-Eosin stain; original magnification X400)

alterations can be detected in the routine diagnostic process by a panel of immuno-histochemical markers, using specific antibodies against IDH1p.R13H (the most common *IDH* mutation), ATRX, and p53. Immunohistochemical staining for IDH1p.R132H and p53 (>10% of tumor nuclei) as well as loss of nuclear staining for ATRX correlate strongly with the presence of *IDH, p53,* and *ATRX* mutations, respectively (Fig. 6.2). If the immunostaining for IDH1p.R132H is negative, sequencing of *IDH1* and *IDH2* mutations can be performed to assess for the very rare non-canonical mutations, which are the less common *IDH1* mutations (IDH1: c.394C > T p.R132C, p.R132G, p.R132S, and p.R132L) or the rare *IDH2* mutations [5].

Molecular analyses have shown key genes that serve to drive tumor grading. Based therefore on the molecular profile, the designation of the highest grade (CNS WHO grade 4) can be applied in tumors showing homozygous deletion of cyclin-dependent kinase inhibitor 2A (*CDKN2A*) and/or cyclin-dependent kinase inhibitor 2A (*CDKN2B*), even in the absence of traditional anaplastic features, such as micro-vascular proliferation or necrosis (Table 6.3) [12, 33].

Several studies have shown that astrocytomas, IDH-mutant with homozygous deletion of *CDKN2A/B* has been associated with aggressive biologic behavior [12, 25, 33]. Other molecular alterations related with worse outcome include homozy-gous deletion of *RB*, amplification of *CDK4* (cyclin-dependent kinase 4), amplifica-tion of PDGFRA (platelet-derived growth factor receptor alpha), and activating point mutations of *PIK3R1* (phosphoinositide-3-kinase regulatory subunit 1 [5, 34].

Very recently, two distinct entities of IDH-mutant astrocytomas with high prog-nostic relevance have been described. *The infratentorial astrocytoma, IDH-mutant* which arises in brainstem or cerebellum and is characterized by the presence of non-canoninal *IDH* mutations [35]. Approximately 80% of *IDH* mutations are of IDH1R132G or IDH2R172S variants. In addition, the frequency of ATRX protein loss, which is typically associated with *IDH* mutations in supratentorial astrocyto-mas, is significantly lower (<50%) in the infratentorial compartment. Moreover, the outcome of patients is worse compared to patients with supratentorial IDH-mutant

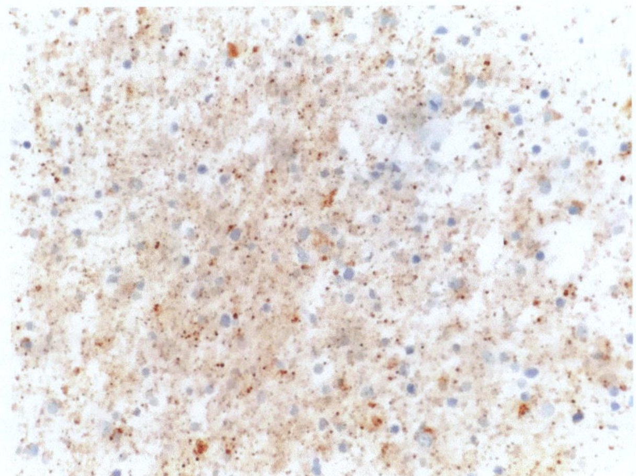

Fig. 6.2 Astrocytoma, IDH-mutant. Immunohistochemical expression for IDH1p. R132H protein exhibiting cytoplasmic staining of tumor cells (Avidin-Biotin-Complex-ABC immunohistochemical method; original magnification X400)

Table 6.3 Criteria for assessing CNS WHO grades in astrocytomas, IDH-mutant

Grade	Criteria
CNS WHO 2	Absence of histologic features of anaplasia Mitotic activity is absent or low microvascular proliferation, necrosis and *CDKN2A/B* homozygous deletion are absent
CNS WHO grade 3	Presence of anaplasia and significant mitotic activity Microvascular proliferation, necrosis and *CDKN2A/B* homozygous deletion are absent
CNS WHO grade 4	Presence of microvascular proliferation or necrosis or *CDKN2A/B* homozygous deletion Or any combination of these features

Abbreviation: *CDKN2A/B* cyclin-dependent kinase inhibitors 2A/B

astrocytomas. Molecular testing is critical for the detection of these tumors since they cannot be identified by IHC. The second new entity is the *primary mismatch repair deficient IDH-mutant astrocytoma,* which is of high histological grade and occurs in children, adolescents and young adults (median age 14 years) with mismatch repair deficiency syndromes (Lynch or Constitutional Mismatch Repair Deficiency Syndrome-CMMRD) [24]. The patients have germline mutations in DNA mismatch repair genes (MLH1, MSH6, or MSH2) along with *p53* mutations, *RB1* and *RTK/PI3K/AKT* (receptor tyrosine kinase/phosphatidylinositol-3-kinase/ protein kinase B) pathways alterations. Diagnosis can be established by DNA-sequencing proving the mismatch repair deficiency or immunohistochemically demonstrating the loss of mismatch repair proteins. Primary mismatch repair-deficient IDH-mutant astrocytomas have the worst clinical outcome with a median survival of 15 months.

6.2.1.2 Oligodendroglioma, IDH-Mutant, and 1p/19q-Codeleted

Oligodendroglioma, IDH-mutant and 1p/19q-codeleted is a diffusely infiltrating glioma with *IDH1* or *IDH2* mutations and codeletion of chromosomes 1p and 19q [5]. The tumor manifests in adults with an average age of 40–50 years and rarely in children and young adults. There is a slight male predominance. Most cases develop sporadically, while germline mutations of the *POT1* (protection of telomere 1) gene, a member of the telombin family that encodes a nuclear protein involved in telomere maintenance, have been recently reported to be associated with familial cases [36].

Histopathology-Molecular Pathology

Oligodendrogliomas are frequently located in frontal and temporal lobes and infiltrate diffusely the cortex, whereas the tumor cells aggregate around neurons or vessels (perineuronal and perivascular satellitosis). In well differentiated tumors (CNS

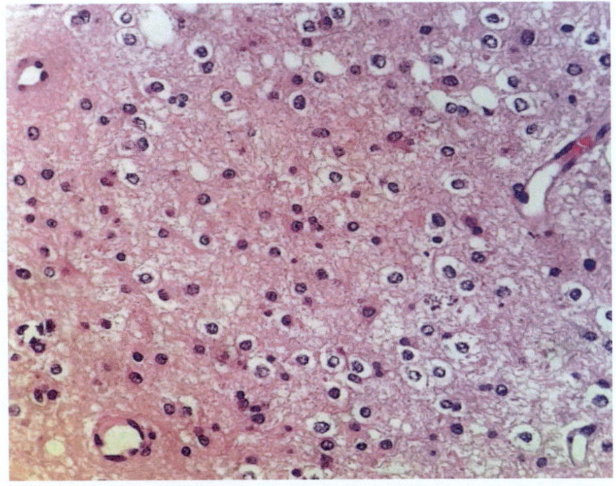

Fig. 6.3 Oligodendroglioma, IDH-mutant and 1p/19q codeteted, CNS WHO grade 2. Tumor cells have round to oval nuclei and clear cytoplasm ("honeycomb" appearance). (Hematoxylin-Eosin stain; original magnification X400)

WHO grade2) the neoplastic cells have round to ovoid nuclei and clear cytoplasm; this is the typical honeycomp or fried-egg appearance which represents an artifact due to tissue fixation in formalin (Fig. 6.3). A subset of tumor cells looks like gemistocytic astrocytes (named "minigemistocytes" or "microgemistocytes"). Microcalcifications are frequent and a dense network of branching small vessels is a typical feature. Histological evidence of high cellularity, significant cytological atypia, increased mitotic activity ($\geq$ 2.5 mitoses/mm^2), microvascular proliferation, and necrosis are consistent with high-grade tumors (CNS WHO grade 3).

Almost all oligodendrogliomas, IDH-mutant and 1p/19q-codeleted have activating mutations of the *TERT* (telomerase reverse transcriptase gene) [37, 38]. *ATRX* mutations are mutually exclusive with 1p/19q codeletion and at the immunohistochemical level this is consistent with the presence of ATRX nuclear staining. *P53* mutations are not common. Homozygous deletion of *CDKN2A* has been reported in few cases of oligodendrogliomas WHO grade 3 and has been correlated with shorter survival [33]. Other abnormalities linked to worse survival in high-grade tumors include *PIK3CA* (phosphatidylinositol-4,5-bisphosphate 3-kinase catalytic subunit alpha) and *TCF12* (transcription factor 12) gene mutations [39, 40].

Oligosarcoma is a distinct group of IDH-mutant gliomas differing from conventional oligodendrogliomas on the histologic, epigenetic, proteomic, molecular, and clinical level [41]. It is a rare aggressive subtype of recurrent oligodendroglioma, with a sarcomatous component and frequent mutations in *TERT* promoter, *p53,* and *NF1* (neurofibromin 1) as well as with *CDKN2A/B* homozygous deletion. Survival of the patients is significantly poorer for oligosarcomas than for grade 3 oligodendrogliomas as first recurrence. The diagnosis can be based on the combined presence of sarcomatous histology, *IDH* mutations, *TERT* promoter mutation, and/or 1p/19q codeletion. In doubtful cases, its characteristic DNA methylation profile is diagnostic.

6.2.1.3   Glioblastoma, IDH-Wildtype

It is defined as a diffuse astrocytic glioma, corresponding to CNS WHO grade 4, that is IDH-wildtype and H3-wildtype and has one or more of the following features: microvascular proliferations, necrosis, *TERT* promoter mutations, *EGFR* gene amplification, and/or + 7/−10 chromosomes copy number changes [5]. Therefore, molecular detection of *TERT* promoter mutations, *EGFR* gene amplification, and/or concurrent +7/−10 in an IDH-wildtype and H3-wildtype diffuse glioma in adults is sufficient for the diagnosis of glioblastoma even in histologically low-grade tumors because they carry a prognosis that is the same as that of histologically diagnosed glioblastoma [5, 42–45].

According to CBTRUS statistical report, glioblastoma accounts for 14.2% of all primary brain and other CNS tumors and 50.1% of primary malignant brain tumors [22]. It is a malignant tumor with the highest number of cases, with 14,190 cases projected in 2022 and 14,490 cases projected in 2023. Glioblastoma affects commonly older adults than children (approximately 2.7% of all brain and other CNS tumors among ages 0–19 years). The reported incidence rate is 3.26 per 100,000 population. The incidence is increased with age, with rates highest in ages 75–84 years. The tumor is 1.6 times more common in males than females and 1.95 times higher among people who are White compared to Black people.

Relative survival estimates for glioblastoma are quite low with a median survival of 8 months; 6.9% of patients survive 5 years post-diagnosis [22]. These survival estimates are somewhat higher for the small number of patients who were diagnosed under the age of 20 years.

Ionizing radiation in the head and neck region is the only validated risk factor for tumor development, while a small subset of tumors occurs in patients with Lynch, Li-Fraumeni, and *NF1* syndromes. Glioblastoma affects all cerebral lobes as a solitary or multiple masses occupying the white and deeper gray matter or extending through the corpus collosum. The tumor is poorly marginated and exhibits extensive hemorrhagic and necrotic areas [5].

Histopathology-Molecular Pathology

Histologically, prominent cellular and nuclear pleomorphism, frequent mitoses, microvascular proliferation, and areas of necrosis are observed (Figs. 6.4, 6.5, 6.6, and 6.7). Cellular pleomorphism includes the presence of undifferentiated, spindled, epithelioid, lipidized or giant cells. Some histological subtypes or patterns have been described, such as epithelioid glioblastoma, small cell glioblastoma, granular cell astrocytoma/glioblastoma, glioblastoma with mesenchymal/epithelial metaplasia, and glioblastoma with primitive neuronal component. Gliosarcoma is a rare histological subtype characterized by a mixture of gliomatous and sarcomatous components.

By IHC, IDH-wildtype glioblastoma does not stain for IDH1R132 and mutations-specific antibodies against H3 histones. ATRX and p53 nuclear staining is observed

Fig. 6.4 Glioblastoma, IDH-wildtype, CNS WHO grade 4. Highly cellular glioma composed of anaplastic cells with nuclear atypia and mitoses (Hematoxylin-Eosin stain; original magnification X400)

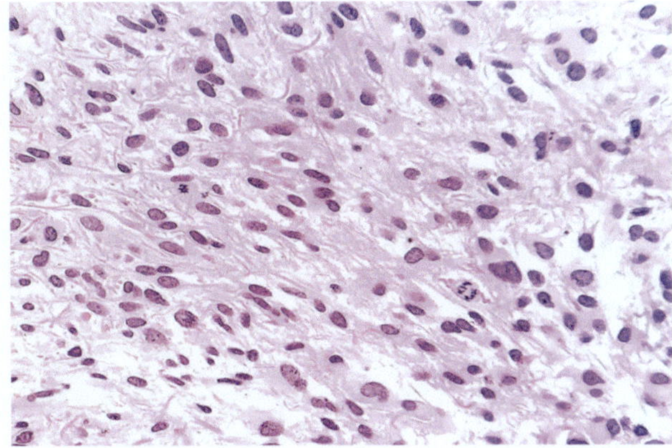

Fig. 6.5 Glioblastoma, IDH-wildtype, CNS WHO grade 4. Apparent microvascular proliferation (Hematoxylin-Eosin stain; original magnification X400)

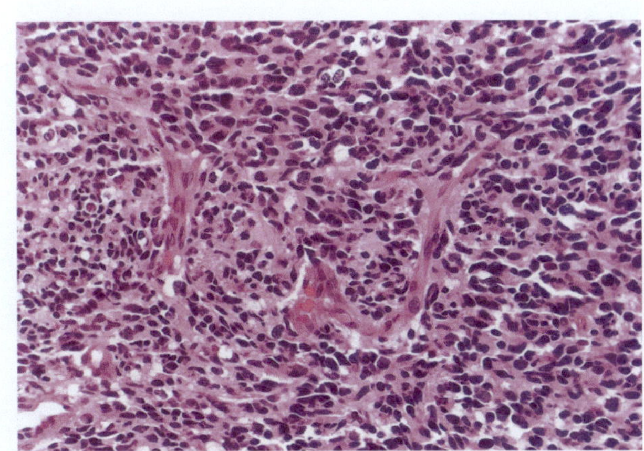

Fig. 6.6 Glioblastoma, IDH-wildtype, CNS WHO grade 4. Necrosis with palisading tumor cells (Hematoxylin-Eosin stain; original magnification X200)

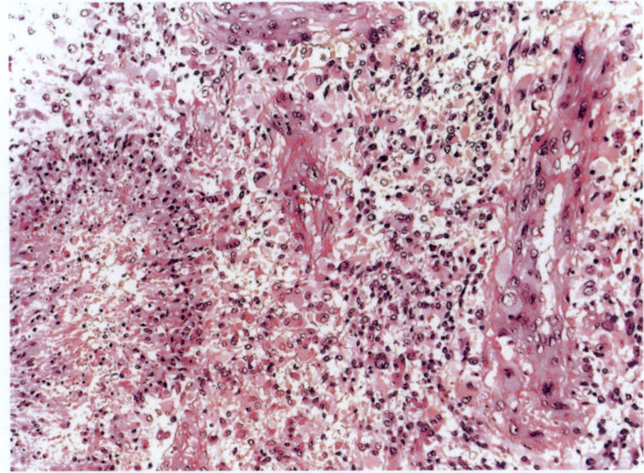

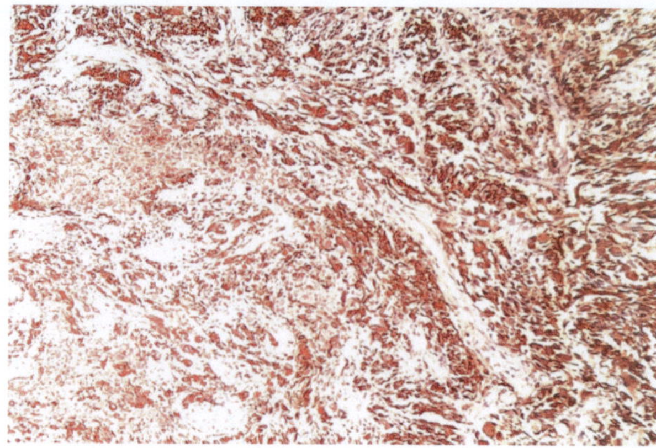

Fig. 6.7 Glioblastoma, CNS WHO grade 4. Immunohistochemistry for GFAP which highlights the glioma cells showing, diffuse cytoplasmic staining (Avidin-Biotin-Complex-ABC immunohistochemical method; original magnification X200)

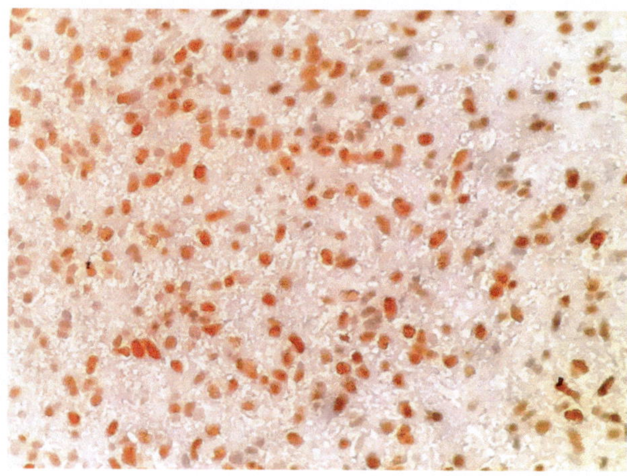

Fig. 6.8 Glioblastoma, IDH-wildtype, CNS WHO grade 4. Diffuse nuclear ATRX immunoreactivity in the nuclei of tumor cells (Avidin-Biotin-Complex-ABC immunohistochemical method; original magnification X400)

in the majority of the cases (Figs. 6.8 and 6.9). Absence of immunostaining for IDH1R132 is sufficient to diagnose IDH-wildtype glioblastoma in patients older than 55 years, without a history of a lower grade glioma and whose tumors are not located in midline structures. In younger patients or in patients with a history of a low-grade glioma, a negative IDH1R132 immunohistochemical result should be followed by sequence for the detection of *IDH* mutations. If the molecular testing is negative, then a diagnosis of glioblastoma, IDH-wildtype can be made. In cases of tumors located in midline structures, testing for histone H3 mutations should also be performed to exclude other types of high-grade gliomas.

Diagnostic molecular alterations of glioblastomas include *TERT* promoter mutations (~80%), *EGFR* amplification, mutation or rearrangement (~60%,), mutations or deletion of *PTEN* (phosphatase and tensin homolog), alterations of the p53 pathway (~90%) through mutation or deletion of *p53* gene (~30%) or alterations involving *CDKN2A* or *MDM2* (MDM2 proto-oncogene) genes, and alterations of the Rb

Fig. 6.9 Glioblastoma, IDH-wildtype, CNS WHO grade 4. High p53 protein expression (Avidin-Biotin-Complex-ABC immunohistochemical method; original magnification X200)

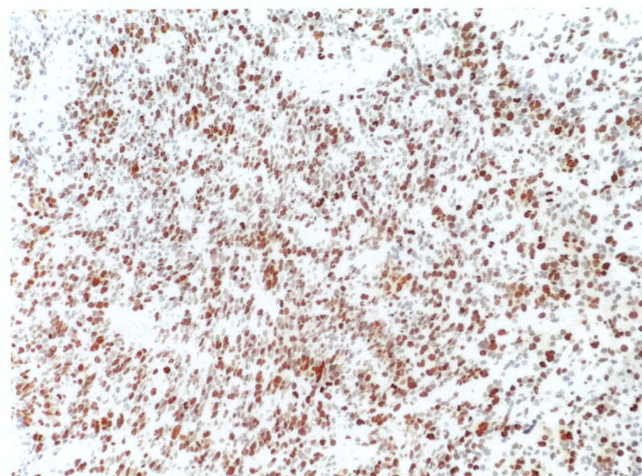

pathway (~80%) through *Rb* mutation or deletion, *CDKN2A* deletion and *CDK4/6* (cyclin-dependent kinases 4/6) amplification [42, 44, 46]. In addition, whole chromosome 7 gain and chromosome 10 loss are the most common numerical chromosome alterations, which frequently occur in combination [44].

MGMT (O-6-methylguanine-DNA methyltransferase) gene promoter methylation is a significant prognostic factor for the patients with glioblastoma and is associated with longer survival when treated with alkylating agents, such as temozolomide [47]. Recently, it has been reported that approximately 3–5% of glioblastomas IDH-wildtype have *FGFR3-TACC3* (fibroblast growth factor receptor 3-transforming acidic coiled-coil containing protein 3) fusions with 4p16.3 tandem duplication [48]. These tumors have unusual morphologic features such as monomorphic round cells with ovoid nuclei, network of "chicken-wire" vessels, microcalcifications, and desmoplastic stroma. The patients have longer survival compared to other glioblastoma patients and *FGFR3-TACC3* fusions may predict response to FGFR (fibroblast growth factor receptor) inhibitor treatment.

6.2.2 Pediatric-Type Diffuse Gliomas

During the last years, it has been clearly shown that gliomas affecting pediatric patients have different clinical course, biology, and genetics in comparison to those occurring in adults [49–54]. Most pediatric gliomas are indolent and slow-growing tumors with rare malignant progression, lack *IDH* mutations, and 1p/19q codeletion, which are the genetic hallmark of adult gliomas, and in addition they have distinct molecular abnormalities, such as alterations of the Ras-Mitogen-activated protein kinase (RAS/MAPK) pathway or mutations in histone genes [49–54]. Therefore, the distinction is of clinical importance since it may lead to appropriate therapeutic options. The incorporation of molecular features with robust prognostic information has led to further classification of pediatric diffuse gliomas, into low-grade and high-grade groups (Table 6.4). Specific entities can be identified only by DNA methylation profile, although methylome profiling methodologies are not recommended as routine diagnostic tools. It should be mentioned that in the updated CNS WHO 2021 classification it is emphasized that, despite the terminology, some pediatric-type gliomas may occur also in adults and vice versa [54].

6.2.2.1 Pediatric-Type Diffuse Low-Grade Gliomas

Pediatric-type diffuse low-grade gliomas (pLGG) represent approximately 10% of all pediatric CNS neoplasms. A significant body of literature has demonstrated that the majority of pLGG are driven by genetic events resulting in up-regulation of the MAPK pathway [55–58]. In this category of tumors four subtypes of gliomas are included: diffuse astrocytoma, MYB or MYBL1-altered; angiocentric glioma; polymorphous low-grade neuroepithelial tumor of the young and diffuse low-grade glioma, MAPK pathway-altered (Table 6.4).

Table 6.4 The most common molecular events in pediatric-type diffuse gliomas [5]

Pediatric-type diffuse low-grade gliomas	Common molecular features
Diffuse astrocytoma, MYB or MYBL1-altered	*MYB* or *MYBL1* fusions
Angiocentric glioma	*MYB-QKI* fusion
Polymorphous low-grade neuroepithelial tumor of the young	MAPK pathway alterations including *BRAF* p.V600E mutations, fusions involving *FGFR2* or *FGFR3*
Diffuse low-grade glioma, MAPK pathway-altered	MAPK pathway alterations, most commonly *BRAF* V600E or alteration of *FGFR1*
Pediatric-type diffuse high-grade gliomas	
Diffuse midline glioma, H3 K27-altered	*H3 K27* mutations or H3 K27 pathway alterations, *EGFR* amplification, EZHIP overexpression
Diffuse hemispheric glioma, H3 G34-mutant	*H3 G34* mutation
Diffuse pediatric-type high-grade glioma, H3-wildtype, and IDH-wildtype	*PDGFRA, EGFR,* and *MYCN* alterations
Infant-type hemispheric glioma	*NRTK* fusions, *ROS1, ALK, MET*

Abbreviations: *MYB* c-myb, *MYBL1* MYB proto-oncogene like 1, *QKI* KH domain RNA binding, MAPK Mitogen-activated protein kinase, *BRAF* v-raf murine sarcoma viral oncogene homolog B1, *FGFR1* fibroblastic growth factor receptor 1, *FGFR2* fibroblastic growth factor receptor 2, *FGFR3* fibroblastic growth factor receptor 3, *H3 K27* histone H3 K27, *EGFR* epidermal growth factor receptor, EZHIP enhancer of zeste homologs inhibitory protein, *H3 G34* histone 3, *PDGFRA* platelet-derived growth factor receptor, *MYCN* MYCN proto-oncogene, bHLH transcription factor, *NRTK* neurotrophic receptor tyrosine kinase, *ROS1* ROS proto-oncogene 1, *ALK* Anaplastic lymphoma kinase, *MET* MET proto-oncogene

Diffuse Astrocytoma, MYB or MYBL1-Altered

Diffuse astrocytoma, *MYB* (c-myb) or *MYBL1* (MYB proto-oncogene like 1)-altered is a rare (<0.5% of all brain tumors) diffusely infiltrating astrocytic tumor, CNS WHO grade 1, that arises in cerebral hemispheres, in both cortical and subcortical areas [5]. Patients present with drug-resistant seizures [59]. Histologically, the tumor consists of monomorphic cells with ovoid or spindled nuclei without evidence of mitoses or signs of anaplasia.

Next generation sequencing (NGS), interphase fluorescence in situ hybridization (FISH) or DNA methylation profiling have demonstrated a fusion between *MYB* or *MYBL1* and a partner gene [5, 60, 61]. The tumor is typically IDH- and H3-wildtype. The available clinical data suggest the benign clinical behavior of the tumor and the low rates of recurrence after surgical excision [55, 56].

Angiocentric Glioma

A diffuse CNS WHO grade 1 glioma occurring in children and young adults with a median age of 17 years [5, 55]. The temporal and frontal lobes are the most commonly affected sites. Microscopically, it is composed of monomorphous elongated cells with bipolar cytoplasmic processes arranged around blood vessels. Signs of anaplasia are absent.

Almost all tumors harbor a *MYB-QKI* (c-myb gene fusion- KH domain RNA binding), a finding that can help confirm the diagnosis [62, 63]. Mutations of *IDH*, histone *H3* genes, *ATRX,* and *p53* genes are lacking. Surgery is curative in most cases.

Polymorphous Low-Grade Neuroepithelial Tumor of the Young

Polymorphous low-grade neuroepithelial tumor of the young (PLNTY) is a CNS WHO grade 1 cerebral neoplasm characterized by refractory seizures [5]. In histological sections, tumor cells exhibit oligodendroglioma-like features such as round nuclei, perinuclear halos, calcifications, and delicate branching capillary network. However, *IDH* mutations and codeletion of 1p/19q are not observed. The mitotic activity is absent or very low and anaplastic features are not evident.

By IHC, glial cells appear positive for CD34 antigen. The main molecular abnormalities of PLNTY are activating genetic alterations of MAPK pathway and especially *BRAF* (v-raf murine sarcoma viral oncogene homolog B1) p.V600E mutations or fusions involving *FGFR2* (fibroblastic growth factor receptor 2) or *FGFR3* (fibroblastic growth factor receptor 3) genes. Although surgery is frequently curative, cases with recurrences or progression to high-grade tumors have been reported [5, 64, 65].

Diffuse Low-Grade Glioma, MAPK Pathway-Altered

A low-grade cerebral tumor with diffuse astrocytic or oligodendroglial morphological appearance which has a diagnostic molecular alteration of the MAPK pathway, most commonly *BRAF* V600E or an alteration of *FGFR1* (fibroblastic growth factor receptor 1) gene along with the absence of an *IDH* or *H3* mutation and *CDKN2A* homozygous deletion [5]. Tumors of this category affect mainly children, but occasionally present in adults [6, 55]. Genes less frequently altered, but involving to MAPK pathway activation, include *NTRK1/2/3, MET, FGFR2*, and *MAP2K1* [66].

The clinical outcome is uncertain, although it seems to depend on various clinicopathological parameters such as patient age, tumor location, histological appearance, and molecular profile. A CNS WHO grade has yet to be assigned [5].

6.2.2.2 Pediatric-Type Diffuse High-Grade Gliomas

High-grade diffuse gliomas (pHGGs) comprise about 10% of pediatric CNS tumors [50, 58, 67]. The majority of the tumors show mutations in histones H3.3 and H3.1 that lead to alterations of chromatin remodeling and transcription [11, 68]. Four pediatric-type diffuse high-grade gliomas are included in this category: diffuse midline glioma H3 K27-altered; diffuse hemispheric glioma H3 G34-mutant; diffuse pediatric-type high-grade glioma H3-wildtype and IDH-wildtype; and infant-type hemispheric glioma [5].

Diffuse Midline Glioma, H3 K27-Altered

Diffuse midline gliomas (DMGs), H3 K27-altered, are infiltrating tumors arising in midline structures, preferentially in the thalamus, brainstem, and spinal cord. They represent approximately 10–15% of all pediatric brain tumors and occur mainly in children with a median age of diagnosis 5–11 years, but they can occur also in adulthood. Histologically, the tumor cells have an astrocytic morphology and may exhibit a variety of nuclear pleomorphism. Most cases have high-grade features characterized by increased number of mitotic figures, microvascular proliferation, and necrosis (CNS WHO grade 4). However, anaplastic morphology is not necessary for the histological diagnosis. In the presence of diffuse infiltration, midline location and *H3 K27* mutations or *H3 K27* pathway alterations, WHO grade 4 is warranted even in the absence of microvascular proliferation or necrosis, due to the aggressive nature of these tumors [5].

By molecular techniques, several subtypes of DMGs have been identified: DMG, H3.3K 27 mutant; DMG, H3.1 K27 mutant; DMG H3 wildtype, enhancer of zeste homologs inhibitory protein (EZHIP) overexpression and DMG, EGFR-mutant [69, 70]. H3 K27 mutant tumors are characterized by somatic mutations in *H3F3A* or *HIST1H3B/C* encoding for histone variants H3.3 and H3.1, respectively. IHC is a robust method for the demonstration of *H3 K27* mutations which result to the loss of H3 K27 mutant protein.

The prognosis of patients with DMGs is poor. The presence of H3 K27M alterations is associated with worse prognosis over wild type diffuse midline gliomas.

Diffuse Hemispheric Glioma, H3 G34-Mutant

pHGGs having H3F3A G34R or G34V mutations (that substitutes glycine to arginine or valine at position 34) arise in cerebral hemispheres and often occur in adolescents and young adults [68, 71, 72]. The histological findings may be similar either with glioblastoma with high cellularity, significant mitotic activity, microvascular proliferation and/or necrosis or with embryonal tumor consisting of small cells with hyperchromatic nuclei and scant cytoplasm. However, even if high-grade features are absent, the presence of an H3 G34R/V mutation confers a CNS WHO grade 4. By IHC, the neoplastic cells are positive for mutation-specific antibodies against H3.3 p. G35R (G34R) and p.G35V (G34V) mutant proteins, but these antibodies are not absolutely specific [73].

The prognosis is generally poor; however, the patients have longer overall survival than those with DMGs [74].

Diffuse Pediatric-Type High-Grade Glioma, H3-Wildtype and IDH-Wildtype

pHGGs, H3-wildtype, and IDH-wildtype are aggressive tumors (CNS WHO grade 4) occurring in children, adolescents, and young adults. The most common affected anatomical sites are the supratentorial brain and the infratentorial/brainstem structures. Histologically, they exhibit glioblastoma-like features or may show an undifferentiated morphology [5].

Based on DNA methylation profile, three subtypes have been identified according to specific alterations in *PDGFRA*, *p53*, *NF1*, *EGFR*, and *MYCN*: diffuse pediatric-type high-grade glioma *RTK1* (receptor tyrosine kinase 1), diffuse pediatric-type high-grade glioma RTK2 (receptor tyrosine kinase 2), and diffuse pediatric-type high-grade glioma MYCN. pHGG RTK*1* *is characterized by PDGFRA amplification,* pHGG RTK2 *by EGFR amplification, and TERT promoter mutations and* pHGG *MYCN is enriched for MYCN amplifications* [75, 76].

Treatment includes total surgical excision followed by radiotherapy and chemotherapy. Patient's prognosis is poor, however, pHGG RTK2 *has a better outcome and* pHGG *MYCN the worst [76].*

Infant-Type Hemispheric Glioma

Infant-type hemispheric glioma is a cerebral astrocytoma that arises mainly in the first years of life. Histologically, it exhibits astrocytic differentiation although cases with ependymal or ganglionic differentiation have also been described [5]. The characteristic molecular alterations include *RTK* fusions involving the neurotrophic receptor tyrosine kinase (*NTRK*) family, or *ROS1, ALK,* and *MET* [77]. According to the underlying molecular abnormality, infant-type hemispheric gliomas are distinguished into the following subtypes: NTRK-altered, ROS1-altered, ALK-altered, and MET-altered.

Survival seems to be worse in tumors with *ROS1* alterations. Studies investigating RTK fusions as therapeutic targets are ongoing.

6.2.3　Circumscribed Astrocytic Gliomas

Some astrocytic gliomas have a more circumscribed growth pattern than diffuse gliomas and tend to have a more indolent clinical course. In this category of tumors, pilocytic astrocytoma, high-grade astrocytoma with piloid features, pleomorphic xanthoastrocytoma, subependymal giant cell astrocytoma, chordoid glioma, and astroblastoma *MN1*-altered are included (Table 6.5).

6.2.3.1　Pilocytic Astrocytoma

Pilocytic astrocytoma (PA) (CNS WHO grade 1) is the most common glioma in children during the first two decades of life, with a median age of diagnosis of 8 years. For children and adolescents of ages 0–19 years, pilocytic astrocytoma accounts for 15.3% of the most common brain and other CNS histopathologies [22]. PAs frequently arise in the cerebellum, midline structures (e.g., brainstem, optic chiasm, basal ganglia) and in the spinal cord. After the age of 20 years, the tumors

Table 6.5 The most common molecular events in circumscribed astrocytic gliomas [5]

Circumscribed astrocytic gliomas	Common molecular features
Pilocytic astrocytoma	*KIAA1549:BRAF* fusion, BRAF p.V600E point mutation, *NF1* mutation *FGFR1* mutation, *FGFR1* fusion, *NTRK* fusions
High-grade astrocytoma with piloid features	*CDKN2A* and/or *CDKN2B* homozygous deletion or mutations; *CDK4* amplification, *KIAA1549:BRAF* fusion, *NF1* mutation, *FGFR1* mutation
Pleomorphic xanthoastrocytoma	*BRAF* V600E mutation, *CDKN2A* and/or *CDKN2B* homozygous deletion
Subependymal giant cell astrocytoma	*TSC1* and *TSC2* alterations
Chordoid glioma	*PRKCA* mutation
Astroblastoma *MN1*-altered	*MN1* fusion, *CDKN2A* homozygous deletion

Abbreviations: *NF1* neurofibromin 1, *FGFR1* fibroblastic growth factor receptor 1, *BRAF* v-raf murine sarcoma viral oncogene homolog, *CDKN2A* cyclin-dependent kinase inhibitor 2A, *CDKN2B* cyclin-dependent kinase inhibitor 2B, *TSC1* tuberous sclerosis complex gene 1, *TSC2* tuberous sclerosis complex gene 2, *NTRK* neurotrophic receptor tyrosine kinase, *PRKCA* protein kinase C alpha, *MN1* anti-meningioma disrupted in balanced translocation1 may arise in the cerebral hemispheres. Most cases develop sporadically, although some tumors are presented in patients with germline mutations in the MAPK pathway genes, including *neurofibromatosis type 1* (*NF1*) [78].

Histologically, PA has a biphasic appearance with dense compact fibrillary areas of bipolar cells alternating with loose or myxoid areas. Typically, Rosenthal fibers or eosinophilic granular bodies are found in compact areas. Hyalinized vessels, gromeruloid microvascular proliferations, and calcifications are common features. Nuclear pleomorphism may be apparent but mitotic activity is absent or very low. Two morphological subtypes of PAs have been described: *pilomyxoid astrocytoma* with a characteristic angiocentric arrangement of tumor cells and *pilocytic astrocytoma with histological features of anaplasia* including significant mitotic activity and palisading necrosis.

Almost all PAs harbor an alteration in the MAPK pathway with the most frequent (~60%) being a rearrangement at chromosome 7q34, resulting in a *KIAA1549:BRAF* fusion [79, 80]. In the appropriate morphological context, this fusion is diagnostic of PAs and is more common in cerebellar tumors. Other genetic alterations seen in a minority of the cases include *BRAF* rearrangements involving other fusion partners, *BRAF* p.V600E point mutations and mutations of *NF1*, *FGFR1*, and *NTRK* family genes [81].

The prognosis of PAs is favorable even after incomplete surgical removal. Therapies targeting BRAF and the MAPK pathway are under investigation in clinical trials.

6.2.3.2 High-Grade Astrocytoma with Piloid Features

High-grade astrocytoma with piloid features is a rare neoplasm arising predominantly in the cerebellum. Histologically, the tumor has a high-grade piloid or a glioblastoma-like appearance [5]. Since the morphological findings are not characteristic for this entity, its diagnostic approach is challenging. The knowledge of tumor DNA methylation profile is necessary since most cases have homozygous deletion or mutations of *CDKN2A* and/or *CDKN2B* or amplification of *CDK4* [82, 83]. Other molecular abnormalities include MAPK pathway gene alterations (e.g., *KIAA1549:BRAF* fusion in ~20% of the cases) and *NF1* and *FGFR1* mutations (~20% and ~17%, respectively) [82].

Prognostic information for the patients with high-grade astrocytoma with piloid features is sparse. The existing data suggest a shorter OS than that of PA and a better survival than that reported for patients with glioblastoma [84].

6.2.3.3 Pleomorphic Xanthoastrocytoma

Pleomorphic xanthoastrocytoma (PXA) is a superficially located cerebral tumor affecting children and young adults. Most patients present with a long history of seizures. Histologically, the tumor consists of large epithelioid pleomorphic cells admixed with multinucleated cells, spindle cells, and xanthomatous cells. Characteristic features include the presence of eosinophilic granular bodies and the prominent reticulin deposition. Cases with low mitotic activity (<2.5 mitoses/mm^2) are classified as CNS WHO grade 2 while those with higher number of mitoses ($\geq$2.5 mitoses/mm^2) and presence of necrosis correspond to CNS WHO grade 3 [5].

The majority of PXAs (up to 80%) harbor *BRAF* V600E mutations. Other common molecular abnormalities include homozygous deletion of *CDKN2A* and/or *CDKN2B* (up to 90%) [85, 86]. Alterations of other genes of the MAPK pathway or *TERT* promoter mutation can also be observed; however, the combination of *BRAF* V600E mutation along with homozygous deletion of *CDKN2A* and/or *CDKN2B* is highly suspicious for tumor diagnosis in morphologically difficult cases.

The prognosis of PXA is generally favorable but recurrence rates are high even in low-grade tumors. Targeted therapies with inhibition of the BRAF and MAPK pathways have been proved beneficial for recurrent/refractory *BRAF* V600E mutant tumors especially when a total surgical resection cannot be achieved [87].

6.2.3.4 Subependymal Giant Cell Astrocytoma

Subependymal giant cell astrocytoma (SEGA) is a slow-growing tumor, corresponding to CNS WHO grade 1 SEGA occurs during the first two decades of life, typically in patients with tuberous sclerosis It characteristically arises in the subependymal areas of the lateral ventricles. On microscopic examination, the tumor consists of large ganglion-like astrocytes arranged in sheets or fascicles into a vascular and rich in inflammatory cells stroma [5].

In morphologically ambiguous cases, the knowledge of the clinical history and the detection of tuberous sclerosis complex genes 1 and 2 (*TSC1* and *TSC2*) alterations are diagnostically helpful [88]. Patients with SEGAs have a good prognosis after complete tumor removal and may respond to treatment with mTOR inhibitors [5].

6.2.3.5 Chordoid Glioma

A rare CNS WHO grade 2 tumor which arises in the wall of the third ventricle The tumor occurs mainly in adults, with a female predominance. Histological features include the presence of cords or clusters of epithelioid cells embedded in a mucinous stroma. High-grade morphological features are absent [5]. By IHC, tumor cells express a variety of markers that possesses overlapping glial, epithelial, endothelial and other elements; therefore the differential diagnosis of chordoid gliomas includes several other tumor entities.

At the molecular level, the detection of a missense mutation in the protein kinase C alpha (*PRKCA* p.D463H) is of diagnostic value [89, 90]. Gross total resection is curative for this type of tumor.

6.2.3.6   Astroblastoma, *MN1*-Altered

Astroblastoma, *MN1*-altered is a rare glial tumor characterized by structural rearrangement in the *MN1* (anti-meningioma disrupted in balanced translocation1) gene at chromosome 22q22.1. The most frequent partners of *MN1* fusions are the BEN domain containing 2 (*BEND2*) and CXXC finger protein 5 (*CXXC5*) [5, 91, 92]. There is a strong female predominance and the reported median age patients is 15 years. Cerebral hemispheres are the most common affected sites.

Histologically, the characteristic finding is the presence of astroblastic rosettes characterized by a radial arrangement of tumor cells around a central vascular structure. Perivascular and pericellular hyalinization is a common feature. Low- and high-grade histological feature may be observed, but up to now no definite histological grading criteria have been established [5].

Gross total resection of low-grade tumors is frequently associated with long survival, without high rates of recurrence. Patients diagnosed after the age of 30 years seem to have worse outcome compared to the outcome of younger patients [5].

6.3   Embryonal Tumors

CNS embryonal tumors comprise a heterogeneous group of malignant neoplasms (mostly WHO grade 4), arising from neural stem cells [5]. They are the most frequently reported brain and other CNS tumors in children of ages 0–4 years, and the fourth most common tumor type overall in children and adolescents aged 0–19 years [22]. They account for 12.2% of all primary brain and other CNS tumors in children aged 0–14 years, 9.2% of tumors in children and adolescents aged 0–19 years, and 0.8% of tumors diagnosed overall. Embryonal tumors are 1.46 times more common in males than females and this sex difference is largest in medulloblastoma [22].

The most common tumor entity of the category of embryonal neoplasms is medulloblastoma. Other CNS embryonal tumors include atypical teratoid/rhabdoid tumor, cribriform neuroepithelial tumor, embryonal tumor with multilayered rosettes, CNS neuroblastoma, *FOXR2*-activated, CNS tumor with *BCOR* internal tandem duplication, and CNS embryonal tumor NEC/NOS. According to CBTRUS statistical report, medulloblastomas, atypical teratoid rhabdoid tumors, and all other embryonal tumors account for 68.3%, 17.2%, and 14.8%, respectively [22].

The spectrum of molecular alterations identified in embryonal tumors has been enlarged dramatically and the demonstration of specific molecular characteristics is now necessary for the accurate diagnostic approach. Among various molecular techniques performed for diagnostic purposes, DNA methylation arrays have become necessary for some tumor types and molecular groups [93, 94].

6.3.1 Medulloblastoma

The vast majority of embryonal tumors are medulloblastomas (MBs) that arise in the posterior fossa, especially in the cerebellum. The incidence of medulloblastoma decreases with age; it is 0.51 per 100,000 population, 0.62 per 100,000 population, 0.32 per 100,000 population, and 0.15 per 100,000 population in children ages groups 0–4, 5–9, 10–14 years, and adolescents ages 15–19 years, respectively [22]. However, some cases have been reported in adults [95]. Most MBs develop sporadically but they may also occur in the setting of several inherited cancer syndromes (e.g., naevoid basal cell carcinoma syndrome/Gorlin syndrome, Li-Fraumeni syndrome, and familial adenomatous polyposis) [96].

The 2021 WHO classification scheme, as in previous 2016 WHO classification, separates MBs into two distinct designations: MB, histologically defined and MB, molecularly defined [5] (Table 6.6).

6.3.1.1 MB, Histologically Defined

Histologically, MBs can be separated into subtypes including classic, desmoplastic/nodular, with extensive nodularity and large cell/anaplastic (Table 6.6). *Classic* MB is the most common subtype and consists of densely packed undifferentiated cells with hyperchromatic nuclei and high mitotic and apoptotic activity. Areas with Homer Wright rosettes can also be observed (Fig. 6.10). *Desmoplastic/nodular* MB is characterized by pale reticulin-free nodular areas surrounded by densely arranged hyperchromatic cells. Homer Wright rosettes are not common. The mitotic activity is higher in the internodular areas. MB *with extensive nodularity* exhibits a lobular architecture with large elongated nodular areas. In the *large/anaplastic* MB there are large anaplastic cells with prominent nuclear pleomorphism, nuclear moulding, cytoplasmic pseudoinclusions, and increased number of mitotic and apoptotic figs [5]. By IHC, most MBs express neural markers and markers for synaptophysin and NeuN while exceptional cases may express GFAP (Fig. 6.11).

Table 6.6 Medulloblastoma classification [5]

Medulloblastomas, histologically defined
Classic
Desmoplastic/nodular
With extensive nodularity
Large cell/anaplastic
Medulloblastomas, molecularly defined
WNT-activated
SHH-activated and *TP53*-wildtype
SHH-activated and *TP53*-mutant
Non-WNT/non-SHH

Abbreviations WNT wingless, *SHH* Sonic hedgehog, *TP53* tumor protein P53

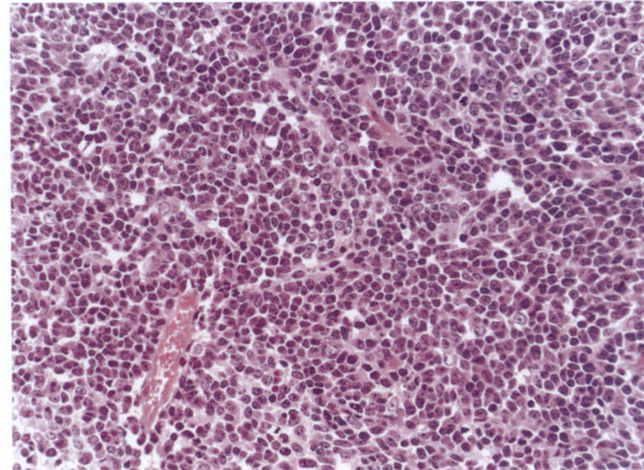

Fig. 6.10 Medulloblastoma, classic subtype, CNS WHO 2021. Densely packed poorly differentiated cells with hyperchromatic nuclei (Hematoxylin-Eosin stain; original magnification X400)

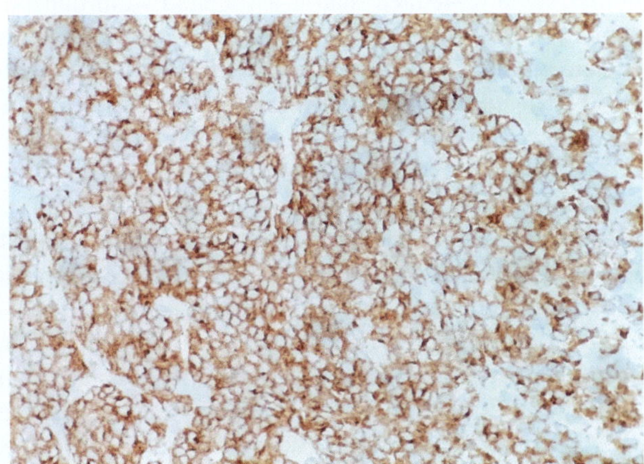

Fig. 6.11 Medulloblastoma, classic subtype, CNS WHO 2021. Strong immunoreactivity of tumor cells for synaptophysin, cells (Avidin-Biotin-Complex-ABC immunohistochemical method; original magnification X400)

6.3.1.2   MB, Molecularly Defined

By using gene expression analysis, MBs are divided into four distinct molecular subgroups: WNT (wingless)-activated, SHH (sonic hedgehog)-activated and *TP53*-wildtype; SHH-activated and *TP53*-mutant and non-WNT/non-SHH [97–102] (Tables 6.6 and 6.7). These subtypes are associated with specific age groups, with *SHH*-activated being most common in infants and adults, and all other groups being more common in childhood.

MB, WNT-activated (~10% of all MBs) is characterized by the activation of the WNT signaling pathway resulting in nuclear accumulation of beta-catenin, as it can be observed by IHC. Most of the tumors harbor somatic mutations in exon 3 of catenin beta 1 (*CTNNB1*) gene, the detection of which is of great diagnostic significance [97]. Other mutated genes include *SMARCA4* (switch/sucrose

Table 6.7 Molecular subgroups of medulloblastoma [5]

Molecular subgroups	Common molecular characteristics
WNT-activated	*CTNNB1, SMARCA4, DDX3X, CSNK2B, KMT2D*
SHH-activated and *TP53*-wildtype	*PTCH1, ELP1, SUFU, SMO, GPR161*
SHH-activated and *TP53*-mutant	*TP53, MYC, MYCN, SUFU, SMO, TERT*
Non-WNT/non-SHH	*MYCN, GFI1 GFI1B*

Abbreviations: *CTNNB1* catenin beta 1, *SMARCA4* switch/sucrose nonfermentable-related matrix-associated actin-dependent regulator of chromatin, subfamily A, member 4, *DDX3X* DEAD-box helicase 3X-linked, *CSNK2B* casein kinase 2 beta, *KMT2D* lysine methyltransferase 2D, *PTCH1* patched 1, *ELP1* elongator acetyltransferase complex subunit 1, *SUFU* sufu negative regulator of hedgehog signaling, *SMO* smoothened, frizzled class receptor, *GPR161* G protein coupled receptor 161, *TP53* tumor protein p53, *MYC* v-Myc avian myelocytomatosis viral oncogene homolog, *MYCN* v-Myc avian myelocytomatosis viral oncogene neuroblastoma-derived homolog, *TERT* telomerase reverse transcriptase, *GFI1* growth factor independent 1 transcriptional repressor 1, *GFI1B* growth factor independent 1 transcriptional repressor 1B

nonfermentable-related matrix-associated actin-dependent regulator of chromatin, subfamily A, member 4), *DDX3X* (DEAD-box helicase 3X-linked), *CSNK2B* (casein kinase 2 beta), and *KMT2D* (lysine methyltransferase 2D). Almost all MBs, WNT-activated are of classic histology. In children, the clinical course is excellent after total surgical removal, but in adults the prognosis may be less favorable [98].

MB, SHH-activated and *TP53*-wildtype (~30% of all MBs) demonstrates activation of the SHH signaling pathway along with a wildtype *TP53* gene. Other genetic alterations include mutations in *PTCH1* (patched 1), *ELP1* (elongator acetyltransferase complex subunit 1), *SUFU* (sufu negative regulator of hedgehog signaling), *SMO* (smoothened, frizzled class receptor), and GPR161 (G protein coupled receptor 161) genes. The tumor occurs predominantly in infants and adulthood, is of desmoplastic/nodular morphology and is associated with favorable prognosis [99, 101]. By DNA methylation and gene expression profiling, four molecular subgroups of MB, SHH-activated have been identified: SHH-1, SHH-2, SSH-3, and SSH-4 with different molecular and prognostic characteristics.

MB, SHH-activated and *TP53*-mutant. Approximately 10–15% of all MBs are SHH-activated and *TP53*-mutant. Other molecular alterations are *MYCN* (v-Myc avian myelocytomatosis viral oncogene neuroblastoma-derived homolog) amplification and mutations in *PTCH1, SUFU, SMO* and *TERT* genes [99–102]. The tumors occur in ages <4 years and >16 years, and morphologically are of large cell/anaplastic phenotype. The prognosis is generally poor.

MB, non-WNT/non-SHH. Non-WNT/non-SHH MBs typically present in the midline structures and are characterized by *MYCN* amplification and mutations of *GFI1* (growth factor independent 1 transcriptional repressor 1) and *GFI1B* (growth factor independent 1 transcriptional repressor 1B) genes [99–102]. Most cases occur in infancy and childhood. Histologically, they are almost always of classic or large cell/anaplastic morphology. The prognosis is poor and metastatic disease is frequently encountered at the time of presentation [100].

6.3.2 Atypical Teratoid/Rhabdoid Tumor

Atypical teratoid/rhabdoid tumor (AT/RT) is a poorly differentiated neoplasm characterized by biallelic inactivation of *SMARCB1* (switch/sucrose nonfermentable-related matrix-associated actin-dependent regulator of chromatin, subfamily B, member 1) or rarely of *SMARCA4*. Defects of *SMARCB1 or SMARCA4* genes result in loss of immunohistochemical nuclear staining for the intact integrase interactor 1 (INI1) or brahma-related gene 1 (BRC1) proteins, respectively [103]. Diagnosis requires either loss of INI1 or BRC1 proteins.

AT/RTs occur mainly in the cerebellum and affect children younger than 4 years. The reported incidence rate is 0.33 per 100,000 population and 0.03 per 100,000 population in children ages 0–4 and 5–9 years, respectively [22]. Histologically, AT/RTs are characterized by rhabdoid cells with high mitotic activity. Areas of necrosis are common. By DNA methylation profiling, three molecular subgroups have been identified: AT/RT-SHH, AT/RT-TYR, and AT/RT-MYC [104]. Although the prognosis of AT/RT is generally poor, patients with germline mutations of *SMARCB1* have worse prognosis compared with those with sporadic tumors. The prognostic value of the molecular subgroups needs to be elucidated.

6.3.3 Cribriform Neuroepithelial Tumor

Cribriform neuroepithelial tumor is defined as a non-rhabdoid neuroectodermal tumor characterized by cribriform strands and ribbons as well as by loss of SMARCB1 nuclear protein expression [5]. There are insufficient literature data about the clinical course of the tumor; however, it seems that it is better than that of AT/RT.

6.3.4 Embryonal Tumor with Multilayered Rosettes

Embryonal tumor with multilayered rosettes (ETMR) comprises three morphological patterns (embryonal tumor with abundant neuropil and true rosettes, ependymoblastoma, and medulloepithelioma). ETMRs most commonly arise in the frontal or parietotemporal lobes and affect children with a median age of 2–3 years [22]. Approximately 90% of the cases, harbor amplification of the *C19MC* (chromosome 19 microRNA cluster) cluster and in the remaining cases a *MIR17HG* (miR-17-92a-1 cluster host gene) amplification or biallelic *DICER1* (Dicer 1 ribonuclease III) gene mutation has been reported [105]. Patients with *DICER1* mutations have a *DICER1* germline predisposition syndrome. ETMRs are aggressive tumors and are associated with a median survival of less than 1 year.

6.3.5 *CNS Neuroblastoma,* **FOXR2-***Activated*

CNS neuroblastoma with structural rearrangement in the forkhead box R2 (*FOXR2*) gene accounts for 10% of tumors, previously classified as CNS primitive neuroectodermal tumors (PNET) [106]. Most cases arise in the cerebral hemispheres. Histologically, the tumor exhibits varying degrees of neuroblastic and/or neuronal differentiation with poorly differentiated cells having high nuclear to cytoplasmic ratio, marked mitotic activity, necrosis, and brain invasion [5]. Survival data are still unknown; however, it seems that the prognosis of patients is better compared to that of the other CNS embryonal tumors [107].

6.3.6 *CNS Tumor with* **BCOR** *Internal Tandem Duplication*

It is defined as a tumor type with BCL6 corepressor (*BCOR*) internal tandem duplication, characterized by solid growth pattern, uniform oval or spindled cells, a capillary network and by the presence of focal pseudorosettes. For the diagnostic approach, a strong nuclear staining of BCOR must be detected [108]. The tumor tends to be large involving multiple lobes or both hemispheres. Survival data are limited.

6.3.7 *CNS Embryonal Tumor NEC/ NOS*

The term CNS embryonal tumor NEC (NEC; not elsewhere classified) is applied for the tumors which do not fulfill any criteria for the diagnosis of a more specific embryonal tumor type [5]. Embryonal tumor NOS (NOS; not otherwise specified) is defined as a tumor with embryonal morphology and immunophenotype, where molecular analyses have not yet or could not be successfully performed. It is strongly recommended that such cases need further molecular analysis to specialized reference centers [5].

6.4 Meningiomas

Meningiomas constitute a heterogeneous group of neoplasms derived from arachnoid cap (meningothelial) cells. They typically arise in the cerebral convexities, skull base, tentorium, and spinal cord. Despite having a benign course in most cases, meningiomas can lead to high recurrence rates and mortality. Recent advances of genomics and epigenomics characteristics suggest that tumor location, grading, and prediction of prognosis or recurrence are associated with specific key mutations and signaling pathways.

Meningiomas are the most common type of primary brain and other CNS tumors in adults (ages 65 years and older), accounting for 40% of tumors overall [22]. The reported incidence rate is 9.51 per 100,000 population [22]. The incidence is greater in females than in males (2.3 times more in females) and significantly higher in Blacks than in Whites [22]. Rare cases may occur in children and adolescents of both sexes and are associated mainly with genetic syndromes [109–112].

Ionizing radiation is the most common risk factor for the development of meningiomas resulting in a six- to tenfold increase in risk [113]. An association with hormone receptors (estrogen, progesterone, and androgen receptors) has also been reported [113–116]. Moreover, several syndromes such as Neurofibromatosis type 2 (NF-2), Gorlin syndrome (or naevoid basal cell carcinoma syndrome) and Cowden syndrome have been associated with an increased risk of meningioma development [109, 110, 117, 118]. Germline mutations in *SMARCB1* and switch/sucrose nonfermentable-related matrix-associated actin-dependent regulator of chromatin subfamily E member 1 (*SMARCE1*), phosphatase and tensin homolog (*PTEN*), Breast Cancer (*BRCA*) 1-associated protein 1 (*BAP1*) have been reported in families with familial meningiomatosis syndromes [109–112, 119, 120].

6.4.1 Histopathology-Molecular Pathology

Grossly, meningiomas are generally round or lobulated, well circumscribed neoplasms attached to the dura. The histological appearance of meningiomas varies widely due to the variety of different morphologically tumor subtypes described (Table 6.8) [5]. Of all the subtypes according to WHO classification of Tumors of the Central Nervous System (CNS), the most common are meningothelial, fibrous, and transitional meningiomas (Figs. 6.12, 6.13, 6.14, 6.15, 6.16, 6.17, 6.18, 6.19, and 6.20).

In morphologically challenging cases, IHC can assist in the differential diagnosis. Meningiomas express markers such as Epithelial Membrane Antigen (EMA) or Vimentin, although their immunoreaction is not always specific (Fig. 6.21). Therefore, diagnosis frequently requires consideration of morphological, immunohistochemical and molecular characteristics.

Most of the tumor subtypes behave in a benign fashion and correspond to WHO grade 1 but there are some variants with an aggressive clinical course in terms of recurrence and overall survival, corresponding to WHO grades 2 and 3 (e.g., atypical and anaplastic meningiomas, respectively) [5]. However, the criteria for diagnosing the higher grade cases can be applied in all meningiomas, regardless of

Table 6.8 Morphological subtypes of meningiomas [5]

Meningioma subtypes	Histological description
Meningothelial	Lobulated growth pattern, epithelioid cells, abundant eosinophilic cytoplasm, round to oval nuclei, intranuclear pseudoinclusions
Fibrous	Storiform or fascicular growth pattern, intercellular collagen bundles, spindle cells
Transitional	Lobulated and fascicular growth patterns, prominent whorls and psammoma bodies
Psammomatous	Numerous psammoma bodies, rare meningothelial cells
Angiomatous	Numerous blood vessels with thick hyalinized walls, rare meningothelial cells, degenerative nuclear atypia
Microcystic	Cysts formed by cells with elongated processes, degenerative nuclear atypia
Secretory	Gland-like spaces with eosinophilic round secretions (pseudopsammoma bodies)
Lymphoplasmacyte-rich	Intense lymphoplasmacytic infiltration, rare meningothelial cells
Metaplastic	Presence of mesenchymal components such as bone, cartilage, fat (as separate components or in combination)
Chordoid	Cords of small epithelioid cells, mucin-rich substrate
Clear cell	Sheets of round clear cells, cytoplasmic glycogen, perivascular or interstitial collagen
Rhabdoid	Rhabdoid cells with eccentric nuclei, prominent nucleoli, eosinophilic paranuclear inclusions
Papillary	Papillary growth pattern, perivascular pseudorosette-like pattern
Atypical	Sheeting growth pattern, small cells with high nucleocytoplasmic ratio, increased mitotic activity
Anaplastic (malignant)	Malignant cellular features, marked mitotic activity

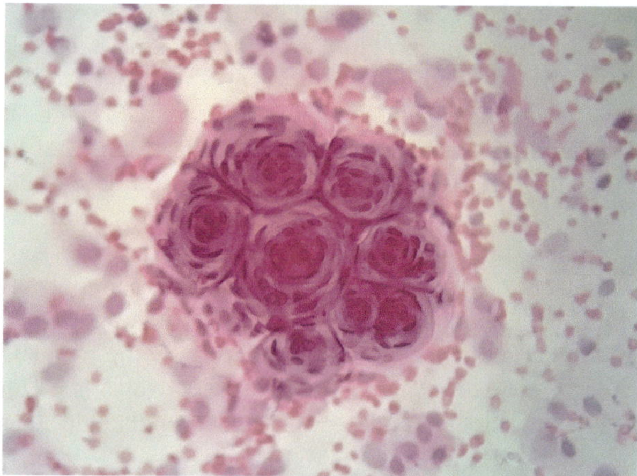

Fig. 6.12 . Meningioma. Intraoperative touch preparation reveals whorls and psammoma bodies

Fig. 6.13 . Meningothelial meningioma. Lobular pattern, nuclear pseudoinclusions (Hematoxylin-Eosin stain, original magnification X400)

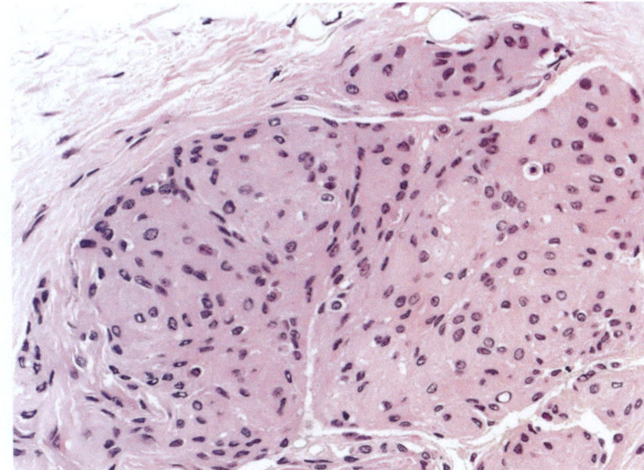

Fig. 6.14 . Fibrous meningioma. Fascicular growth pattern, spindle cells, collageneous substrate (Hematoxylin-Eosin stain, original magnification X400)

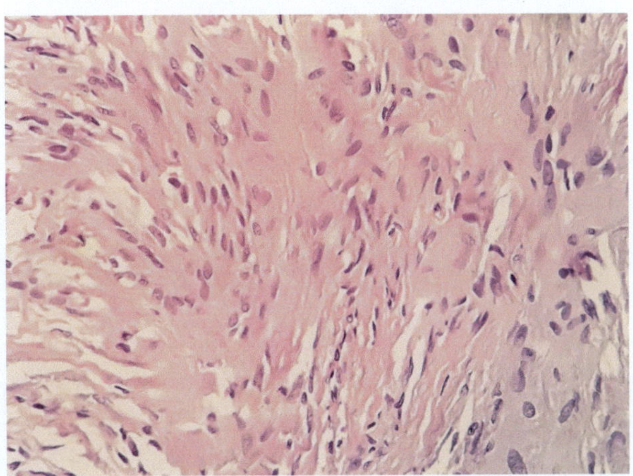

subtyping. Specific molecular alterations have been recently incorporated in the morphology for the diagnosis of WHO grade 3 meningiomas (Table 6.9). Interestingly, the presence of *TERT* promoter mutations has been associated with higher grades and increased recurrence rate [121–126]. Alterations of *CDKN2A* and *CDKN2B* were found more frequently in recurrent meningiomas and were associated with poor prognosis [112, 127–129]. Moreover, it has been reported that high expression levels of the proliferation associated marker Ki67 are correlated with high recurrence rates (Fig. 6.22). A higher cut-off value (>4%) was of significance for prediction of prognosis and a Ki67 index more than 20% was related with high mortality, like that of WHO grade 3 tumors [130]. Until now, however, Ki67 is not considered as an independent indicator for grading.

Fig. 6.15 Transitional meningioma. Fascicular growth pattern and whorls formation (Hematoxylin-Eosin stain, original magnification X400)

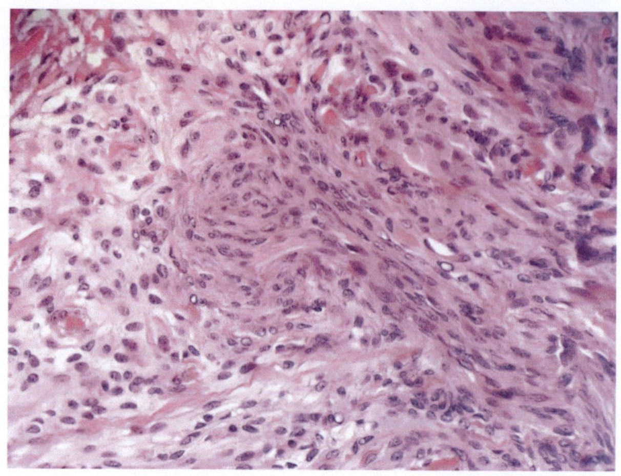

Fig. 6.16 . Psammomatous meningioma. Numerous psammomatous calcifications (psammoma bodies) (Hematoxylin-Eosin stain, original magnification X400)

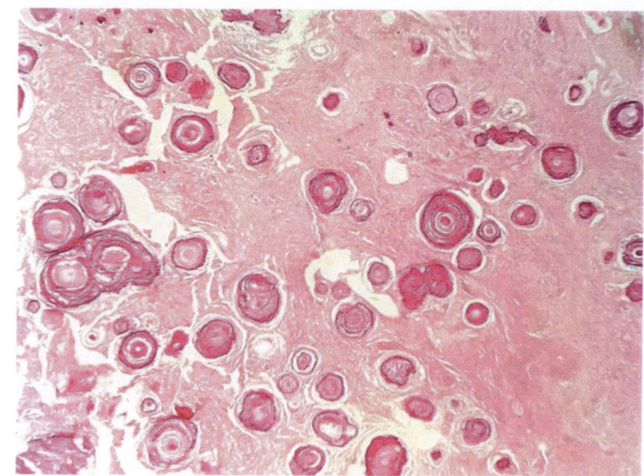

Fig. 6.17 Secretory meningioma. Glandular-like spaces filled with eosinophilic material, called pseudopsammoma bodies (Hematoxylin-Eosin stain, original magnification X400)

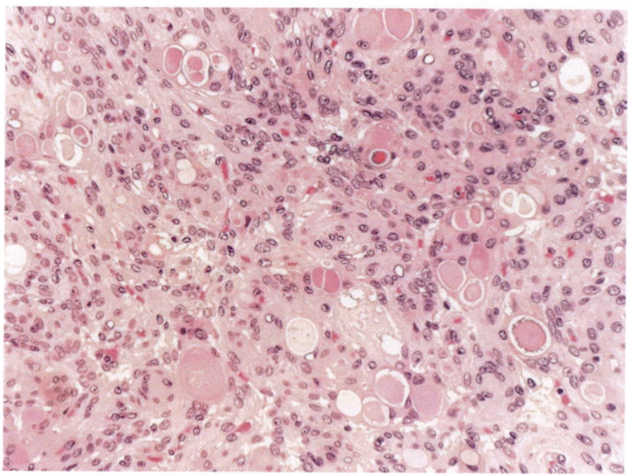

Fig. 6.18 Secretory meningioma. The pseudopsammoma bodies are positive for cytokeratin (Avidin-Biotin Complex-ABC, immunohistochemical method, original magnification X400)

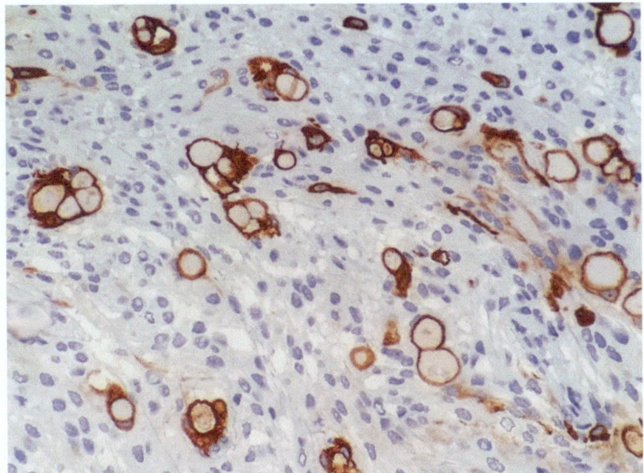

Fig. 6.19 Anaplastic (malignant) meningioma. Morphologically malignant cells resembling carcinoma, increased mitotic activity. (Hematoxylin-Eosin stain, original magnification X400)

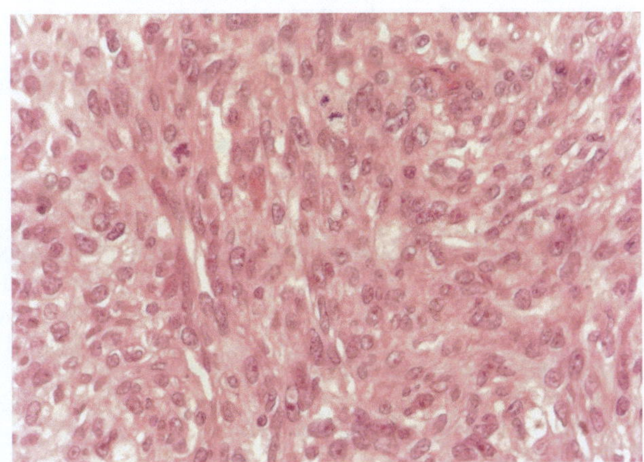

Fig. 6.20 Anaplastic (malignant) meningioma. Focus of necrosis (Hematoxylin-Eosin stain, original magnification X400)

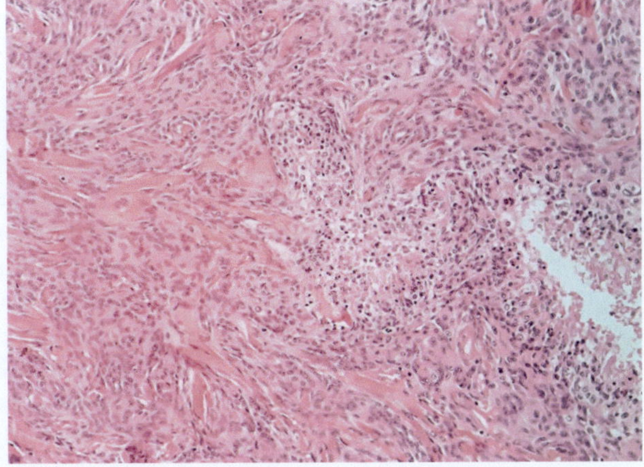

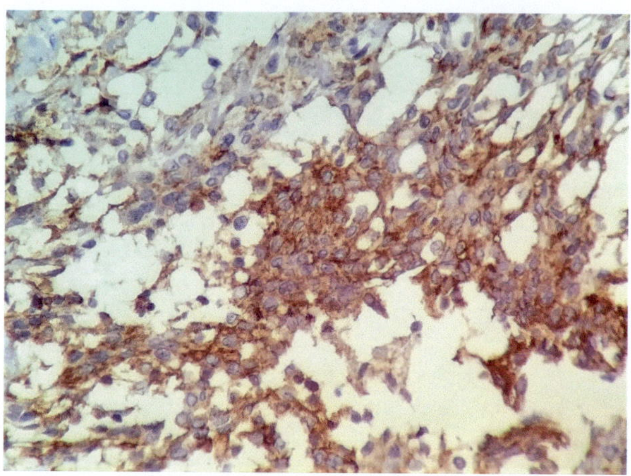

Fig. 6.21 Immunohistochemical expression of tumor cells for EMA (Avidin-Biotin Complex-ABC immunohistochemical method, original magnification X400)

Table 6.9 Criteria for assessing WHO grades 2 and 3 meningiomas [5]

WHO grade 2	WHO grade 3
4–19 mitoses/10 high power fields (HPF)[a]	>20 mitoses/10 high power fields (HPF)[a]
Brain invasion	Morphology like carcinoma, high-grade sarcoma or melanoma
Chordoid or clear cell morphology	Specific molecular alterations: • *TERT* mutations and/or • *CDKN2A* and/or *CDKN2B* homozygous deletion
At least three of the below features: • Increased cellularity • Small cells with high nucleocytoplasmic (N/C) ratio • Prominent nucleoli • Sheeting growth pattern • Necrosis (spontaneous)	

[a]HPF of 0.16mm^2

Several molecular alterations have been described in meningiomas, some of them with diagnostic, prognostic, and potential clinical value. Mutations in the *NF-2* gene, which is located in chromosome 22q, are observed in most cases associated with NF-2 as well as in about 60% of sporadic meningiomas [9, 131, 132]. In most cases, NF-2 meningiomas are more aggressive tumors corresponding to atypical and anaplastic subtypes [133]. Other alterations correlated with higher tumor grade and high recurrence rates include deletion of 1p (the second more common abnormality), 6q, 9p, 10, 14q, and 18q [134–136]. Next generation sequencing revealed a variety of molecular alterations, especially in NF-2 non mutated meningiomas, such as mutations of *AKT1* (AKT serine/threonine kinase 1), *KLF4*

Fig. 6.22 High imunohistochemical expression of proliferation marker Ki67 (Avidin-Biotin Complex-ABC immunohistochemical method, original magnification X200)

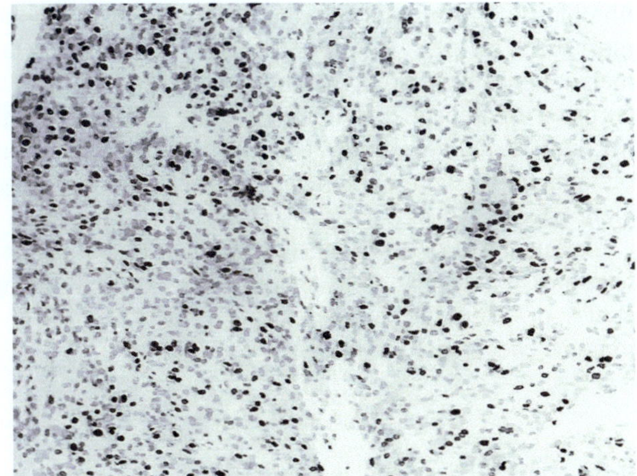

(Kruppel-like factor 4), smoothened, *SMO*, *TRAF 7*(tumor necrosis factor receptor-associated factor 7), *PIK3CA*, *SMARC*, and *BAP1* [129, 137–141].

Mutation status has been correlated with tumor location and histologic subtypes. Therefore, tumors located at the convexity are frequently characterized by *NF-2* and *SMARCB1* mutations and are mainly of transitional or fibroblastic subtypes [9, 137–140, 142–144]. Meningiomas of the base of the skull have mutations of *AKT1*, *KLF4*, *TRAF7*, *SMO,* and *PIK3CA* and are frequently of meningothelial, secretory or microcystic subtypes. Spinal cord tumors harbor *SMARCE1* mutations associated with clear cell histology [145, 146]. *AKT1* mutations are detected predominantly in meningothelial and transitional [142, 143], inactivating mutations of the PBAF complex gene (*PBRM1*) in papillary meningiomas [147], *POLR2A* gene mutations in meningiomas of meningothelial histology [148, 149], while *BAP1* mutations are found in the aggressive rhabdoid meningiomas [141].

Growing evidence suggests that mutation status is correlated with patients' prognosis as well. Meningiomas with *TERT* promoter mutations have a tendency for malignancy, high recurrence rate and short overall survival [121–125]. Therefore, these meningiomas should have a very close follow-up or an aggressive treatment. Alterations of *CDKN2A* and/or *CDKN2B* are more often found in recurrent and progressive tumors and confer a poor prognosis [127–129]. The 2021 WHO classification of CNS tumors incorporates the above molecular events for assessing the histological grading. Therefore, anaplastic meningiomas are now diagnosed if *TERT* promoter mutations and/or *CDKN2A/B* homozygous deletion occur, even in the absence of histological features consistent with anaplasia (Table 6.8) [5].

Recent studies suggest that by DNA methylation profiling, meningiomas may be classified in separate tumor subgroups with different prognosis in terms of recurrence-free survival and clinical outcome [111, 150–152]. In the study of Sahm et al., six methylation classes have been identified [150]. Among them, three classes were benign (MC ben-1, MC ben-2, MC ben-3), two intermediate (MC int-A, MC int-B) and one malignant (MC mal). In the MC ben-1 class, meningiomas of fibroblastic and psammomatous histology were included, in the MC ben-2 class most cases were secretory meningiomas and in the class MC ben-3 angiomatous meningiomas were predominantly clustered. MC int-A and MC int-B groups were enriched for atypical meningiomas while anaplastic meningiomas were found in the MC mal class. Interestingly, benign (grade 1) meningiomas with intermediate level of methylation status exhibited more aggressive behavior than those with low methylation levels [150].

During the last years, clinical trials investigating targetable genetic abnormalities in aggressive meningiomas are ongoing. Potential therapeutic targets include molecules of major signaling pathways (mTOR, MEK, CDK/p16/Rb) as well as immune checkpoint inhibitors [153–158].

6.5 Conclusions

During the last decades, the results from genomic and epigenomic studies have shed light in our understanding of CNS tumors' biology. WHO CNS5 classification moved molecular diagnostics forward and the suggested integrated pathological diagnostic approach is one of the most important changes. Incorporating histopathology with molecular and genetic characteristics will undoubtedly improve the diagnostic accuracy, classification, and grading. The adoption of specific molecular features into the everyday practice will change dramatically the patients' therapeutic approach, especially when Pathologists are faced with histologically similar but distinct at the molecular level tumors.

References

1. Kristensen BW, Priesterbach-Ackley LP, Petersen JK, Wesseling P. Molecular pathology of tumors of the central nervous system. Ann Oncol. 2019;30:1265–78.
2. Gonzalez Castro LN, Wesseling P. The cIMPACT-NOW updates and their significance to current neuro-oncology practice. Neurooncol Pract. 2020;8:4–10.
3. Sonoda Y. Clinical impact of revisions to the WHO classification of diffuse gliomas and associated future problems. Int J Clin Oncol. 2020;25:1004–9.
4. Wen PY, Packer RJ. The 2021 WHO Classification of Tumors of the Central Nervous System: clinical implications. Neuro Oncol. 2021;23:1215–7.
5. WHO Classification of Tumours Editorial Board. WHO classification of tumours of the central nervous system. 5th ed. Lyon: International Agency for Research in Cancer; 2021.
6. Louis DN, Perry A, Wesseling P, Brat DJ, Cree IA, Figarella-Branger D, et al. The 2021 WHO classification of tumors of the central nervous system: a summary. Neuro Oncol. 2021;23:1231–51.
7. Whitfield BT, Huse JT. Classification of adult-type diffuse gliomas: impact of the World Health Organization 2021 update. Brain Pathol. 2022;32:e13062.
8. Brat DJ, Aldape K, Bridge JA, Canoll P, Colman H, Hameed MR, Harris BT, Hattab EM, Huse JT, Jenkins RB, Lopez-Terrada DH, McDonald WC, Rodriguez FJ, Souter LH, Colasacco C,

Thomas NE, Yount MH, van den Bent MJ, Perry A. Molecular biomarker testing for the diagnosis of diffuse gliomas. Arch Pathol Lab Med. 2022;146:547–74.

9. Gritsch S, Batchelor TT, Gonzalez Castro LN. Diagnostic, therapeutic, and prognostic implications of the 2021 World Health Organization classification of tumors of the central nervous system. Cancer. 2022;128:47–58.

10. Komori T. The 2021 WHO classification of tumors, 5th edition, central nervous system tumors: the 10 basic principles. Brain Tumor Pathol. 2022;39:47–50.

11. Louis DN, Giannini C, Capper D, Paulus W, Figarella-Branger D, Lopes MB, et al. cIMPACT-NOW update 2: diagnostic clarifications for diffuse midline glioma, H3 K27M-mutant and diffuse astrocytoma/anaplastic astrocytoma, IDH-mutant. Acta Neuropathol. 2018;135:639–42.

12. Brat DJ, Aldape K, Colman H, Figrarella-Branger D, Fuller GN, Giannini C, et al. cIMPACT-NOW update 5: recommended grading criteria and terminologies for IDH-mutant astrocytomas. Acta Neuropathol. 2020;139:603–8.

13. Louis DN, Wesseling P, Aldape K, Brat DJ, Capper D, Cree IA, et al. cIMPACT-NOW update 6: new entity and diagnostic principal recommendations of the cIMPACT-Utrecht meeting on the future CNS classification and grading. Brain Pathol. 2020;30:844–56.

14. Reus DE, Sahm F, Schrimpf D, Wiestler B, Capper D, Koelsche C, et al. ATRX and IDH1-R132H immunohistochemistry with subsequent copy number analysis and IDH sequencing as a basis for an "integrated" diagnostic approach for adult astrocytoma, oligodendroglioma and glioblastoma. Acta Neuropathol. 2015;129:133–46.

15. Meredith DM. Advances in diagnostic immunohistochemistry for primary tumors of the central nervous system. Adv Anat Pathol. 2020;27:206–9.

16. Tian Y, Rich BE, Vena N, Craig JM, Macconaill LE, Rajaram V, et al. Detection of KIAA1549-BRAF fusion transcripts in formalin-fixed paraffin-embedded pediatric low-grade gliomas. J Mol Diagn. 2011;13:669–77.

17. Surrey LF, MacFarland SP, Chang F, Cao K, Rathi KS, Akgumus GT, et al. Clinical utility of custom designed NGS panel testing in pediatric tumors. Genome Med. 2019;11:32.

18. Capper D, Jones DTW, Sill M, Hovestadt V, Schrimpf D, Sturm D, et al. DNA methylation-based classification of central nervous system tumours. Nature. 2018;555:469–74.

19. Capper D, Stichel D, Sahm F, Jones DTW, Schrimpf D, Sill M, et al. Practical implementation of DNA methylation and copy-number-based CNS tumor diagnostics: the Heidelberg experience. Acta Neuropathol. 2018;136:181–210.

20. Jaunmuktane Z, Capper D, Jones DTW, Schrimpf D, Sill M, Dutt M, et al. Methylation array profiling of adult brain tumours: diagnostic outcomes in a large, single centre. Acta Neuropathol Commun. 2019;20:24.

21. Ostrom QT, Cioffi G, Waite K, Kruchko C, Barnholtz-Sloan JS. CBTRUS statistical report: primary brain and other central nervous system tumors diagnosed in the United States in 2014–2018. Neuro Oncol. 2021;23:iii1–iii105.

22. Ostrom QT, Price M, Neff C, Cioffi G, Waite KA, Kruchko C, et al. CBTRUS statistical report: primary brain and other central nervous system tumors diagnosed in the United States in 2015–2019. Neuro Oncol. 2022;24:v1–v95.

23. Sloan EA, Hilz S, Gupta R, Cadwell C, Ramani B, Hofmann J, et al. Gliomas arising in the setting of Li-Fraumeni syndrome stratify into two molecular subgroups with divergent clinicopathologic features. Acta Neuropathol. 2020;139:953–7.

24. Suwala AK, Stichel D, Schrimpf D, Kloor M, Wefers AK, Reinhardt A, et al. Primary mismatch repair deficient IDH-mutant astrocytoma (PMMRDIA) is a distinct type with a poor prognosis. Acta Neuropathol. 2021;141:85–100.

25. Shirahata M, Ono T, Stichel D, Schrimpf D, Reus DF, Sahm F, et al. Novel, improved grading system(s) for IDH-mutant astrocytic gliomas. Acta Neuropathol. 2018;136:153–66.

26. Komori T. Updating the grading criteria for adult diffuse gliomas: beyond the WHO2016 CNS classifcation. Brain Tumor Pathol. 2020;37:1–4.

27. Yan H, Parsons DW, Jin G, McLendon R, Rasheed BA, Yuan W, et al. IDH1 and IDH2 mutations in gliomas. N Engl J Med. 2009;360:765–73.

28. Dang L, White DW, Gross S, Bennett BD, Bittinger MA, Driggers EM, et al. Cancer-associated IDH1 mutations produce 2-hydroxyglutarate. Nature. 2009;462:739–44.

29. Gross S, Cairns RA, Minden MD, Driggers EM, Bittinger MA, Jang HG, Sasaki M. Cancer-associated metabolite 2-hydroxyglutarate accumulates in acute myelogenous leukemia with isocitrate dehydrogenase 1 and 2 mutations. J Exp Med. 2010;207:339–44.

30. Jiao Y, Killela PJ, Reitman ZJ, Rasheed AB, Heaphy CM, de Wilde RF, et al. Frequent ATRX, CIC, FUBP1 and IDH1 mutations refine the classification of malignant gliomas. Oncotarget. 2012;3:709–22.

31. Liu XY, Gerges N, Korsunov A, Sabha N, Khuong-Quang D-A, Fontebasso AM, et al. Frequent ATRX mutations and loss of expression in adult diffuse astrocytic tumors carrying IDH1/IDH2 and TP53 mutations. Acta Neuropathol. 2012;124:615–25.

32. Abedalthagafi M, Phillips JJ, Kim GE, Mueller S, Haas-Kogen DA, Marshall RE, et al. The alternative lengthening of telomere phenotype is significantly associated with loss of ATRX expression in high-grade pediatric and adult astrocytomas: a multi-institutional study of 214 astrocytomas. Mod Pathol. 2013;26:1425–32.

33. Appay R, Dehais C, Maurage C-A, Alentorn A, Carpentier C, Colin C, et al. CDKN2A homozygous deletion is a strong adverse prognosis factor in diffuse malignant IDH-mutant gliomas. Neuro Oncol. 2019;21:1519–28.

34. Tesileanu MS, Vallentgoed WR, French PJ, van den Bent MJ. Molecular markers related to patient outcome in patients with IDH-mutant astrocytomas grade 2 to 4: a systematic review C. Eur J Cancer 2022; 175: 214–223. Neuro Oncol. 2020;(22):515–23.

35. Banan R, Stichel D, Bleck A, Hong B, Lehman U, Suwala A, et al. Infratentorial IDH-mutant astrocytoma is a distinct subtype. Acta Neuropathol. 2020;140:569–81.

36. Bainbridge MN, Armstrong GN, Gramatges MM, Bertuch AA, Jhangiani SN, Doddapaneni H, et al. Germline mutations in shelterin complex genes are associated with familial glioma. J Natl Cancer Inst. 2015:107, 384.

37. Wesseling P, van den Bent M, Perry A. Oligodendroglioma: pathology, molecular mechanisms, and markers. Acta Neuropathol. 2015;129(6):809–27.

38. Arita H, Matsushita Y, Machida R, Yamasaki K, Hata N, Ohno M, et al. TERT promoter mutation confers favorable prognosis regardless of 1p/19q status in adult difuse gliomas with IDH1/2 mutations. Acta Neuropathol Commun. 2020;143:263–81.

39. Broderick DK, Di C, Parrett TJ, Samuels YR, Cummins JM, McLendon RE, et al. Advances in brief mutations of PIK3CA in anaplastic oligodendrogliomas, high-grade astrocytomas, and medulloblastomas. Cancer Res. 2004;64:5048–50.

40. Labreche V, Simeonova I, Kamoun A, Gleize V. TCF12 is mutated in anaplastic oligodendroglioma. Nat Commun. 2015;6:7207.

41. Oligosarcoma Suwala AK, Felix M, Friedel D, Stichel D, Schrimpf D, Hinz F, et al. Oligosarcomas, IDH-mutant are distinct and aggressive. Acta Neuropathol. 2022;143:263–81.

42. Killela PJ, Pirozzi CJ, Healy P, Reitman ZJ, Lipp E, Rasheed BA, et al. Mutations in IDH1, IDH2, and in the TERT promoter define clinically distinct subgroups of adult malignant gliomas. Oncotarget. 2014;5:1515–25.

43. Aldape K, Zadeh G, Mansouri S, Reifenberger G, von Deimling A. Glioblastoma: pathology, molecular mechanisms, and markers. Acta Neuropathol. 2015;129:829–48.

44. Stichel D, Ebrahimi A, Reuss D, Schrimpf D, Ono T, Shirahata M, et al. Distribution of EGFR amplification, combined chromosome 7 gain and chromosome 10 loss, and TERT promoter mutation in brain tumors and their potential for the reclassification of IDHwt astrocytoma to glioblastoma. Acta Neuropathol. 2018;136:793–803.

45. Tesileanu CMS, Dirven L, Wijnenga MMJ, Koekkoek JAF, Vincent AJPE, Dubbink HJ, et al. Survival of diffuse astrocytic glioma, IDH1/2 wildtype, with molecular features of glioblastoma, WHO grade IV: a confirmation of the cIMPACT-NOW criteria. Neuro Oncol. 2020;22:515–23.

46. Donehower LA, Soussi T, Korkut A, Liu Y, Schultz A, Cardenas M, et al. Integrated analysis of TP53 gene and pathway alterations in the Cancer Genome Atlas. Cell Rep. 2019;28:1370–84.
47. Hegi ME, Diserens A-C, Gorlia T, Hamou M-F, de Tribolet N, Weller M, et al. MGMT gene silencing and benefit from temozolomide in glioblastoma. N Engl J Med. 2005;352:997–1003.
48. Bielle F, Di Stefano A-L, Meyronet D, Picca A, Villa C, Bernier M, et al. Diffuse gliomas with FGFR3-TACC3 fusion have characteristic histopathological and molecular features. Brain Pathol. 2018;28:674–83.
49. Sturm D, Pfister SM, Jones DTW. Pediatric gliomas: Current concepts on diagnosis, biology, and clinical management. J Clin Oncol. 2017;35:2370–7.
50. Ostrom QT, Fahmideh MA, Cote DJ, Muskens IS, Schraw JM, Scheuer ME, Bondy ML. Risk factors for childhood and adult primary brain tumors. Neuro Oncol. 2019;21:1357–75.
51. Cacciotti C, Fleming A, Ramaswamy V. Advances in the molecular classification of pediatric brain tumors: A guide to the galaxy. J Pathol. 2020;251:249–61.
52. Mahajan S, Sharma MC, Sarkar C, Suri V. Approach to integrating molecular markers for assessment of pediatric gliomas. Int J Neurooncol. 2021;4:166–74.
53. Funakoshi Y, Hata N, Kuga D, Hatae R, Sangatsuda Y, Fujioka Y, et al. Pediatric glioma: an update of diagnosis, biology, and treatment. Cancers. 2021;13:758.
54. Komori T. The molecular framework of pediatric-type diffuse gliomas: shifting toward the revision of the WHO classifcation of tumors of the central nervous system. Brain Tumor Pathol. 2021;38:1–3.
55. Ellison DW, Hawkins C, Jones DTW, Onar-Thomas A, Pfister SM, Reifenberger G, et al. cIMPACT-NOW update 4: diffuse gliomas characterized by MYB, MYBL1, or FGFR1 alterations or BRAF(V600E) mutation. Acta Neuropathol. 2019;137:683–7.
56. Wefers AK, Stichel D, Schrimpf D, Coras R, Pages M, Tauziede-Espariat A, et al. Isomorphic diffuse glioma is a morphologically and molecularly distinct tumour entity with recurrent gene fusions of MYBL1 or MYB and a benign disease course. Acta Neuropathol. 2020;139:193–209.
57. Ryall S, Tabori U, Hawkins C. Pediatric low-grade glioma in the era of molecular diagnostics. Acta Neuropathol Commun. 2020;8:30.
58. Cole BL. Neuropathology of pediatric brain tumors. A concise review. Neurosurgery. 2022;90:7–15.
59. Bale TA, Rosenblum MK. The 2021 WHO classification of tumors of the central nervous system: An update on pediatric low-grade gliomas and glioneuronal tumors. Brain Pathol. 2022;32:e13060.
60. Ramkissoon LA, Horowitz PM, Craig JM, Ramkissoon SH, Rich BE, Schumacher SE, et al. Genomic analysis of diffuse pediatric low-grade gliomas identifies recurrent oncogenic truncating rearrangements in the transcription factor MYBL1. Proc Natl Acad Sci U S A. 2013;110:8188–93.
61. Chiang J, Harreld JH, Tinkle CL, Moreira DC, Li X, Acharya S, et al. A single-center study of the clinicopathologic correlates of gliomas with a MYB or MYBL1 alteration. Acta Neuropathol. 2019;138:1091.
62. Bandopadhayay P, Ramkissoon LA, Jain P, , Bergthold G, Wala J, Zeid R et al. MYB-QKI rearrangements in angiocentric glioma drive tumorigenicity through a tripartite mechanism. Nat Genet 2016; 48:273.
63. Han GQ, Zhang JS, Ma Y, Gui QP, Yin S. Clinical characteristics, treatment and prognosis of angiocentric glioma. Oncol Lett. 2020;20:1641–8.
64. Huse JT, Snuderl M, Jones DT, Brathwaite CD, Altman N, Lavi E, et al. Polymorphous low-grade neuroepithelial tumor of the young (PLNTY): an epileptogenic neoplasm with oligodendroglioma-like components, aberrant CD34 expression, and genetic alterations involving the MAP kinase pathway. Acta Neuropathol. 2017;133:417.
65. Bale TA, Sait SF, Benhamida J, Benhamida J, Ptashkin R, Haquue S, et al. Malignant transformation of a polymorphous low grade neuroepithelial tumor of the young (PLNTY). Acta Neuropathol. 2021;141:123.

66. Ryall S, Zapotocky M, Fukuoka K, Nobre L, Guerreiro Stucklin A, Bennett J, et al. Integrated molecular and clinical analysis of 1,000 pediatric low-grade gliomas. Cancer Cell. 2020;37(4):569–83 e5.
67. Chatwin HV, Cruz JC, Green AL. Pediatric high-grade glioma: moving toward subtype-specific multimodal therapy. FEBS J. 2021;288:6127–41.
68. Lucas CG, Mueller S, Reddy A, Taylor JW, Oberheim Bush NA, Clarke JL, et al. Diffuse hemispheric glioma, H3 G34-mutant: genomic landscape of a new tumor entity and prospects for targeted therapy. Neuro Oncol. 2021;23:1974.
69. Castel D, Kergrohen T, Tauziède-Espariat A, Mackay A, Ghermaoui S, Lechapt E, et al. Histone H3 wild-type DIPG/DMG overexpressing EZHIP extend the spectrum diffuse midline gliomas with PRC2 inhibition beyond H3-K27M mutation. Acta Neuropathol. 2020;139:1109–13.
70. Mondal G, Lee JC, Ravindranathan A, Villanueva-Meyer JE, Tran QT, Allen SJ, et al. Pediatric bithalamic gliomas have a distinct epigenetic signature and frequent EGFR exon 20 insertions resulting in potential sensitivity to targeted kinase inhibition. Acta Neuropathol. 2020;139:1071–88.
71. Korshunov A, Capper D, Reuss D, et al. Histologically distinct neuroepithelial tumors with histone 3 G34 mutation are molecularly similar and comprise a single nosologic entity. Acta Neuropathol. 2016;131:137.
72. Haase S, Nuñez FM, Gauss JC, Thompson S, Brumley E, Lowenstein P, et al. Hemispherical pediatric high-grade glioma: Molecular basis and therapeutic opportunities. Int J Mol Sci. 2020;21:9654.
73. Haque F, Varlet P, Puntonet J, Storer L, Bountali A, Rahman R, et al. Evaluation of a novel antibody to define histone 3.3 G34R mutant brain tumours. Acta Neuropathol Commun. 2017;5:45.
74. Coleman C, Stoller S, Grotzer M, Stucklin AG, Nazarian J, Mueller S. Pediatric hemispheric high-grade glioma: targeting the future. Cancer Metastasis Rev. 2020;39:245–60.
75. Korshunov A, Schrimpf D, Ryzhova M, Sturm D, Chavez L, Hovestadt V, et al. H3-/IDH-wild type pediatric glioblastoma is comprised of molecularly and prognostically distinct subtypes with associated oncogenic drivers. Acta Neuropathol. 2017;134:507–16.
76. Clarke M, Mackay A, Ismer B, Pickles JC, Tatevossian RG, Newman S, et al. Infant high-grade gliomas comprise multiple subgroups characterized by novel targetable gene fusions and favorable outcomes. Cancer Discov. 2020;10:942–63.
77. Guereiro Stucklin AS, Ryall S, Fukuoka K, Zapotocky M, Lassaletta A, Li C, et al. Alterations in ALK/ROS1/NTRK/MET drive a group of infantile hemispheric gliomas. Nat Commun. 2019;10:4343.
78. Gutmann DH, McLellan MD, Hussain I, Wallis JW, Fulton LL, Fulton RS, Magrini V, et al. Somatic neurofibromatosis type 1 (NF1) inactivation characterizes NF1-associated pilocytic astrocytoma. Genome Res. 2013;23:431–9.
79. Hawkins C, Walker E, Mohamed N, Zhang C, Jacob K, Shirinian M, et al. BRAF-KIAA1549 fusion predicts better clinical outcome in pediatric low-grade astrocytoma. Clin Cancer Res. 2011;17:4790–8.
80. Lassaletta A, Zapotocky M, Bouffet E, Hawkins C, Tabori U. An integrative molecular and genomic analysis of pediatric hemispheric low-grade gliomas: an update. Childs Nerv Syst. 2016;32(10):1789–97.
81. Jones DT, Hutter B, Jager N, Korshunov A, Kool M, Warnatz H-J, et al. Recurrent somatic alterations of FGFR1 and NTRK2 in pilocytic astrocytoma. Nat Genet. 2013;45:927–32.
82. Reinhardt A, Stichel D, Schrimpf D, Sahm F, Korshunov A, Reuss DE, et al. Anaplastic astrocytoma with piloid features, a novel molecular class of IDH wildtype glioma with recurrent MAPK pathway, CDKN2A/B and ATRX alterations. Acta Neuropathol. 2018;136:273–91.
83. Bender K, Perez E, Chirica M, Onken J, Kahn J, Brenner W, et al. High-grade astrocytoma with piloid features (HGAP): the Charite experience with a new central nervous system tumor entity. J Neurooncol. 2021;153:109–20.

84. Rodriguez FJ, Scheithauer BW, Burger PC, Jenkins S, Giannini C. Anaplasia in pilocytic astrocytoma predicts aggressive behavior. Am J Surg Pathol. 2010;34:147–60.
85. Dias-Santagata D, Lam Q, Vernovsky K, Vena N, Lennerz JK, Borger DR, Batchelor TT. BRAF V600E mutations are common in pleomorphic xanthoastrocytoma: diagnostic and therapeutic implications. PLoS One. 2011;6(3):e17948.
86. Shaikh N, Brahmbhatt N, Kruser TJ, Kam KL, Appin CL, Wadhwani N, Chandler J, Kumthekar P, Lukas RV. Pleomorphic xanthoastrocytoma: a brief review. CNS Oncol. 2019;8:CNS39.
87. Phillips JJ, Gong H, Chen K, Joseph NM, van Ziffle J, Bastian BC, et al. The genetic landscape of anaplastic pleomorphic xanthoastrocytoma. Brain Pathol. 2019;29:85–96.
88. Bongaarts A, Giannikou K, Reinten RJ, Anink JJ, Mills JD, Jansen FE, Spliet GMW. Subependymal giant cell astrocytomas in tuberous sclerosis complex have consistent TSC1/TSC2 biallelic inactivation, and no BRAF mutations. Oncotarget. 2017;8(56):95516–29.
89. Rosenberg S, Simeonova I, Bielle F, Verreault M, Bance B, Le Roux I, et al. A recurrent point mutation in PRKCA is a hallmark of chordoid gliomas. Nat Commun. 2018;9:2371.
90. Yao K, Duan Z, Du Z, Fan X, Qu Y, Zhang M, et al. PRKCA D463H mutation in chordoid glioma of the third ventricle: a cohort of 16 cases, including two cases harboring BRAFV600E mutation. J Neuropathol Exp Neurol. 2020;79:1183–92.
91. Hirose T, Nobusawa S, Sugiyama K, Amatva VJ, Fujimoto N, Sasaki A, et al. Astroblastoma: a distinct tumor entity characterized by alterations of the X chromosome and MN1 rearrangement. Brain Pathol. 2018;28:684–94.
92. Mhatre R, Sugur HS, Nandeesh BN, Chickabasaviah Y, Saini J, Santosh V. MN1 rearrangement in astroblastoma: study of eight cases and review of literature. Brain Tumor Pathol. 2019;36:112–20.
93. Andrey K, Felix S, Olga Z, Andrey G, Damian S, Daniel S, et al. DNA methylation profiling is a method of choice for molecular verification of pediatric WNT-activated medulloblastomas. Neuro Oncol. 2019;21:214–21.
94. Orr BA. Pathology, diagnostics, and classification of medulloblastoma. Brain Pathol. 2020;30:664–78.
95. Merchant TE, Pollack IF, Loeffler JS. Brain tumors across the age spectrum: biology, therapy, and late effects. Semin Radiat Oncol. 2010;20:58–66.
96. Smith MJ, Beetz C, Williams SG, Bhaskar SS, O'Sullivan J, Anderson B, et al. Germline mutations in SUFU cause Gorlin syndrome-associated childhood medulloblastoma and redefine the risk associated with PTCH1 mutations. J Clin Oncol. 2014;32:4155.
97. Jones DT, Jäger N, Kool M, Zichner T, Hutter B, Sultan M, et al. Dissecting the genomic complexity underlying medulloblastoma. Nature. 2012;488:100–5.
98. Goschzik T, Schwalbe EC, Hicks D, Smith A, Zur Muehlen A, Figarella-Branger D, et al. Prognostic effect of whole chromosomal aberration signatures in standard-risk, non-WNT/non-SHH medulloblastoma: a retrospective, molecular analysis of the HIT-SIOP PNET 4 trial. Lancet Oncol. 2018;19:1602–16.
99. Northcott PA, Buchhalter I, Morrissy AS, Hovestadt V, Weischenfeldt J, Ehrenberger T, et al. The whole-genome landscape of medulloblastoma subtypes. Nature. 2017;547:311–7.
100. Schwalbe EC, Lindsey JC, Nakjang S, Crosier S, Smith AJ, Hicks D, et al. Novel molecular subgroups for clinical classification and outcome prediction in childhood medulloblastoma: a cohort study. Lancet Oncol. 2017;18:958–71.
101. Juraschka K, Taylor MD. Medulloblatoma in the age of molecular subgroups: a review. J Neurosurg Pediatr. 2019;24:353–63.
102. Sharma T, Schwalbe EC, Williamson D, Sill M, Hovestadt V, Mynarek M, et al. Second-generation molecular subgrouping of medulloblastoma: an international meta-analysis of Group 3 and Group 4 subtypes. Acta Neuropathol. 2019;138(2):309–26.

103. Miller S, Ward JH, Rogers HA, Lowe J, Grundy RG. Loss of INI1 protein expression defines a subgroup of aggressive central nervous system primitive neuroectodermal tumors. Brain Pathol. 2013;23:19–27.
104. Ho B, Johann PD, Grabovska Y, De Dieu Andrianteranagna MJ, Yao F, Frühwald M, Hasselblatt M, et al. Molecular subgrouping of atypicalteratoid/rhabdoid tumors-a reinvestigation and current consensus. Neuro Oncol. 2020;22(5):613–24.
105. Korshunov A, Sturm D, Ryzhova M, Hovestadt V, Gessi M, Jones DTW, et al. Embryonal tumor with abundant neuropil and true rosettes (ETANTR), ependymoblastoma, and medulloepithelioma share molecular similarity and comprise a single clinicopathological entity. Acta Neuropathol. 2014;128(2):279–89.
106. Sturm D, Orr BA, Toprak UH, et al. New brain tumor entities emerge from molecular classification of CNS-PNETs. Cell. 2016;164:1060–72.
107. von Hoff K, et al. Therapeutic implications of improved molecular diagnostics for rare CNS embryonal tumor entities: results of an international, retrospective study. Neuro Oncol. 2021;23(9):1597–611.
108. Mardi L, Tauziede-Espariat A, Guillemot D, Pierron G, Gigant P, Mehdi L, Charlotte Berthaud C, et al. BCOR immunohistochemistry, but not SATB2 immunohistochemistry, is a sensitive and specific diagnostic biomarker for central nervous system tumours with BCOR internal tandem duplication. Histopathology. 2021;79(5):891–4.
109. Zwerdling T, Dothage J. Meningiomas in children and adolescents. J Pediatr Hematol Oncol. 2002;24:199–204.
110. Kerr K, Qualmann K, Esquenazi Y, Hagan J, Kim DH. Familial syndromes involving meningiomas provide mechanistic insight into sporadic disease. Neurosurgery. 2018;83:1107–18.
111. Huntoon K, Toland AMS, Dahiya S. Meningioma: a review of clinicopathological and molecular aspects. Front Oncol. 2020;10:579599.
112. Ogasawara C, Philbrick BD, Adamson DC. Meningioma: a review of epidemiology, pathology, diagnosis, treatment, and future directions. Biomedicines. 2021;9:319.
113. Wiemels J, Wrensch M, Claus EB. Epidemiology and etiology of meningioma. J Neurooncol. 2010;99:307–14.
114. Korhonen K, Salminen T, Raitanen J, Auvinen A, Isola J, Haapasalo H. Female predominance in meningiomas can not be explained by differences in progesterone, estrogen, or androgen receptor expression. J Neurooncol. 2006;80:1–7.
115. Qi ZY, Shao C, Huang YL, Hui GZ, Zhou YX, Wan Z. Reproductive and exogenous hormone factors in relation to risk of meningioma in women: a meta-analysis. PLoS One. 2013;8:e83261.
116. Wu W, Zhou Y, Wang Y, Liu L, Lou J, Deng Y, et al. Clinical significance of somatostatin receptor (SSTR) 2 in meningioma. Front Oncol. 2020;10:1633.
117. Wang N, Osswald M. Meningiomas: overview and new directions in therapy. Semin Neurol. 2018;38:112–20.
118. Pereira BJA, Oba-Shinjo SM, de Almeida AN, Marie SKN. Molecular Alterations in Meningiomas: Literature Review. Clin Neurol Neurosurg. 2019;176:89–96.
119. Smith MJ. Germline and somatic mutations in meningiomas. Cancer Genet. 2015;208:107–14.
120. Shankar GM, Santagata S. BAP1 mutations in high-grade meningioma: implications for patient care. Neuro Oncol. 2017;19:1447–56.
121. Sahm F, Schrimpf D, Olar A, Koelsche C, Reuss D, Bissel J, et al. TERT promoter mutations and risk of recurrence in meningioma. J Natl Cancer Inst. 2016;108:djv370.
122. Proctor DT, Ramachandran S, Lama S, Sutherland GR. Towards molecular classification of meningioma: evolving treatment and diagnostic paradigms. World Neurosurg. 2018;119:366–73.
123. Mirian C, Duun-Henriksen AK, Juratli T, Sahm F, Spiegl-Kreinecker S, Peyre M, et al. Poor prognosis associated with TERT gene alterations in meningioma is independent of the WHO classification: an individual patient data meta-analysis. J Neurol Neurosurg Psychiatry. 2020;91:378–87.

124. Lee YS, Lee YS. Molecular characteristics of meningiomas. J Pathol Transl Med. 2020;54:45–63.
125. Mirian C, Grell K, Juratli TA, Sahm F, Spiegl-Kreinecker S, Peyre M, et al. Implementation of TERT promoter mutations improve prognostication of the WHO classification in meningioma. Neuropathol Appl Neurobiol. 2022;48:e12773.
126. Pellerino A, Bruno F, Palmiero R, Pronello E, Bertero L, Riccardo Soffietti R, Rudà R. Clinical significance of molecular alterations and systemic therapy for meningiomas: where do we stand? Cancers (Basel). 2022;14:2256.
127. Guyot A, Duchesne M, Robert S, Lia AS, Derouault P, Scaon E, et al. Analysis of CDKN2A gene alterations in recurrent and non-recurrent meningioma. J Neurooncol. 2019;145:449–59.
128. Sievers P, Hielscher T, Schrimpf D, Stichel D, Reuss DE, Berghof AS, et al. CDKN2A/B homozygous deletion is associated with early recurrence in meningiomas. Acta Neuropathol. 2020;140:409–13.
129. Robert SM, Vesta S, Nadar A, Vasandani S, Youngblood MW, Gorelick E, et al. The integrated multiomic diagnosis of sporadic meningiomas: a review of its clinical implications. J Neuro Oncol. 2022;156:205–14.
130. Liu N, Song S-Y, Jiang J-B, Wang T-J, Yan C-X. The prognostic role of Ki-67/MIB-1 in meningioma. A systematic review with meta-analysis. Medicine (Baltimore). 2020;99:e18644.
131. Merlin P-SN. The NF2 gene product. Pathol Oncol Res. 2013;19:365–73.
132. Afshar-Oromieh A, Wolf MB, Kratochwil C, Giesel FL, Combs SE, Dimitrakopoulou-Strauss A, et al. Comparison of (6)(8) Ga-DOTATOC-PET/CT and PET/MRI hybrid systems in patients with cranial meningioma: Initial results. Neuro Oncol. 2015;17:312–9.
133. Weber RG, Boströ J, Wolter M, Baudis M, Collins VP, Reifenberger G, Lichter P. Analysis of genomic alterations in benign, atypical, and anaplastic meningiomas: toward a genetic model of meningioma progression. Proc Natl Acad Sci U S A. 1997;94:14719–24.
134. Lamszus K. Meningioma pathology, genetics, and biology. J Neuropathol Exp Neurol. 2004;63:275–86.
135. Mawrin C, Perry A. Pathological classification and molecular genetics of meningiomas. J Neurooncol. 2010;99:379–91.
136. Och W, Szmuda T, Sikorska B, Springer J, Jaskólski D, Zakrzewska M, Liberski PP. Recurrence-associated chromosomal anomalies in meningiomas: single-institution study and a systematic review with meta-analysis. Neurol Neurochir Pol. 2016;50:439–48.
137. Brastianos PK, Horowitz PM, Santagata S, Jones RT, McKenna A, Getz G, et al. Genomic sequencing of meningiomas identifes oncogenic SMO and AKT1 mutations. Nat Genet. 2013;45:285–9.
138. Clark VE, Erson-Omay EZ, Serin A, Yin J, Cotney J, Ozduman K, et al. Genomic analysis of non- NF2 meningiomas reveals mutations in TRAF7, KLF4, AKT1, and SMO. Science. 2013;339:1077–80.
139. Reuss DE, Piro RM, Jones DTW, Simon M, Ketter R, Kool M, et al. Secretory meningiomas are defined by combined KLF4K409Q and TRAF7 mutations. Acta Neuropathol. 2013;125:351–8.
140. Abedalthagafi M, Bi WL, Aizer AA, Merrill PH, Brewster R, Pankaj K, et al. Oncogenic PI3K mutations are as common as AKT1 and SMO mutations in meningioma. Neuro Oncol. 2016;18:649–55.
141. Shankar GM, Abedalthagafi M, Vaubel RA, Merrill PH, Nayyar N, Gill CM, et al. Germline and somatic BAP1 mutations in high- grade rhabdoid meningiomas. Neuro Oncol. 2017;19:535–45.
142. Sahm F, Bissel J, Koelsche C, Schweizer L, Capper D, Reus D, et al. AKT1E17K mutations cluster with meningothelial and transitional meningiomas and can be detected by SFRP1 immunohistochemistry. Acta Neuropathol. 2013;126:757–62.
143. Strickland MR, Gill CM, Nayyar N, D'Andrea MR, Thiede CH, Juratli TA, Schackert G. Targeted sequencing of SMO and AKT1 in anterior skull base meningiomas. J Neurosurg. 2017;127:438–44.

144. Boetto J, Bielle F, Sanson M, Peyre M, Kalamarides M. SMO mutation status defines a distinct and frequent molecular subgroup in olfactory groove meningiomas. Neuro Oncol. 2017;19:345–51.
145. Smith MJ, O'Sullivan J, Bhaskar SS, Hadfield KD, Poke G, Caird J, et al. Loss-of-function mutations in SMARCE1 cause an inherited disorder of multiple spinal meningiomas. Nat Genet. 2013;45:295–8.
146. Smith MJ, Wallace AJ, Bennett C, Hasselblatt M, Elert-Dobkowska E, Evans LT, et al. Germline SMARCE1 mutations predispose to both spinal and cranial clear cell meningiomas. J Pathol. 2014;234:436–40.
147. Williams EA, Wakimoto H, Shankar GM, Barker FG 2nd, Brastianos PK, Santagata S, et al. Frequent inactivating mutations of the PBAF complex gene PBRM1 in meningioma with papillary features. Acta Neuropathol. 2020;140:89–93.
148. Ji Y, Rankin C, Grunberg S, Sherrod AE, Ahmadi J, Townsend JJ, et al. Unresectable meningioma: SWOG S9005. J Clin Oncol. 2015;33:4093–8.
149. Clark VE, Harmanci AS, Bai H, Youngblood MW, Lee TI, Baranoski JF, et al. Recurrent somatic mutations in POLR2A define a distinct subset of meningiomas. Nat Genet. 2016;48:1253–9.
150. Sahm F, Schrimpf D, Stichel D, Jones DTW, Hielscher T, Schefzyk S, et al. DNA methylation-based classification and grading system for meningioma: a multicentre, retrospective analysis. Lancet Oncol. 2017;18:682–94.
151. Olar A, Wani KM, Wilson CD, Zadeh G, DeMonte F, Jones DT, et al. Global epigenetic profiling identifies methylation subgroups associated with recurrence-free survival in meningioma. Acta Neuropathol. 2017;133:431–44.
152. Nassiri F, Mamatjan Y, Suppiah S, Badhiwala JH, Mansouri S, Karimi S, et al. DNA methylation profiling to predict recurrence risk in meningioma: development and validation of a nomogram to optimize clinical management. Neuro Oncol. 2019;21:901–10.
153. Du Z, Abedalthagafi M, Aizer AA, McHenry AR, Sun HH, Bray M-A, et al. Increased expression of the immune modulatory molecule PD-L1 (CD274) in anaplastic meningioma. Oncotarget. 2014;6:4704–16.
154. Nebot-Bral L, Brandao D, Verlingue L, Rouleau E, Caron O, Despras E, et al. Hypermutated tumours in the era of immunotherapy: the paradigm of personalised medicine. Eur J Cancer. 2017;84:290–303.
155. Preusser M, Brastianos PK, Mawrin C. Advances in meningioma genetics: novel therapeutic opportunities. Nat Rev Neurol. 2018;14:106–15.
156. Graillon T, Sanson M, Campello C, Idbaih A, Peyre M, Peyrière H, et al. Everolimus and octreotide for patients with recurrent meningioma: results from the phase II CEVOREM trial. Clin Cancer Res. 2020;26:552–7.
157. Juric V, Murphy B. Cyclin-dependent kinase inhibitors in brain cancer: Current state and future directions. Cancer Drug Resist. 2020;3:48–62.
158. Bi WL, Nayak L, Meredith DM, Driver J, Du Z, Hoffman S, et al. Activity of PD-1 blockade with nivolumab among patients with recurrent atypical/anaplastic meningioma: phase II trial results. Neuro Oncol. 2021;2:101–11.

Chapter 7
Current Methods for Intraoperative Application

Marcos Vinicius D'Amato Figueiredo and Roberta Rehder

7.1 Introduction

Central nervous system tumors represent approximately 1% of newly diagnosed cancers in the USA, in which two-thirds of brain tumors are benign. Malignant tumors include high grade gliomas, representing approximately 80% of all malignant brain tumors [1–3].

High-grade gliomas are very aggressive, in which the overall survival in 1-year and 5-year in high-grade gliomas is 37.4% and 5%, respectively, despite treatment. Prognostic factors include age, performance status, tumor grade, histology, and extent of surgical resection [4–7]. Current intraoperative methods for tumor resection have been developed to improve safety and minimize postoperative morbidity.

Among the different methods, flow cytometry analysis has been considered a promise tool to assess tumor samples intraoperatively. Flow cytometry is the gold standard laser-based technique to analyze and measure cell features. It is an indispensable method in basic research, using a flow cytometer and specific reagents, including fluorescein and data analysis [8–10]. Such a technique enables one to perform rapid cell analysis with high reproducibility.

Flow cytometry has been widely used in hematological malignancies, including therapy guiding and follow-up disease progression [9–11]. It consists of a fast and accurate data collection method from a fluid mixture containing cells and their

M. V. D'Amato Figueiredo
Hospital do Coração, São Paulo, Brazil

R. Rehder (✉)
Hospital do Coração, São Paulo, Brazil

Division of Pediatric Neurosurgery, Department of Neurosurgery, Hospital Santa Marcelina, São Paulo, Brazil

G. Alexiou, G. Vartholomatos (eds.), *Intraoperative Flow Cytometry*, https://doi.org/10.1007/978-3-031-33517-4_7

particles that can provide information on pathological findings. The samples for flow cytometry may include fresh and formalin-fixed cells, frozen specimens, and paraffin-embedded tissues.

Early cancer detection improves treatment and optimizes patient outcomes and survival. Intraoperative flow cytometry has recently emerged as a novel method for cancer diagnosis and treatment, particularly in central nervous system tumor surgery. The present chapter presents intraoperative flow cytometry as a novel and adjunct method in brain tumors to standard histopathological and frozen diagnosis.

7.2 The Cell Cycle

The cell cycle has different stages, including G1, S, G2, and M. The G1 is the stage that the cell is preparing to divide. The next stage is the S phase, known as synthesis, in which the cell copies all the DNA. The following stage is known as the G2, where the cell organizes and condenses the genetic material and prepares to divide. The next stage is the M stage, known as mitosis, where the cell partitions the two copies of the genetic material into the two daughter cells [10–12]. As the M phase completes and the cell division occurs, the cell cycle starts over again (Fig. 7.1).

Flow cytometry provides a valuable tool to assess cells in G0/G1 phase, S phase, G2/M, and polyploidy, which holds prognostic significance. An important parameter that quantifies cancer cell proliferation in cancer cells is tumor index, which is the proportion of cells in the S and G2/M phases. Tumor index is associated with the degree of tumor malignancy [13–15]. An additional index described is that of DNA index (DI) that includes the ploidy of cancer with an abnormal number of chromosomes as well as cancer cells.

Fig. 7.1 Different stages of the cell cycle

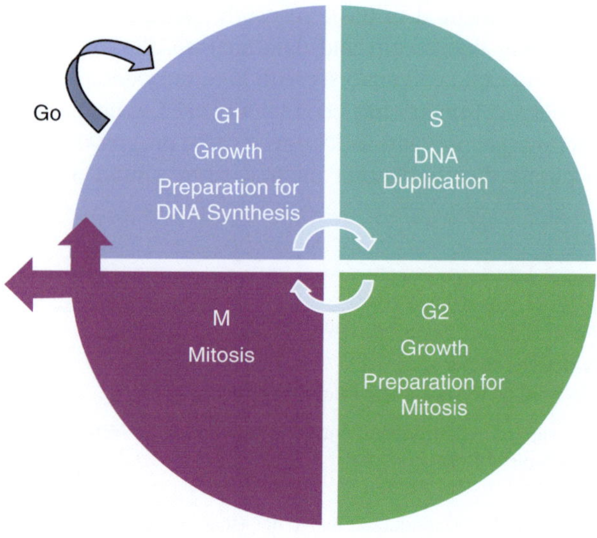

7.3 Brain Tumors Intraoperative Techniques

Central nervous system tumors are the leading cause of cancer death among females younger than 19 years and among males younger than 39 years. Intracranial gliomas are frequent lesions, in which high-grade gliomas are the most malignant primary brain tumor in adults with a median survival of approximately 15 months [4, 5, 16]. Current treatment includes maximal surgical resection, followed by radiotherapy and concomitant temozolomide chemotherapy.

Maximal safe resection is the mainstay treatment of low- and high-grade gliomas. A comprehensive understanding of tumor anatomy, as well as the location of the eloquent cortex and subcortical pathways, is required to maximize the extent of resection and preserve the neurological status, which affects overall survival [5, 17–20].

The extent of tumor resection is one of the most important prognostic factors for patients with gliomas. Current techniques of intraoperative brain tumor surgery provide a means to improve the extent of resection with safety, minimizing postoperative morbidity and optimizing surgical resection. Intraoperative methods in neurosurgery for tumor surgery include intraoperative neurophysiological monitoring, intraoperative magnetic resonance image (MRI), neuronavigation system, minimally invasive techniques, intraoperative ultrasound, intraoperative frozen section evaluation, and the use of 5-aminolevulinic acid (5-ALA) [21–24].

7.3.1 Intraoperative Neurophysiological Monitoring

Intraoperative neurophysiological monitoring enables the surgeon to optimize the extent of resection in eloquent locations, minimizing postoperative morbidity. Continuous motor and sensory evoked potentials as well as cortical and subcortical stimulation have been implemented intraoperatively to prevent neurological deficits [23, 25]. Neurophysiological mapping techniques enable the surgeon to identify cortical anatomical landmarks, including the central sulcus, the primary sensory and motor areas, and the frontal and temporal regions related to language. Such a technique is helpful in identifying eloquent structures, assisting the neurosurgeon to maximize tumor resection within functional boundaries [26].

7.3.2 Intraoperative MRI

The success of oncologic surgery is associated with the extent of tumor resection. Maximal safe resection has a significant prognostic benefit by improving overall survival. Intraoperative MRI is a useful method to maximize tumor resection [23].

　　　　　　　　　　　　　　　　　　　　　　　M. V. D'Amato Figueiredo and R. Rehder

Although it is expensive and time-consuming, intraoperative MRI has been used as a surgical adjunct in brain tumor resection. Several studies have reported the benefits of using intraoperative MRI in detecting residual tumor intraoperatively leading to extended tumor resections [26–29].

Intraoperative MRI provides near real-time information about the dynamic changes known as the brain shift phenomenon, which is often observed in patients with hydrocephalus, edema, brain atrophy, and lesions with mass effect. It is currently the gold standard method when determining the extent of resection, providing the surgeon with an accurate assessment of residual tumor.

7.3.3   Neuronavigation

Neuronavigation system provides intraoperative information on tumor localization using multimodal image fusion, assisting neurosurgeon on tumor guidance and orientation with a high level of accuracy and precision. Disadvantages of the technique include cost and intraoperative brain shift [23, 26, 30]. Currently, frameless neuronavigation methods for tumor localization yield positional accuracy within 2–3 mm during surgery, which is equivalent to the accuracy of frame-based stereotaxic.

7.3.4   Minimally Invasive Techniques

Minimally invasive techniques have improved over time surgical resection with minimal exposure and high-definition imaging. Advances in endoscope-assisted microsurgery have improved the ability to assess the extent of resection and reduce the risk of surgery-related complications [31–33]. Novel instruments in neuroendoscopy have enabled neurosurgeons to maximize tumor resection with minimal approaches, thus optimizing postoperative recovery and patient's survival [31, 34].

7.3.5   5-ALA

The 5-Aminolevulinic Acid Hydrochloride (5-ALA), a precursor of the heme biosynthesis pathway in human cell, accumulates in high amounts within malignant glial cell. It is converted into a fluorescent metabolite known as protoporphyrin IX, which can be stimulated by blue light during surgery. Such a property enables neurosurgeon to visualize residual tumor intraoperatively, thus improving the extent of tumor resection and minimizing normal brain tissue injury [21, 22].

7.3.6 Frozen Section

Frozen section analysis is the gold standard method to assess tumor margin resection and confirm tumor sample intraoperatively. Among few limitations include the pathologist's expertise and tissue sample quality and preparation.

7.3.7 Mass Spectrometry

Recently desorption electrospray ionization-mass spectrometry imaging (DESI-MS) has been a promising tool for intraoperative analysis of tumor margins resection. Such a technique may distinguish tumor and adjacent normal tissue based on the detection of different lipid and metabolites profiles [28, 35].

7.3.8 Intraoperative Flow Cytometry

Another promising tool for tumor diagnosis includes intraoperative flow cytometry. It was first introduced in an early work by Mesiwala et al., in which flow cytometry supported the analysis of fresh beef-brain tissue samples. The experiment included an ultrasound aspiration that was utilized removal and homogenization of pathological tissue of brain tumors, which was followed by DNA staining and in situ automatic DNA quantification [36].

Alexiou GA et al. reported normal brain tissue from epilepsy samples has a G0/G1 phase fraction of 97.1 ± 0.5%, S phase of 1.7 ± 0.5%, and G2/M fraction of 1.25 ± 0.5% [13, 14, 37]. Therefore, higher S and G2/M phase fractions correlate with high-grade lesions. Diploid DNA content and low proliferative index are observed in benign tumors, including meningiomas, pituitary adenomas, low-grade gliomas, and inflammatory lesions. In contrast, more aggressive lesions often present aneuploid populations and/or a higher proliferation index [13, 14, 37, 38].

Different intraoperative flow cytometry protocols have been developed recently for brain tumor analysis. Shioyama et al. described a detailed flow cytometry protocol for tumor DNA analysis within 10 min based on the malignancy index [39]. The Ioannina protocol based on rapid cell cycle analysis categorized tumor samples in low- and high-grade lesions, tumor margins, and primary central nervous system lymphoma within 6 min (Fig. 7.2) [14, 37, 38].

Alexiou et al. described the association between G0/G1 and S phases and tumor prognosis [14]. Patients with G0/G1 phase lower than 70% and S phase greater than 6% presented a worse prognosis. Interestingly, such findings were also observed in meningiomas grades I, II/III in G0/G1 phase, S phase, and G2/M phase fractions.

In pediatric brain tumors, including ependymomas, medulloblastomas, atypical teratoid/rhabdoid tumors, astrocytoma, and PNETs, higher G0/G1 phase fraction and significantly lower G2/M phase fraction were observed in low-grade lesions [37, 40]. Particularly in ependymomas and medulloblastomas, a significant correlation between S phase fraction and Ki-67 index was observed.

Shioyama et al. reported the malignancy index (MI) in flow cytometry in patients with high-grade gliomas surgically treated followed by radiotherapy and temozolomide [39]. The MI is calculated based on the predominance of a cell type on the histogram and determined by the ratio of the number of cells with greater than normal DNA content and the total cell number. In the presence of DNA aneuploidy, the DNA index was calculated as the ratio of DNA content in the aneuploid cells and the abnormal number of chromosomes to those in G0/G1 cells. The MI values over 26% are correlated with patient survival and IDH1 mutation status [39].

The CD45, a glycoprotein expressed in lymphohematopoietic cells, is diagnostic of primary central nervous system lymphoma (PCNSL). The expression of CD20 in PCNSL is considered a prognostic and therapeutic marker, in which treatment with rituximab, a monoclonal antibody against the CD20 antigen, has improved survival. Therefore, flow cytometry may have an additional role as a therapeutic strategy in PCNSL patients [14, 38].

The NCAM, known as CD56, and its isoforms (NCAM120, NCAM-140, and NCAM-180) are expressed in several brain tumors, including medulloblastomas, gliomas, and ependymomas. The analysis of CD56 expression can be done using flow cytometry. According to the studies, high-grade lesions present lower CD56 expression than low-grade tumors [14, 37, 38].

In intracranial meningiomas, flow cytometry analysis is a promising tool in prognosis and diagnosis. The malignancy of these lesions has been associated with proliferative potential and aneuploidy as well as with cerebral edema [14].

Fig. 7.2 (**a**) Glioblastoma case in a 63-year-old female patient. (**b**) Intraoperative sampling. (**c**) DNA content and cell cycle distribution analysis using intraoperative flow cytometry (iFC) in a glioblastoma case. Typical cell cycle distributions as analyzed by iFC are presented for a center and three margin samples. Markers M1, M2, and M3 represent G0/G1, S, and G2/M cell cycle phases, respectively. M4 marker contains normal diploid cells. First row: iFC analysis of cancer cells and cells from a positive margin. Second row: iFC analysis of a positive margin and a negative margin. Third row: overlays of cancer cells with a positive margin and a negative margin, respectively (Courtesy of the Editors)

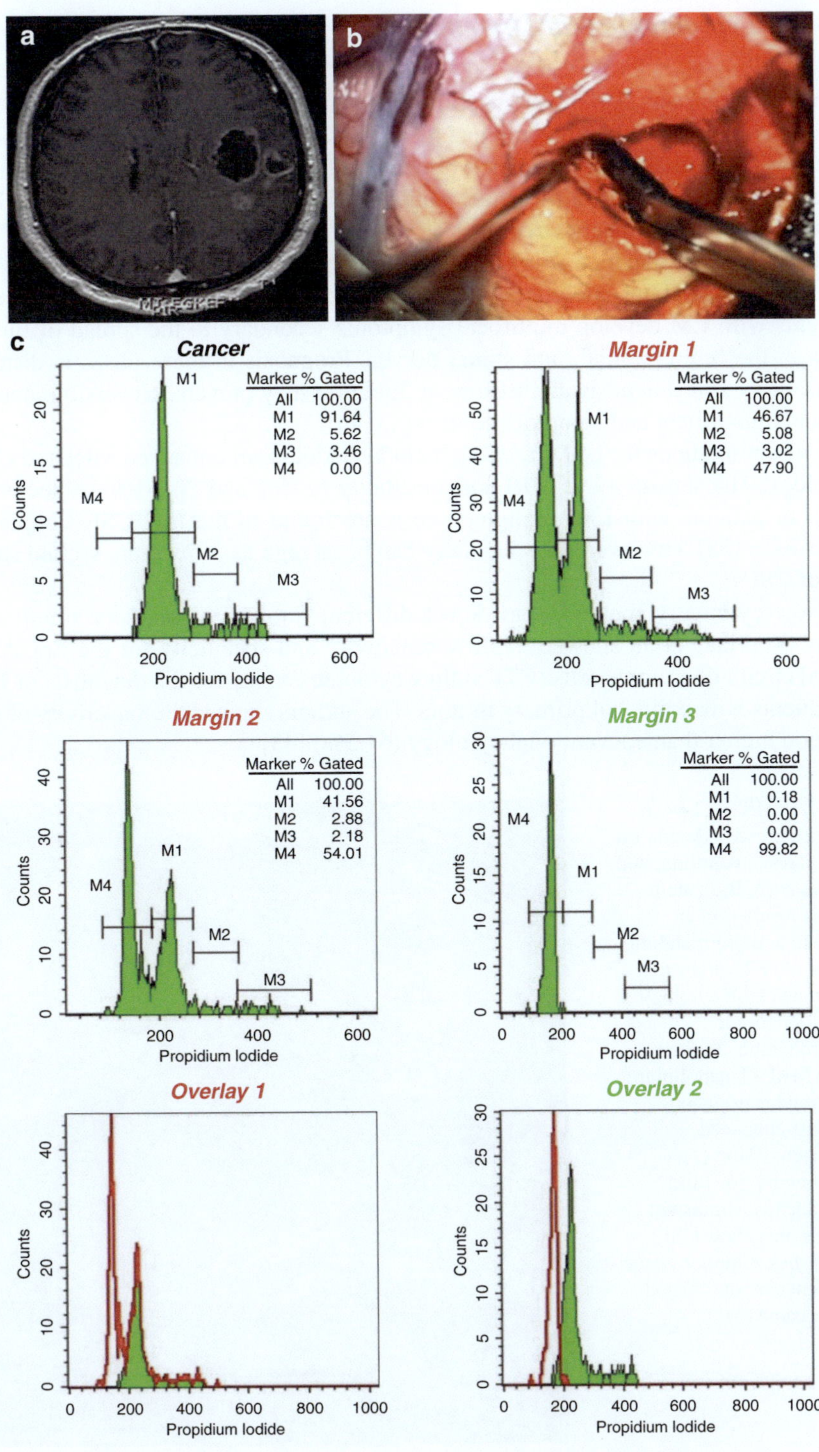
a
b
c
Cancer
M1
Counts
M4
M2
M3
Marker % Gated
All   100.00
M1   91.64
M2   5.62
M3   3.46
M4   0.00
Propidium Iodide
Margin 1
M1
Counts
M4
M2
M3
Marker % Gated
All   100.00
M1   46.67
M2   5.08
M3   3.02
M4   47.90
Propidium Iodide
Margin 2
M1
Counts
M4
M2
M3
Marker % Gated
All   100.00
M1   41.56
M2   2.88
M3   2.18
M4   54.01
Propidium Iodide
Margin 3
M4
M1
Counts
M2
M3
Marker % Gated
All   100.00
M1   0.18
M2   0.00
M3   0.00
M4   99.82
Propidium Iodide
Overlay 1
Counts
Propidium Iodide
Overlay 2
Counts
Propidium Iodide

7.3.9 Leptomeningeal Dissemination

Flow cytometry has also proved useful in the analysis of cerebrospinal fluid (CSF) tumor dissemination. Leptomeningeal metastases (LM), known as meningeal carcinomatosis, is a diffuse dissemination of tumor cells into the CSF and leptomeninges (Fig. 7.3). Almost 5–10% of cancer patients with solid tumors will develop LM during their lifetime despite treatment [41–43].

The most common tumors to develop LM include patients with melanoma, breast cancer, small cell lung carcinoma, and non-small cell lung carcinoma. Consequently, patients with LM develop multifocal symptoms secondary to the spread of tumor cells in the brain, cranial, and spinal nerves. Prognosis in these cases is dismal. Thus, early LM diagnosis and treatment initiation may prevent irreversible neurological impairment and symptom control [43, 44].

Current methods for LM screening include Gadolinium-enhanced MRI and CSF cytology. The sensitivity of MRI and specificity is 75% and 20–91%, respectively [37]. In patients with LM, malignant cells are found in the first CSF sample in 50%–67% [38]. However, the specificity can be as high as 80% in the second sample of CSF.

Flow cytometry methods can detect different fluorescent markers simultaneously. Kerklaan et al. showed a 100% sensitivity and specificity for the EpCAM-based circulating tumor cells (CTCs) flow cytometry assay for the diagnosis of LM in patients with epithelial primary tumors. The authors showed the sensitivity of the method higher than conventional cytology (61.5%) [43].

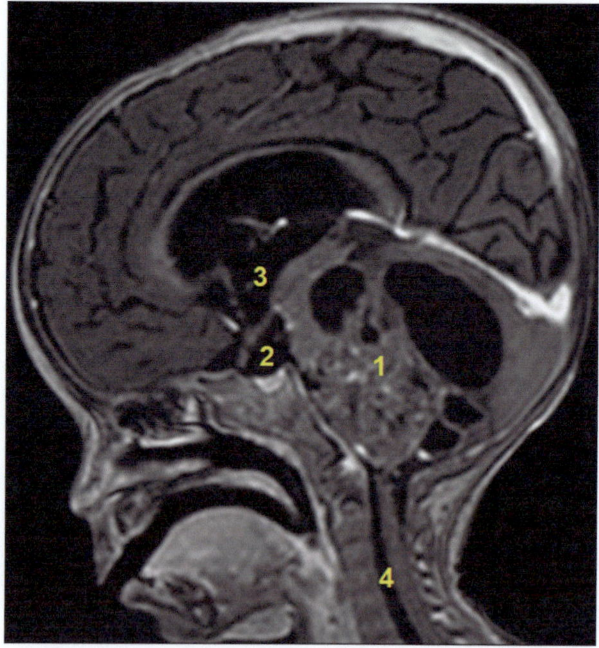

Fig. 7.3 MSS, a 1-year-old girl, presented with left hemiparesis, vomiting, and somnolence. Brainstem biopsy resulted in an atypical teratoid rhabdoid tumor (ATRT) brainstem lesion and CSF cytology identified tumor dissemination. Sagittal brain MRI T1-gadolinium showing heterogenous contrast-enhanced brainstem lesion (1), compressing the third ventricle (3). Brainstem lesions may show CSF tumor dissemination to the adjacent cisterns (2) and spinal canal (4)

Patients with undiagnosed LM for solid tumors may benefit from flow cytometry methods. Such a method may reduce the diagnostic uncertainty of LM and unnecessary lumbar punctures can be prevented. Flow cytometry facilitates information on diagnosis and prognosis on patients with LM, optimizing treatment initiation and improving patient survival and quality of life [41, 43, 44].

In conclusion, iFC can be proved useful in all aspects of analysis of malignant cells from brain tumors with a high diagnostic impact [45].

7.4 Conclusion

Advances in intraoperative monitoring and surgical techniques have improved tumor diagnosis and resection with safety. Novel intraoperative methods in neurosurgical procedures, including neuronavigation system, neurophysiological monitoring, minimally invasive techniques, and intraoperative MRI, have enabled neurosurgeons to improve tumor resection and patient's functional outcome. In addition, molecular analysis using flow cytometry have improved tumor diagnosis in real time. Such a technique is an attractive alternative or adjunct to frozen analysis, especially in time-sensitive scenarios like an intraoperative assessment of oncology procedures. Flow cytometry is a promising technique that can provide substantial information on tumor analysis and, consequently, maximize cancer treatment and expedite patient's survival.

References

1. Altieri R, Agnoletti A, Quattrucci F, Garbossa D, Calamo Specchia FM, Bozzaro M, et al. Molecular biology of gliomas: present and future challenges. Transl Med UniSa. 2014;10:29–37.
2. Louis DN, Perry A, Reifenberger G, von Deimling A, Figarella-Branger D, Cavenee WK, et al. The 2016 World Health Organization classification of tumors of the central nervous system: a summary. Acta Neuropathol. 2016;131(6):803–20.
3. Prabhu SP, Poussaint TY. Pediatric brain tumors. 2016:613–633.
4. Ohgaki H, Kleihues P. Epidemiology and etiology of gliomas. Acta Neuropathol. 2005;109(1):93–108.
5. Fisher JL, Schwartzbaum JA, Wrensch M, Wiemels JL. Epidemiology of brain tumors. Neurol Clin. 2007;25(4):867–90, vii.
6. Ostrom QT, Gittleman H, Farah P, Ondracek A, Chen Y, Wolinsky Y, et al. CBTRUS statistical report: primary brain and central nervous system tumors diagnosed in the United States in 2006-2010. Neuro Oncol. 2013;15 Suppl 2:ii1–56.
7. Ostrom QT, Gittleman H, Fulop J, Liu M, Blanda R, Kromer C, et al. CBTRUS statistical report: primary brain and central nervous system tumors diagnosed in the United States in 2008-2012. Neuro Oncol. 2015;17 Suppl 4:iv1–iv62.
8. Giaretti W. Origins of ... Flow cytometry and applications in oncology. J Clin Pathol. 1997;50(4):275–7.

9. Varma N, Naseem S. Application of flow cytometry in pediatric hematology-oncology. Pediatr Blood Cancer. 2011;57(1):18–29.

10. Betters DM. Use of flow cytometry in clinical practice. J Adv Pract Oncol. 2015;6(5):435–40.

11. Dong Q, Huang J, Zhou Y, Li L, Bao G, Feng J, Sha H. Hematogenous dissemination of lung cancer cells during surgery: quantitative detection by flow cytometry and prognostic significance. Lung Cancer. 2002;37(3):293–301.

12. McKinnon KM. Flow cytometry: an overview. Curr Protoc Immunol. 2018;120:5.1.1–5.1.11.

13. Vartholomatos G, Basiari L, Exarchakos G, Kastanioudakis I, Komnos I, Michali M, et al. Intraoperative flow cytometry for head and neck lesions. Assessment of malignancy and tumour-free resection margins. Oral Oncol. 2019;99:104344.

14. Alexiou GA, Vartholomatos G, Kobayashi T, Voulgaris S, Kyritsis AP. The emerging role of intraoperative flow cytometry in intracranial tumor surgery. Clin Neurol Neurosurg. 2020;192:105742.

15. Markopoulos GS, Glantzounis GK, Goussia AC, Lianos GD, Karampa A, Alexiou GA, et al. Touch imprint intraoperative flow cytometry as a complementary tool for detailed assessment of resection margins and tumor biology in liver surgery for primary and metastatic liver neoplasms. Methods Protoc. 2021;4(3):66.

16. Johnson KJ, Cullen J, Barnholtz-Sloan JS, Ostrom QT, Langer CE, Turner MC, et al. Childhood brain tumor epidemiology: a brain tumor epidemiology consortium review. Cancer Epidemiol Biomark Prev. 2014;23(12):2716–36.

17. Pollack IF, Hoffman HJ, Humphreys RP, Becker L. The long-term outcome after surgical treatment of dorsally exophytic brain-stem gliomas. J Neurosurg. 1993;78(6):859.

18. Stupp R, Tonn JC, Brada M, Pentheroudakis G, ESMO Guidelines Working Group. High-grade malignant glioma: ESMO clinical practice guidelines for diagnosis, treatment and follow-up. Ann Oncol. 2010;21(Suppl 5):v190–3.

19. Pollack IF. Multidisciplinary management of childhood brain tumors: a review of outcomes, recent advances, and challenges. J Neurosurg Pediatr. 2011;8(2):135–48.

20. Klimo P Jr, Pai Panandiker AS, Thompson CJ, Boop FA, Qaddoumi I, Gajjar A, et al. Management and outcome of focal low-grade brainstem tumors in pediatric patients: the St. Jude experience. J Neurosurg Pediatr. 2013;11(3):274–81.

21. Coburger J, Wirtz CR. Fluorescence guided surgery by 5-ALA and intraoperative MRI in high grade glioma: a systematic review. J Neuro-Oncol. 2019;141(3):533–46.

22. Golub D, Hyde J, Dogra S, Nicholson J, Kirkwood KA, Gohel P, et al. Intraoperative MRI versus 5-ALA in high-grade glioma resection: a network meta-analysis. J Neurosurg. 2020:1–15.

23. Senft C, Forster MT, Bink A, Mittelbronn M, Franz K, Seifert V, et al. Optimizing the extent of resection in eloquently located gliomas by combining intraoperative MRI guidance with intraoperative neurophysiological monitoring. J Neuro-Oncol. 2012;109(1):81–90.

24. Abolfotoh M, Bi WL, Hong CK, Almefty KK, Boskovitz A, Dunn IF, et al. The combined microscopic-endoscopic technique for radical resection of cerebellopontine angle tumors. J Neurosurg. 2015;123(5):1301–11.

25. Sala F, Krzan MJ, Deletis V. Intraoperative neurophysiological monitoring in pediatric neurosurgery: why, when, how? Childs Nerv Syst. 2002;18(6–7):264–87.

26. Wu K, Bi WL, Essayed W, Patel V, Kadri P, Al-Mefty O. Integration of microanatomy, neuronavigation, dynamic neurophysiologic monitoring, and intraoperative multimodality imaging for the safe removal of an insular glioma: 2-dimensional operative video. Oper Neurosurg (Hagerstown). 2021;21(1):E28–E9.

27. Rykkje AM, Li D, Skjoth-Rasmussen J, Larsen VA, Nielsen MB, Hansen AE, et al. Surgically induced contrast enhancements on intraoperative and early postoperative MRI following high-grade glioma surgery: a systematic review. Diagnostics (Basel). 2021;11(8):1344.

28. Pirro V, Alfaro CM, Jarmusch AK, Hattab EM, Cohen-Gadol AA, Cooks RG. Intraoperative assessment of tumor margins during glioma resection by desorption electrospray ionization-mass spectrometry. Proc Natl Acad Sci U S A. 2017;114(26):6700–5.

29. Bettmann MA. Intraoperative MRI for treatment of high-grade glioma: is it cost-effective? Radiology. 2019;291(3):698–9.
30. Rohde V, Krombach GA, Struffert T, Gilsbach JM. Virtual MRI endoscopy: detection of anomalies of the ventricular anatomy and its possible role as a presurgical planning tool for endoscopic third ventriculostomy. Acta Neurochir. 2001;143(11):1085–91.
31. Abd-El-Barr MM, Cohen AR. The origin and evolution of neuroendoscopy. Childs Nerv Syst. 2013;29(5):727–37.
32. Dlouhy BJ, Chae MP, Teo C. The supraorbital eyebrow approach in children: clinical outcomes, cosmetic results, and complications. J Neurosurg Pediatr. 2015;15(1):12–9.
33. Waran V, Narayanan V, Karuppiah R, Thambynayagam HC, Muthusamy KA, Rahman ZA, et al. Neurosurgical endoscopic training via a realistic 3-dimensional model with pathology. Simul Healthc. 2015;10(1):43–8.
34. Esposito F, Cappabianca P. Neuroendoscopy: general aspects and principles. World Neurosurg. 2013;79(2):S14.e7.
35. Gholami B, Norton I, Tannenbaum AR, Agar NY. Recursive feature elimination for brain tumor classification using desorption electrospray ionization mass spectrometry imaging. Annu Int Conf IEEE Eng Med Biol Soc. 2012;2012:5258–61.
36. Mesiwala AH, Scampavia LD, Rabinovitch PS, Ruzicka J, Rostomily RC. On-line flow cytometry for real-time surgical guidance. Neurosurgery. 2004;55(3):551–60; discussion 60–1.
37. Alexiou GA, Vartholomatos G, Stefanaki K, Lykoudis EG, Patereli A, Tseka G, et al. The role of fast cell cycle analysis in pediatric brain tumors. Pediatr Neurosurg. 2015;50(5):257–63.
38. Vartholomatos E, Vartholomatos G, Alexiou GA, Markopoulos GS. The past, present and future of flow cytometry in central nervous system malignancies. Methods Protoc. 2021;4(1):11.
39. Shioyama T, Muragaki Y, Maruyama T, Komori T, Iseki H. Intraoperative flow cytometry analysis of glioma tissue for rapid determination of tumor presence and its histopathological grade: clinical article. J Neurosurg. 2013;118(6):1232–8.
40. Saito T, Muragaki Y, Shioyama T, Komori T, Maruyama T, Nitta M, et al. Malignancy index using intraoperative flow cytometry is a valuable prognostic factor for glioblastoma treated with radiotherapy and concomitant Temozolomide. Neurosurgery. 2019;84(3):662–72.
41. Subira D, Simo M, Illan J, Serrano C, Castanon S, Gonzalo R, et al. Diagnostic and prognostic significance of flow cytometry immunophenotyping in patients with leptomeningeal carcinomatosis. Clin Exp Metastasis. 2015;32(4):383–91.
42. Huang HB, Ge MJ. The effects of different surgical approaches on the perioperative level of circulating tumor cells in patients with non-small cell lung cancer. Thorac Cardiovasc Surg. 2016;64(6):515–9.
43. Milojkovic Kerklaan B, Pluim D, Bol M, Hofland I, Westerga J, van Tinteren H, et al. EpCAM-based flow cytometry in cerebrospinal fluid greatly improves diagnostic accuracy of leptomeningeal metastases from epithelial tumors. Neuro Oncol. 2016;18(6):855–62.
44. Subira D, Serrano C, Castanon S, Gonzalo R, Illan J, Pardo J, et al. Role of flow cytometry immunophenotyping in the diagnosis of leptomeningeal carcinomatosis. Neuro Oncol. 2012;14(1):43–52.
45. D'Amato Figueiredo MV, Alexiou GA, Vartholomatos G, Rehder R. Advances in intraoperative flow cytometry. Int J Mol Sci. 2022;23(21):13430. https://doi.org/10.3390/ijms232113430.

Chapter 8
Intraoperative Flow Cytometry in Gliomas

Georgios Vartholomatos, Georgios Alexiou, and Spyridon Voulgaris

8.1 Introduction

The incidence rate of all primary malignant and non-malignant central nervous system (CNS) tumors in the USA was 24.23 cases per 100,000. Among them, glioblastoma constitute the most common malignant CNS tumor in adults (14.3% of all tumors and 49.1% of malignant tumors) and is more common in men [1]. The World Health Organization (WHO) Classification of CNS Tumors published in 2021 classify tumors into more biologically and molecularly defined entities [2].

Flow cytometry is an indispensable method in hematology to quantify rare events and monitor residual disease. Furthermore, it is the method of choice for detecting circulating endothelial, rare events, and tumor cells. However, its role as a valid research tool in solid tumors remained until recently unexplored and underreported. Flow cytometry permits the identification of aneuploidy, which is associated with poor prognosis in several cancers [3, 4]. In the past, analysis of the DNA content was performed on paraffin embedded tissues and required substantial time for analysis [5]. Over the last years two research groups, one from Tokyo, Japan, and the other from Ioannina, Greece, working independently, developed protocols for fast DNA content analysis and implemented flow cytometry intraoperatively [3, 6]. Herewith, we present the role of intraoperative flow cytometry in gliomas.

G. Vartholomatos (✉)
Unit of Molecular Biology and Translational Flow Cytometry,
University Hospital of Ioannina, Ioannina, Greece

G. Alexiou · S. Voulgaris
Department of Neurosurgery, University of Ioannina, Ioannina, Greece

G. Alexiou, G. Vartholomatos (eds.), *Intraoperative Flow Cytometry*,
https://doi.org/10.1007/978-3-031-33517-4_8

123

8.2 Glioma Grade

Flow cytometry may permit assessment of glioma grade intraoperatively within minutes (Fig. 8.1). Studies on brain tissue that was excised in epilepsy surgery revealed that normal brain tissue has a G0/G1phase fraction of 97.1 ± 0.5%, S phase of 1.7 ± 0.5%, and G2/M fraction of 1.25 ± 0.5% [7]. Thus, neoplastic tissue

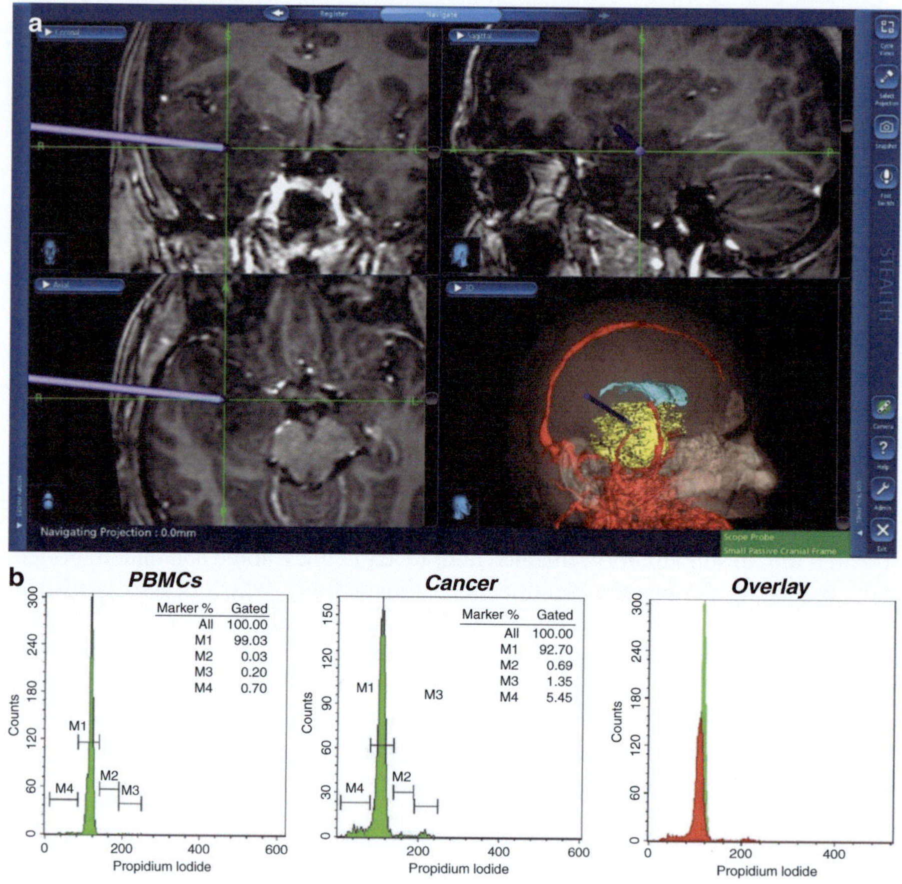

Fig. 8.1 (**a**) Neuronavigation (Medronic Inc., USA) photo during resection of a low-grade glioma. The blue line corresponds to the site of biopsy taken. (**b**) Cell cycle distribution analysis using intraoperative flow cytometry (iFC) reveals a low-grade tumor. Markers M1, M2, M3, and M4 represent G0/G1, S, G2/M cell cycle phases and apoptosis, respectively. On the left of each figure the cell cycle distribution of peripheral blood mononuclear cells (PBMCs) is presented as control. The presented case is diploid, with a DNA index of 1. In the overlay histogram the G0/G1 peak of cancer cells in red is discernible from that of normal cells in green. Tumor index (i.e., percentage of proliferative cells) was calculated at ~7%. Pathology revealed the presence of an oligode-dronglioma (WHO grade 2)

exhibits lower G0/G1 values and higher malignant index, namely S and G2/M phase fractions. Shioyama et al. analyzed by IFC328 biopsy specimens that were obtained during the excision of 81 intracranial gliomas. There were 29 low-grade gliomas and 52 high-grade gliomas. The ratio derived from the number of cells with higher-than-normal DNA content to the total number of cells was defined as malignancy index. Significant differences in the malignancy index were found between grade 2, 3, and 4 gliomas. The malignant index for grade 2 gliomas was 13.3% ± 11.0%, for grade 3 35.0% ± 21.8%, and for glioblastoma the malignancy index was 46.6% ± 23.1%. Furthermore, aneuploidy was more common in high-grade tumors. In detail, aneuploidy was observed in 1/3 of grade 2 tumors, in nearly half of grade 3 tumors and in 58.6% of glioblastomas [6]. Alexiou et al. showed that high-grade gliomas exhibited a mean G0/G1 phase fraction of 60.8 ± 17.9%, a S phase of 13.9 ± 15.4%, and G2/M phase fraction of 18.6 ± 15.5%, whereas a pilocytic astrocytoma (WHO grade I) had a 87.1% G0/G1 phase fraction, a S phase fraction of 2%, and 4% G2/M phase fraction [3].

8.3 Glioma Margins

Gliomas are diffusely infiltrative brain tumors and cure by surgical resection alone cannot be performed. Historical reports performing even hemispherectomies failed to cure patients [8]. The surgical goal is macroscopical total excision without neurological compromise of the patient, since glioma cells can be detected histologically in uninvolved regions on MRI, far enough from the contrast-enhancing rim. Several techniques such as intraoperative MRI and 5-aminolevulinic acid-induced fluorescence have been shown to increase extent of resection and to improve survival [9]. However, when 5-ALA is used there might not be fluorescence in low-grade tumors and in high-grade there might also be some tumor unrecognized [10]. Shioyama et al. in a study that included 328 biopsy specimens that were obtained during the excision of 81 intracranial gliomas showed that the malignancy index differed significantly between cancerous and perilesional brain tissue. A threshold of 6.8% in the malignancy index had a 88% sensitivity, 88% specificity, 97% positive predictive value, 60% negative predictive value, and 88% diagnostic accuracy [6]. Alexiou et al. analyzed nine glioblastoma surgical margins and found a significant difference in the G0/G1 phase between glioma core and perilesional tissue (median 58.3% versus 81.1%) and also a significant difference for the median S phase and mitoses fraction between glioma core and perilesional tissue (12.8% versus 4.6% and 19.3% versus 6.8%, respectively) (Fig. 8.2). Using cut-off values tumor burden excision can be maximized [3]. In case the tumor is aneuploid then the identification of glioma cells is much more simple since two distinct cell populations appear, a normal diploid and a malignant aneuploid. A device combining an ultrasonic aspirator with a real-time flow cytometer has been proposed and could revolutionize glioma excision [11].

G. Vartholomatos et al.

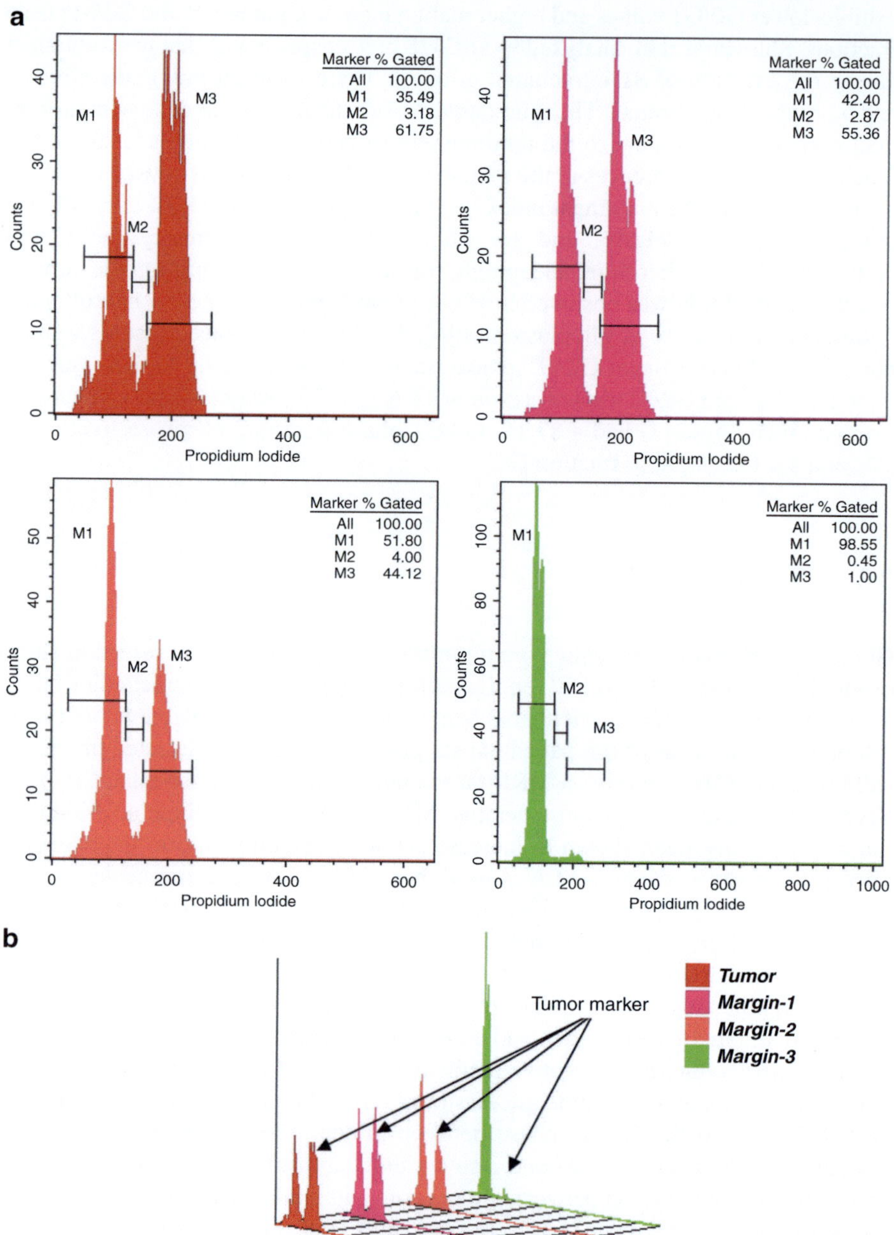

Fig. 8.2 (**a**) A glioblastoma case (red histogram) and specimens analyzed during resection (histogram purple, orange, and green). (**b**) 3D plot of the four histograms, from tumor core (red) and perilesional tissue (purple, orange, green), demonstrating the transition of tumor marker (S phase and mitosis fraction) toward more benign pathology (green)

8.4   Stereotactic Biopsy

Intraoperative flow cytometry requires for analysis very small tissue sample. Cell cycle analysis requires 3–5 minutes thus this technique is ideal for biopsies. During stereotactic biopsy procedures a fast and reliable technique to identify the presence of neoplastic tissue would be of paramount importance. Frozen section consultation which is the gold standard takes substantial time for interpretation, its impractical when there is a need to analyze several samples at different time points and has several limitations [12]. Thus, there is a need for other methods that would diminish duration of surgery and the need for additional biopsies that may increase the risk of a catastrophic hemorrhage. Intraoperative flow cytometry has been shown capable of identifying neoplastic tissue within minutes and the results were verified after histopathological examination (Fig. 8.3) [13].

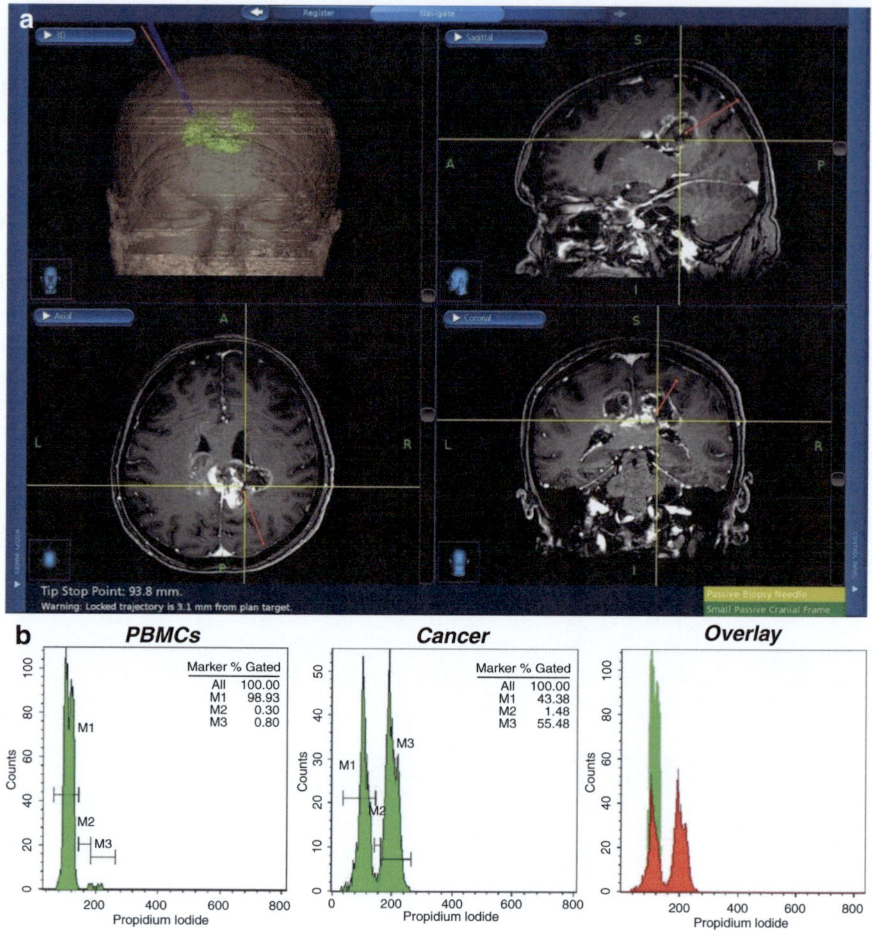

Fig. 8.3 (**a**) Stereotactic biopsy (Passive Biopsy Needle Kit, Medtronic, Louisville, Colorado, USA) of a tumor that infiltrated corpus callosum. (**b**) Cell cycle distribution analysis using iFC reveals a high-grade tumor. Markers M1, M2, and M3 represent G0/G1, S, and G2/M cell cycle phases, respectively. On the left of each figure the cell cycle distribution of peripheral blood mononuclear cells (PBMCs) is presented as control. The presented case is diploid, with a DNA index of 1. In the overlay histogram the G0/G1 peak of cancer cells in red is discernible from that of normal cells in green. Tumor index (i.e., percentage of proliferative cells) was calculated at 57%. Pathology revealed the presence of a glioblastoma (WHO grade 4)

8.5 Survival

Regarding prognostic markers deletions in the short arm of chromosome 1 and the long arm of chromosome 19 in oligodendrogliomas is associated with better outcome. Furthermore, mutations in the isocitrate dehydrogenase 1 (*IDH1*) and in isocitrate dehydrogenase 2 (*IDH2*) has been also associated with increased survival. Increased methylation of the promotor region of the gene O-6-methylguanine-DNA methyltransferase (*MGMT*) is another alteration that predicts better prognosis. However, the results for these biomarkers have been mainly obtained from analyses of resected samples after surgery. From the perspective of surgical strategy, pre- or more rapid intraoperative prediction of sensitivity to radiochemotherapy is desirable for improving the clinical management of GBM patients, particularly that are located in eloquent areas of the brain [14].

Flow cytometry has been also utilized for the assessment of prognosis in glioma patients. In a study that used standard protocol of DNA content analysis on 20 glioma patients (14 glioblastomas, 3 anaplastic astrocytomas, and 3 low-grade gliomas) the G0/G1 and S phase fractions showed significant correlations with patients' survival. Patient's with G0/G1 phase fraction more than 69% had significant higher survival than patients with lower than 69% G0/G1 phase fraction (22 versus 12.5 months). When S phase fraction was used a cut-off value of 6% had also prognostic significance. In detail, patients with high proliferation tumors had lower survival when compared with patients with lower that 6% S phase fraction (22 vs. 11 months) [3].

Regarding intraoperative DNA content analysis Suzuki et al. evaluated 102 consecutive cases of newly diagnosed WHO grade II supratentorial gliomas. Aneuploidy was found in 33% of cases. The presence of aneuploidy suggests more aggressive tumor, thus worse survival. Aneuploidy was more common in diffuse astrocytomas that oligodendrogliomas and was associated with more frequent progression and dedifferentiation to glioblastoma. On the contrary, diploid tumors displayed significantly longer progression free and overall survival. The presence of aneuploidy may guide the most suitable postoperative adjuvant therapy in low grade gliomas [15].

Concerning high-grade gliomas Sato et al. studied 102 patients with glioblastoma who underwent iFC analysis and received the standard treatment protocol. The authors calculated the malignant index in all samples. The results showed that high malignant index correlated significantly with better survival only among glioblastoma patients underwent radiotherapy plus concomitant and adjuvant chemotherapy with temozolomide. Furthermore, malignant index correlated with *IDH1* mutation status [16].

Using "Ioannina Protocol" we analyzed tissue samples from 43 glioblastoma patients (28 males, 15 females, mean age 60.7 ± 11.5). All patients received postoperative standard chemoradiotherapy according to Stupp protocol. Cell cycle fractions were defined as the number of cells in G0/G1, S, and G2/M phase. Tumor index was defined as the sum of S and G2/M phase fractions. The mean Ki-67 in tumors was 44.7% (range 5–85%). A total of 20 tumors were diploids and 23 aneuploids. We found that a cut-off tumor index (S + G2/M) value of 40% as best predicting survival. Patients with tumor index lower than 40% differed significantly from those with tumor index higher than 40% and were associated with better survival (18 vs. 8 months, respectively; $p = 0.0012$) (Fig. 8.4). Extent of resection had also a prognostic significance. In multivariate analysis tumor index was the most

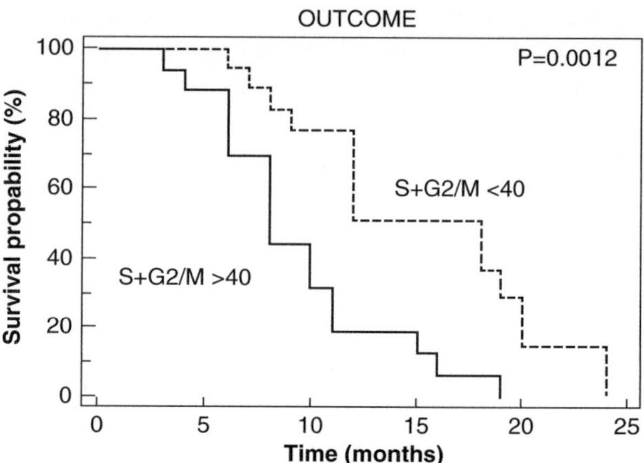

Fig. 8.4 Survival analysis of glioblastoma cases

significant prognostic factor ($p = 0.001$, 95% CI 0.0088–0.2958). Based on that iFC is an easily performed technique that additional holds prognostic information.

8.6 Immunophenotypic Analysis

Immunophenotypic analysis has diagnostic implications for brain tumors both in adults and children [17]. A metastatic tumor is expected usually to have increased cytokeratin expression. Cytokeratins, belonging to the intermediate filament (IF) protein family, are particularly useful tools in oncology diagnostics. A central nervous system lymphoma is expected to exhibit expression of cluster of differentiation (CD) molecule CD45. CD45 is a transmembrane protein tyrosine phosphatase located on most haematopoietic cells. Gliomas express the glial fibrillary acidic protein (GFAP) in increased levels. GFAP is a monomeric intermediate filament protein found in the astroglial cytoskeleton, while it is not expressed outside the CNS. Increased GFAP immunoreactivity (or astrocytic activation) is usually viewed as an index of gliosis (Fig. 8.5).

Vartholomatos et al. showed that the diagnosis of central nervous system lymphoma can be conformed within 5 min intraoperatively, by analyzing the expression of CD molecules CD45, CD3, CD19, and CD20. CD3 is a protein complex and T cell co-receptor that is involved in activating both the cytotoxic T cell and T helper cells, while CD19 is B-Lymphocyte Surface Antigen B4, a transmembrane protein that in humans is expressed in all B lineage cells. CD20 is a transmembrane protein, originally identified as a B cell surface marker, expressed in the resected specimens. Additionally, the level of CD20 expression holds prognostic and therapeutic role. Rituximab is an anti-CD20 monoclonal antibody that increase survival of patients with diffuse large B cell lymphomas [18]. Koriyama et al. showed that even tumor's aneuploidy status and S phase fraction can differentiate glioblastoma from primary central nervous system lymphoma [19].

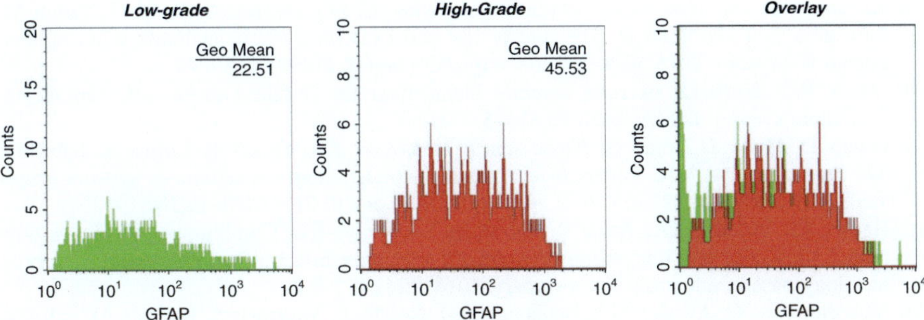

Fig. 8.5 GFAP expression in a low-grade tumor (oligodendroglioma) and in a high-grade tumor (glioblastoma). The overlay histogram revealed that glioblastoma had significant higher GFAP expression

8.7   Conclusion

In conclusion, intraoperative flow cytometry is a novel and promising technique that can be implemented during glioma surgery and may become a reliable adjunct to the standard histopathological diagnosis. Based on the evidence so far, intraoperative flow cytometry provides information on glioma grade and margins, presence of neoplastic tissue during biopsies and several of its metrics are of prognostic significance.

References

1. Ostrom QT, Cioffi G, Waite K, Kruchko C, Barnholtz-Sloan JS. CBTRUS statistical report: primary brain and other central nervous system tumors diagnosed in the United States in 2014-2018. Neuro Oncol. 2021;23(12 Suppl 2):iii1–iii105. https://doi.org/10.1093/neuonc/noab200.
2. Louis DN, Perry A, Wesseling P, Brat DJ, Cree IA, Figarella-Branger D, Hawkins C, Ng HK, Pfister SM, Reifenberger G, Soffietti R, von Deimling A, Ellison DW. The 2021 WHO classification of tumors of the central nervous system: a summary. Neuro Oncol. 2021;23(8):1231–51. https://doi.org/10.1093/neuonc/noab106.
3. Alexiou GA, Vartholomatos G, Goussia A, Batistatou A, Tsamis K, Voulgaris S, Kyritsis AP. Fast cell cycle analysis for intraoperative characterization of brain tumor margins and malignancy. J Clin Neurosci. 2015;22(1):129–32. https://doi.org/10.1016/j.jocn.2014.05.029.
4. Alexiou GA, Vartholomatos E, Goussia A, Dova L, Karamoutsios A, Fotakopoulos G, Kyritsis AP, Voulgaris S. DNA content is associated with malignancy of intracranial neoplasms. Clin Neurol Neurosurg. 2013;115(9):1784–7. https://doi.org/10.1016/j.clineuro.2013.04.015.
5. Vartholomatos E, Vartholomatos G, Alexiou GA, Markopoulos GS. The past, present and future of flow cytometry in central nervous system malignancies. Methods Protoc. 2021;4(1):11. https://doi.org/10.3390/mps4010011.
6. Shioyama T, Muragaki Y, Maruyama T, Komori T, Iseki H. Intraoperative flow cytometry analysis of glioma tissue for rapid determination of tumor presence and its histopathological grade: clinical article. J Neurosurg. 2013;118(6):1232–8. https://doi.org/10.3171/2013.1.JNS12681.

7. Alexiou GA, Vartholomatos G, Stefanaki K, Lykoudis EG, Patereli A, Tseka G, Tzoufi M, Sfakianos G, Prodromou N. The role of fast cell cycle analysis in pediatric brain tumors. Pediatr Neurosurg. 2015;50(5):257–63. https://doi.org/10.1159/000439029.

8. Dandy WE. Removal of right cerebral hemisphere for certain tumors with hemiplegia. Preliminary report. JAMA. 1928;90:823–5.

9. Golub D, Hyde J, Dogra S, Nicholson J, Kirkwood KA, Gohel P, Loftus S, Schwartz TH. Intraoperative MRI versus 5-ALA in high-grade glioma resection: a network meta-analysis. J Neurosurg. 2020 Feb;21:1–15. https://doi.org/10.3171/2019.12.JNS191203.

10. Hauser SB, Kockro RA, Actor B, Sarnthein J, Bernays RL. Combining 5-aminolevulinic acid fluorescence and intraoperative magnetic resonance imaging inglioblastoma surgery: a histology-based evaluation. Neurosurgery. 2016;78(4):475–83.

11. Vartholomatos G, Alexiou GA, Batistatou A, Lykoudis E, Voulgaris S, Kyritsis AP. GV/GA Sarissa-lancet: a proposed real-time flow cytometer for intraoperative identification of glioma margins. Surg Innov. 2016;23(1):104–5. https://doi.org/10.1177/1553350615589860.

12. Alexiou GA, Vartholomatos G, Goussia A, Voulgaris S, Kyritsis AP. Letter: is intraoperative pathology needed if 5-Aminolevulinic-acid-induced tissue fluorescence is found in stereotactic brain tumor biopsy? Neurosurgery. 2020;87(3):E425–6.

13. Alexiou GA, Vartholomatos G, Kobayashi T, Voulgaris S, Kyritsis AP. The emerging role of intraoperative flow cytometry in intracranial tumor surgery. Clin Neurol Neurosurg. 2020;192:105742. https://doi.org/10.1016/j.clineuro.2020.105742.

14. El Khayari A, Bouchmaa N, Taib B, Wei Z, Zeng A, El Fatimy R. Metabolic rewiring in glioblastoma cancer: EGFR, IDH and beyond. Front Oncol. 2022;12:901951. https://doi.org/10.3389/fonc.2022.901951.

15. Suzuki A, Maruyama T, Nitta M, Komori T, Ikuta S, Chernov M, Tamura M, Kawamata T, Muragaki Y. Evaluation of DNA ploidy with intraoperative flow cytometry may predict long-term survival of patients with supratentorial low-grade gliomas: analysis of 102 cases. Clin Neurol Neurosurg. 2018;168:46–53. https://doi.org/10.1016/j.clineuro.2018.02.027.

16. Saito T, Muragaki Y, Shioyama T, Komori T, Maruyama T, Nitta M, Yasuda T, Hosono J, Okamoto S, Kawamata T. Malignancy index using intraoperative flow cytometry is a valuable prognostic factor for glioblastoma treated with radiotherapy and concomitant Temozolomide. Neurosurgery. 2019;84(3):662–72. https://doi.org/10.1093/neuros/nyy089.

17. Alexiou G, Vartholomatos G. Intraoperative flow cytometry in pediatric brain tumors. In: Alexiou G, Prodromou N, editors. Pediatric neurosurgery for clinicians. Cham: Springer; 2022. https://doi.org/10.1007/978-3-030-80522-7_51.

18. Vartholomatos G, Alexiou GA, Voulgaris S, Kyritsis AP. Intraoperative Immunophenotypic analysis for diagnosis and classification of primary central nervous system lymphomas. World Neurosurg. 2018;117:464–5. https://doi.org/10.1016/j.wneu.2018.03.022.

19. Koriyama S, Nitta M, Shioyama T, Komori T, Maruyama T, Kawamata T, Muragaki Y. Intraoperative flow cytometry enables the differentiation of primary central nervous system lymphoma from glioblastoma. World Neurosurg. 2018;112:e261–8. https://doi.org/10.1016/j.wneu.2018.01.033.

Chapter 9
Intraoperative Flow Cytometry in Meningiomas

Georgios Alexiou, Spyridon Voulgaris, and Georgios Vartholomatos

9.1 Introduction

Meningiomas are usually benign extra-axial neoplasms arising from the meningo-thelial cells of the arachnoid. Meningiomas constitute the most frequent central nervous system tumor in adults (38.3% of all tumors) with an incidence of 8.81 cases per 100,000 population [1]. Meningiomas are more common in females (male: female ratio is 1:1.8) and the incidence increases with age. Meningiomas in children are exceedingly rare [2]. Based on the World Health Organization (WHO) 2021 classification meningiomas can be grade 1, 2, and 3. There are 15 meningioma sub-types and several molecular biomarkers, such as *BAP1* and homozygous deletion of *CDKN2A/B*, which are also used for meningioma grading [3]. Tumor recurrence is frequent in grade 3 meningiomas (60–94%), whereas for grade 2, the chance of recurrence is 29–59%, and for grade 1 tumors, 7–25% will recur [4]. The most sig-nificant factor for the prevention of meningioma recurrence is the extent of surgical resection [5]. Herewith, we discuss the role of intraoperative flow cytometry on meningiomas.

G. Alexiou (✉) · S. Voulgaris
Department of Neurosurgery, University of Ioannina, Ioannina, Greece
e-mail: galexiou@uoi.gr

G. Vartholomatos
Haematology Laboratory, Unit of Molecular Biology and Translational Flow Cytometry,
University Hospital of Ioannina, Ioannina, Greece

G. Alexiou, G. Vartholomatos (eds.), *Intraoperative Flow Cytometry*,
https://doi.org/10.1007/978-3-031-33517-4_9

9.2 Flow Cytometry in Meningiomas

Flow cytometry has been previously performed in meningiomas mainly in paraffin-embedded or frozen tissue (Table 9.1) [6–14]. Cell cycle analysis was not oriented toward intraoperative use and analysis protocols had a long duration, usually more than an hour long [13]. Ironside et al. studied 39 meningiomas by flow cytometry. A total of 16 meningioma were aneuploid. The majority of meningiomas exhibited S and G2/M phase fractions under 10%. Nevertheless, grade 3 tumors exhibited more than 25% S and G2/M phases. No relationship was detected between the ploidy status and the results of cell cycle analysis. No relationships were found between the

Table 9.1 Flow cytometry studies on meningiomas before the use of intraoperative protocols

Study	Year	No of meningiomas	Tissue	I vs. II/II	Aneuploidy	Main findings
Ironside et al. [6]	1987	39	Frozen tissue	36/3	40%	Grade 3 tumors had >25% S + G2/M
Crone et al. [7]	1988	20	Frozen tissue	17/3	30%	Increased S + G2/M is associated with increased periturmoral edema
May et al. [8]	1989	40	Paraffin-embedded	38/2	n/a	S + G2/M predict recurrence of grade 1 tumors
Zellner et al. [9]	1998	135	Frozen tissue	105/30	30.3%	Aneuploid tumors higher mitotic activity S-phase fraction significant higher in recurrent tumors and with high mitotic activity
Perry et al. [10]	1998	425	Paraffin-embedded	344/81	33%	S-phase fraction equal to 10.15% was associated with decreased recurrence free survival
Mailo et al. [11]	1999	105	Fresh tissue	93/12	14%	S-phase cells associated with lower mean age, aggressive histology and a significantly shorter disease-free survival
Alexiou et al. [12]	2013	25	Fresh tissue	19/6	16%	Differentiation of grade 1 from grade 2/3 based on G0/G1, S, and G2/M phase fractions
Lin et al. [13]	2015	43	Fresh tissue	27/16	n/a	Differentiation of grade 1 from grade 2/3 based on G2/M phase and S + G2/M phase fractions Ki-67 index and recurrence were correlated with G2/M phase and S1 + G2/M phase fractions

Abbreviations: n/a = not available

results of cell cycle and ploidy analysis and the age and sex of the patients or the location of the meningioma [6]. On the contrary the study by Mailo et al. reported that aneuploidy is associated with a higher incidence of aggressive histopathologic subtypes, older patients and location at the cerebral convexity [11]. Zellner et al. in a study that included 135 tumors reported that aneuploid tumors had a higher rate of infiltration of dura mater and a higher mitotic activity. Recurrent meningiomas and tumors with higher mitotic rate had significant higher S-phase fractions. Tumors infiltrating the cortex or exhibiting focal necrosis had no significant differences in respect to S-phase fraction [9]. In a study that included 425 meningioma patients, flow cytometry was performed in paraffin-embedded tissue. Ploidy status was not significantly associated with recurrence free survival, whereas an S-phase fraction equal to 10.15% was associated with decreased recurrence free survival. No correlation was also found between S-phase fraction and MIB-1 or mitotic index [10]. High proportion of S-phase cells was significant associated with shorter disease-free survival by another study [11].

Peritumoral brain edema can be found in more than 50% of meningiomas and is associated with neurological deficits and influences surgical outcome. Meningiomas with severe edema exhibit significantly higher S + G2/M phase fractions than those with moderate or minimal oedema [7]. Regarding meningioma grade, differentiation between grade 1 and grade 2/3 tumors can be performed by cell cycle analysis. A G0/G1 cut-off value of 85.5% had 87.5% sensitivity and 100% specificity. A G2/M phase fraction of 6% also had 81.2% sensitivity and 100% specificity [12]. Lin et al. in a study of 43 meningioma cases reported that the optimal cut-off values of G2/M phase and S + G2/M phase fractions were 5.12% and 7.52% for the distinction of grade 1 from grade 2/3 meningiomas [13]. Additionally, G2/M phase and S + G2/M phase fractions were correlated significant with Ki-67 index and the histopathological features such as focal necrosis, infiltration of dura mater, and mitotic activity [13].

Regarding the correlation of imaging techniques metrics with flow cytometry parameters, only one study has been performed to date using single-photon emission computed tomography (SPECT). Alexiou et al. performed brain SPECT using [99mTc]-Tetrofosmin, a tumor seeking agent in ten meningioma cases. The radiotracer accumulation was quantified by calculating the lesion-to-normal (L/N) uptake ratio. There was a significant correlation between [99mTc]-Tetrofosmin uptake and the S-phase phase fraction. There was also a positive correlation between [99mTc]-Tetrofosmin uptake and aneuploidy status and tumor grade [14].

9.3 Intraoperative Flow Cytometry in Meningiomas

Intraoperative identification of meningioma grade might modify treatment strategy concerning extent of resection and removal of tumor from neighboring structures such as brain, nerves, and vessels, which might increase the risk for postoperative complications. Intraoperative pathological evaluation through frozen section analysis usually cannot establish meningioma grade. Thus, an intraoperative technique that would permit meningioma grading would be of importance.

Matsuoka et al. performed intraoperative flow cytometry in 117 meningioma cases. The sample had a volume of approximately 2 mm and the analysis required 9 min. The authors evaluated the ratio of the number of cells with a higher than normal DNA content to the total number of cells, called malignant index (MI). The authors grouped together meningioma grade 2 and 3. A cut-off value of 8% could differentiate grade 1 from grade 2/3 meningiomas with 64.7% sensitivity and 85.0% specificity [15].

MI as assessed by rapid flow cytometry correlates with meningioma's Ki-67 proliferation index and with annual growth rate, as calculated by serial MR imaging preoperative that were performed more than twice with an interval of 6 months or longer [15]. Intratumoral heterogeneity of MI, as assessed by analyzing samples from attached, central, and peripheral section of the tumor, was linked to tumor biological characteristics such as annual growth rate and the development of pial feeders [16].

Another fast cell cycle analysis protocol named "Ioannina Protocol" was created by a group in Ioannina, Greece. This protocol permitted cell cycle analysis within 6 minutes. In a study that included 15 benign and 1 anaplastic meningioma, the latter exhibited lower mean G0/G1 phase fraction (49.7% versus 83.4 ± 14.6%). Anaplastic meningioma had higher S-phase and G2/M phase fraction than grade 1 meningiomas (13.1% versus 4.1 ± 4%, and 25.2% versus 5.9 ± 5.7%, respectively) (Figs. 9.1 and 9.2) [17].

Advanced magnetic resonance imaging (MRI) techniques namely, diffusion, perfusion, and spectroscopy are currently used for the evaluation of intracranial lesion and can improve diagnostic accuracy. Diffusion tensor imaging (DTI) metrics, such as apparent diffusion coefficient (ADC) and fractional anisotropy (FA) and dynamic susceptibility perfusion imaging (DSC) metrics, such as relative

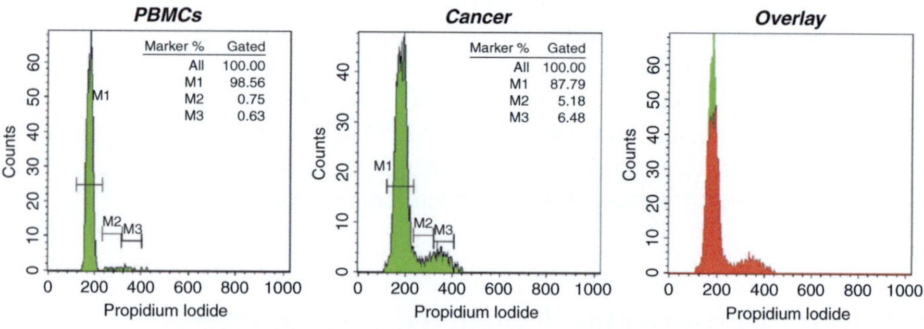

Fig. 9.1 Cell cycle distribution analysis using intraoperative flow cytometry in a grade 2 meningioma. Markers M1, M2, and M3 represent G0/G1, S, and G2/M cell cycle phases, respectively. On the left of each figure the cell cycle distribution of peripheral blood mononuclear cells (PBMCs) is presented as control. The presented case is diploid, with a DNA index = 1. In the overlay histogram the G0/G1 peak of cancer cells in red is discernible from that of normal cells in green. Tumor index (i.e., percentage of proliferative cells) was calculated at ~11.5%

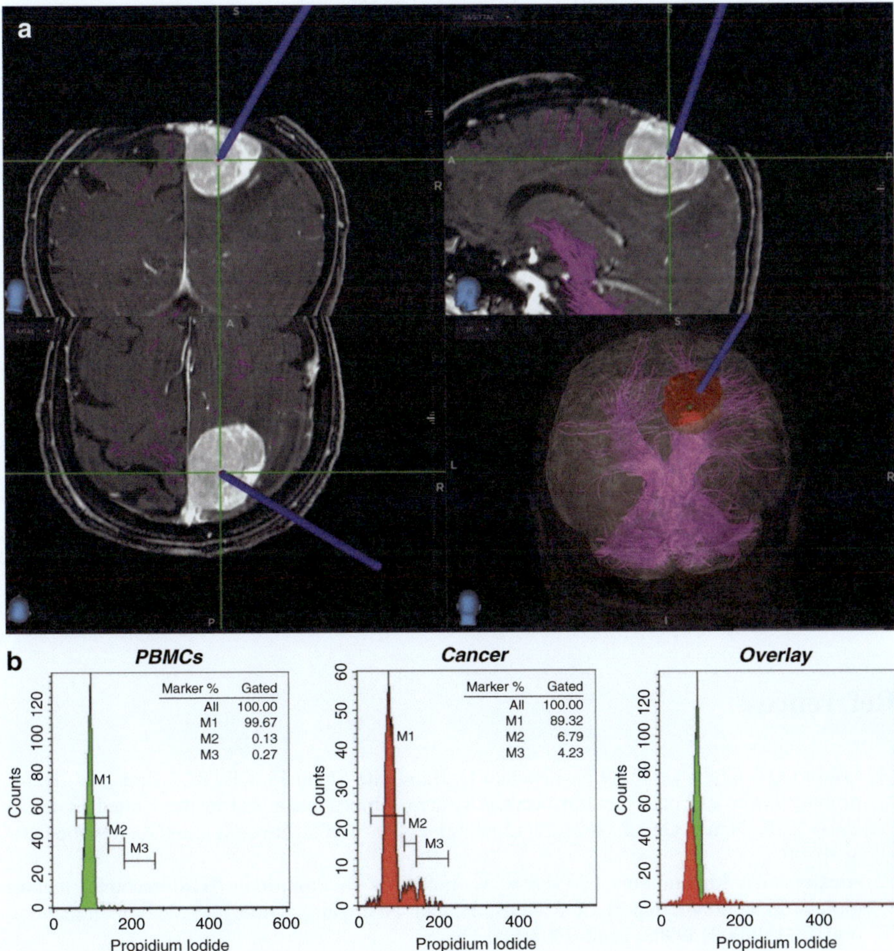

Fig. 9.2 (a) Intraoperative neuronavigation (Medronic Inc., USA) during resection of a parasagittal meningioma. The blue line corresponds to the site of biopsy taken for DNA content analysis in the three planes. In the right corner whole brain tractography can be seen. (b) Cell cycle distribution analysis using intraoperative flow cytometry in the meningioma. Markers M1, M2, and M3 represent G0/G1, S, G2/M cell cycle phases, respectively. On the left of each figure the cell cycle distribution of peripheral blood mononuclear cells (PBMCs) is presented as control. The presented case is hypoploid, with a DNA index = 0.9. In the overlay histogram the G0/G1 peak of cancer cells in red is discernible from that of normal cells in green. Tumor index (i.e., percentage of proliferative cells) was calculated at ~11%. Pathology revealed the presence of a grade 2 meningioma.

cerebral blood volume (rCBV), were correlated with the proliferative potentials of meningiomas as assessed by intraoperative flow cytometry protocol. ADC has been reported to inversely correlate with tumor grade and high-grade tumors that exhibit high cellular density have decreased ADC values [18]. Blood vessels are more abundant within tumors than in normal brain tissue. The rCBV measurements have been correlated with tumor grade and histologic findings of increased tumor vascularity [19]. In a study that included 14 meningiomas, 9 grade I and 5 grade II, all grade I meningiomas were diploid and 3/5 grade II meningiomas were aneuploid. Meningiomas that exhibited increased perfusion, as assessed by rCBV, had significant lower G0/G1phase fraction and increased G2/M phase fraction. A significant correlation was also observed between FA ratio and G0/G1 phase fraction. No significant difference was found between diploid and aneuploid tumors with respect to rCBV, ADC, and FA values [20].

9.4　Conclusion

Flow cytometry has been performed in meningiomas mainly for the assessment of tumor grade and risk of recurrence. The majority of studies had been performed on paraffin-embedded or frozen tissue. Intraoperative flow cytometry may permit identification of meningioma grade, thus notifying the surgeon to modify his strategy if needed. Preoperative imaging findings might be correlated with meningioma cell cycle analysis metrics and ploidy status.

References

1. Ostrom QT, Cioffi G, Waite K, Kruchko C, Barnholtz-Sloan JS. CBTRUS statistical report: primary brain and other central nervous system tumors diagnosed in the United States in 2014-2018. Neuro Oncol. 2021;23(12 Suppl 2):iii1–iii105. https://doi.org/10.1093/neuonc/noab200.
2. Alexiou GA, Mpairamidis E, Psarros A, Sfakianos G, Prodromou N. Intracranial meningiomas in children: report of 8 cases. Pediatr Neurosurg. 2008;44(5):373–5. https://doi.org/10.1159/000149903; Epub 2008 Aug 15.
3. Louis DN, Perry A, Wesseling P, Brat DJ, Cree IA, Figarella-Branger D, Hawkins C, Ng HK, Pfister SM, Reifenberger G, Soffietti R, von Deimling A, Ellison DW. The 2021 WHO classification of tumors of the central nervous system: a summary. Neuro-Oncology. 2021;23(8):1231–51. https://doi.org/10.1093/neuonc/noab106.
4. Marciscano AE, Stemmer-Rachamimov AO, Niemierko A, Larvie M, Curry WT, Barker FG, et al. Benign meningiomas (WHO grade I) with atypical histological features: correlation of histopathological features with clinical outcomes. J Neurosurg. 2016;124:106–14.
5. Alexiou GA, Gogou P, Markoula S, Kyritsis AP. Management of meningiomas. Clin Neurol Neurosurg. 2010;112(3):177–82. https://doi.org/10.1016/j.clineuro.2009.12.011.
6. Ironside JW, Battersby RD, Lawry J, Loomes RS, Day CA, Timperley WR. DNA in meningioma tissues and explant cell cultures. A flow cytometric study with clinicopathological correlates. J Neurosurg. 1987;66(4):588–94. https://doi.org/10.3171/jns.1987.66.4.0588.
7. Crone KR, Challa VR, Kute TE, Moody DM, Kelly DL Jr. Relationship between flow cytometric features and clinical behavior of meningiomas. Neurosurgery. 1988;23(6):720–4. https://doi.org/10.1227/00006123-198812000-00006.
8. May PL, Broome JC, Lawry J, Buxton RA, Battersby RD. The prediction of recurrence in meningiomas. A flow cytometric study of paraffin-embedded archival material. J Neurosurg. 1989;71(3):347–51.

9. Zellner A, Meixensberger J, Roggendorf W, Janka M, Hoehn H, Roosen K. DNA ploidy and cell-cycle analysis in intracranial meningiomas and hemangiopericytomas: a study with high-resolution DNA flow cytometry. Int J Cancer. 1998;79(2):116–20.

10. Perry A, Stafford SL, Scheithauer BW, Suman VJ, Lohse CM. The prognostic significance of MIB-1, p53, and DNA flow cytometry in completely resected primary meningiomas. Cancer. 1998;82(11):2262–9.

11. Maíllo A, Díaz P, Blanco A, López A, Ciudad J, Hernández J, Morales F, Pérez-Simón JA, Orfao A. Proportion of S-phase tumor cells measured by flow cytometry is an independent prognostic factor in meningioma tumors. Cytometry. 1999;38(3):118–23.

12. Alexiou GA, Vartholomatos E, Goussia A, Dova L, Karamoutsios A, Fotakopoulos G, Kyritsis AP, Voulgaris S. DNA content is associated with malignancy of intracranial neoplasms. Clin Neurol Neurosurg. 2013;115(9):1784–7. https://doi.org/10.1016/j.clineuro.2013.04.015.

13. Lin YW, Tai SH, Huang YH, Chang CC, Juan WS, Chao LC, Wen MJ, Hung YC, Lee EJ. The application of flow cytometry for evaluating biological aggressiveness of intracranial meningiomas. Cytometry B Clin Cytom. 2015;88(5):312–9. https://doi.org/10.1002/cyto.b.21202.

14. Alexiou GA, Vartholomatos G, Tsiouris S, Papadopoulos A, Kyritsis AP, Polyzoidis KS, Voulgaris S, Fotopoulos AD. Evaluation of meningioma aggressiveness by (99m) Tc-Tetrofosmin SPECT. Clin Neurol Neurosurg. 2008;110(7):645–8.

15. Matsuoka G, Eguchi S, Anami H, Ishikawa T, Yamaguchi K, Nitta M, Muragaki Y, Kawamata T. Ultrarapid evaluation of meningioma malignancy by intraoperative flow cytometry. World Neurosurg. 2018;120:320–7. https://doi.org/10.1016/j.wneu.2018.08.084.

16. Oya S, Yoshida S, Tsuchiya T, Fujisawa N, Mukasa A, Nakatomi H, Saito N, Matsui T. Intraoperative quantification of meningioma cell proliferation potential using rapid flow cytometry reveals intratumoral heterogeneity. Cancer Med. 2019;8(6):2793–801. https://doi.org/10.1002/cam4.2178.

17. Alexiou GA, Vartholomatos G, Goussia A, Batistatou A, Tsamis K, Voulgaris S, Kyritsis AP. Fast cell cycle analysis for intraoperative characterization of brain tumor margins and malignancy. J Clin Neurosci. 2015;22(1):129–32. https://doi.org/10.1016/j.jocn.2014.05.029.

18. Yamasaki F, Kurisu K, Satoh K, et al. Apparent diffusion coefficient of human brain tumors at MR imaging. Radiology. 2005;235:985–91.

19. Law M, Yang S, Wang H, et al. Glioma grading: sensitivity, specificity, and predictive values of perfusion MR imaging and proton MR spectroscopic imaging compared with conventional MR imaging. AJNR Am J Neuroradiol. 2003;24:1989–98.

20. Alexiou AG, Zikou KA, Vartholomatos G, Goussia A, Voulgaris S, Kyritsis AP, Argyropoulou MI. Correlation of DNA ploidy and cell cycle analysis with diffusion tensor and dynamic susceptibility contrast MRI metrics in meningiomas. Hell J Radiol. 2018;3(3):1–6.

Chapter 10
Intraoperative Flow Cytometry in Pediatric Brain Tumors

Georgios Alexiou and Georgios Vartholomatos

10.1 Introduction

The most common malignancies in children are leukemia, lymphoma, and brain tumors. In the USA the incidence of pediatric brain tumors (birth to 14 years) is 5.65/100.000 population [1]. The supratentorial compartment with the pituitary and craniopharyngeal duct was the most common localization in children and adolescents. Gliomas followed by embryonal tumors are the most frequent. Among gliomas, pilocytic astrocytoma is the most common and is associated with favorable prognosis. Medulloblastoma is the most frequent embryonal tumor [1, 2]. Contrary to adults, meningeal tumors constitute the 3% of all tumors in childhood and adolescence [3]. The latest 2021 World Health Organization (WHO) classification of brain tumors introduced new tumor types and subtypes and a better biologically and molecularly definition of several tumors [4].

Flow cytometry is an indispensable tool for basic research. In the clinical setting flow cytometry is essential for the hematological practice. This technique uses a laser-based technology that can count, sort, and study the fluorescent features of the cells. Analysis requires the sample to be on a liquid form. Up-to-date several applications are widely used. The value of flow cytometry in solid tumors has not been extensively studied, since a cell suspension must be prepared before analysis. Measurement of cellular DNA content and cell cycle analysis were among the first applications of flow cytometry [5, 6]. However, cell cycle analysis required

G. Alexiou (✉)
Department of Neurosurgery, University of Ioannina, Ioannina, Greece
e-mail: galexiou@uoi.gr

G. Vartholomatos
Haematology Laboratory, Unit of Molecular Biology and Translational Flow Cytometry,
University Hospital of Ioannina, Ioannina, Greece

© The Author(s), under exclusive license to Springer Nature Switzerland AG 2023
G. Alexiou, G. Vartholomatos (eds.), *Intraoperative Flow Cytometry*,
https://doi.org/10.1007/978-3-031-33517-4_10

substantial time. By developing fast cell cycle analysis protocols intraoperative flow cytometry emerged with promising results [7, 8]. Herewith, we present the current role of intraoperative flow cytometry for pediatric brain tumor surgery.

10.2 Intraoperative Techniques

Surgical resection is a mainstay in the treatment of brain tumors in children. Apart from frozen section analysis, which has several shortcomings, several other intraoperative techniques, for pediatric brain tumor surgery, have been developed. The majority of studies have been focused on resection margins assessment, since differentiation of neoplastic from normal brain tumor using microscopic visualization and intraoperative navigation may not be possible. Raman spectroscopy is a fast, non-destructive imaging technique based on the Raman effect and can be used to image fresh ex vivo tissue. In a recent study, tissue samples of 2–4 mm were evaluated with this technique from 29 children who underwent resection of brain tumors or epilepsy surgery. In total 160 samples were evaluated. Raman spectroscopy could differentiate neoplastic from non-neoplastic tissue with an accuracy of 89.8%, sensitivity of 84.9%, and specificity of 92.3%. For the differentiation between low-grade glioma and normal brain this technique had an accuracy of 86.2%, sensitivity of 91.3%, and specificity of 81.2% [9]. The intraoperative MRI (iMRI) is another method for intraoperative use but is associated with high cost and is available only in selected centers. Furthermore, it might be technically cumbersome requiring repeat imaging. A recent meta-analysis that evaluated the role of iMRI in extent of resection and safety outcomes during pediatric brain tumor surgery found that the rate of gross-total resection in both low and high-grade tumors was 78.5%. The mean rate of gross-total resection in iMRI-assisted low-grade glioma surgery was 74.3% [10]. Fluorescence guided surgery with 5-aminolevulinic acid (5-ALA) is another technique for maximizing resection and improve survival in high-grade glioma in adults. In children, although there is fluorescence in high-grade gliomas, in pilocytic astrocytomas (WHO grade 1) and medulloblastomas (WHO grade 4) the 5-ALA was found helpful only in 12% and 22% of cases respectively [11].

10.3 Flow Cytometry in Pediatric Brain Tumors

Cell cycle analysis by flow cytometry using conventional protocols and in paraffin-embedded specimens has been evaluated in the past. DNA content analysis entails evaluation of ploidy status, meaning the number of chromosomes. Diploid tumors have a DNA index equal to 1, whereas aneuploid tumors are those with DNA index more (hyperploid) or less (hypoploid) than 1. Cell cycle analysis evaluates G0/G1, S, and G2/M phase fractions. The higher the malignancy the lower the G0/G1 and higher the S and G2/M phase fractions. Studies on paraffin-embedded medulloblastoma specimens revealed that about half of tumors were aneuploids, usually hyperdiploids or tetraploids [12]. Arush et al. evaluated 30 children with diagnosed gliomas. Nine tumors were aneuploids and 21 diploids. Of the patients with diploid tumors, 81% survived, whereas only 33% of patietns survived with the aneuploid tumors [13]. Regarding ependymomas, the third most common brain tumor in children, in a study that performed cell cycle analysis in 17 paraffin-embedded tumors from patients aged 7 months to 16 years, proliferation fractions ranged between 1% and 17% and seven tumors were aneuploids. Unfavorable prognosis was found for diploid tumors, high proliferative status and young age [14].

10.4 Fast Cell Cycle Analysis

Rapid DNA analysis protocols that permitted intraoperative use have been reported by Shioyama et al. and Alexiou et al. [7, 8]. Both protocols were first evaluated for intracranial tumors in adults as presented in the previous chapters. Fast cell cycle analysis has also been evaluated in pediatric brain tumor cases [15]. Alexiou et al. focused on the analysis of cell cycle fractions, namely G0/G1, S, and G2/M and ploidy status in pediatric intracranial tumors. The fast analysis protocol was named "Ioannina Protocol" and could be performed within 6 min from sample acquisition. The sample requirements are minimum in the range of 1–2 mm^3 [7]. A total of 68 pediatric brain tumors samples, which were histopathologically verified and well preserved in RNA later solution, were analyzed by the rapid flow cytometry protocol. The histological diagnoses were 26 medulloblastomas, 12 atypical teratoid/rhabdoid tumors, 14 anaplastic ependymomas, 3 glioblastomas, 1 anaplastic xanthoastrocytoma, 2 diffuse astrocytomas, 1 pilocytic astrocytoma, and other less frequent pathologies. Tumors were categorized into grades of malignancy. As control, samples obtained during surgery for epilepsy were used. First, for the differentiation of normal from neoplastic tissue, flow cytometry analysis had 100% sensitivity and specificity using cut-off values for G0/G1 (89%) and mitosis (2%) phase fractions. Low-grade tumors exhibited significantly higher G0/G1 and significantly lower mitosis fractions compared to high-grade tumors, permitting an intraoperative grading of tumor within minutes. Tumors with an S-phase fraction higher than 10% or G2/M fraction more than 13% were always high grade. Thirty-three tumors were diploid and 35 were aneuploid (20% hypoploid, 68.6% hyperploid, and 11.4% tetraploid). Aneuploid tumors exhibited more aggressive characteristics, such as higher S and G2/M phase fractions. In the subgroup analysis, large-cell medulloblastomas, which are associated with unfavorable prognosis, had more aggressive characteristics in cell cycle analysis compared to other subtypes. The S-phase fraction was directly correlated with the immunohistochemically evaluated Ki-67/MIB-1 proliferation index (Fig. 10.1).

Atypical teratoid/rhabdoid tumors, one of the most frequent and aggressive brain tumors of early childhood, had high S-phase and G2/M phase fractions. Ependymomas exhibited a less aggressive cell cycle features (Fig. 10.2) [15].

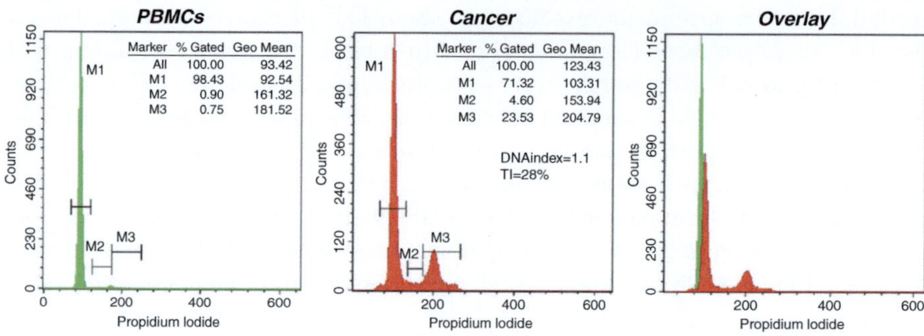

Fig. 10.1 Cell cycle distribution analysis using Intraoperative Flow cytometry (iFC) reveals a high-grade tumor. Markers M1, M2, and M3 represent G0/G1, S, and G2/M cell cycle phases, respectively. On the left of each figure the cell cycle distribution of peripheral blood mononuclear cells (PBMCs) is presented as control. The presented case is aneuploid, with a DNA index of 1.1. In the overlay histogram the G0/G1 peak of cancer cells in red is discernible from that of normal cells in green. Tumor index (i.e., percentage of proliferative cells) was calculated at 28%. Pathology revealed the presence of a medulloblastoma (WHO grade 4)

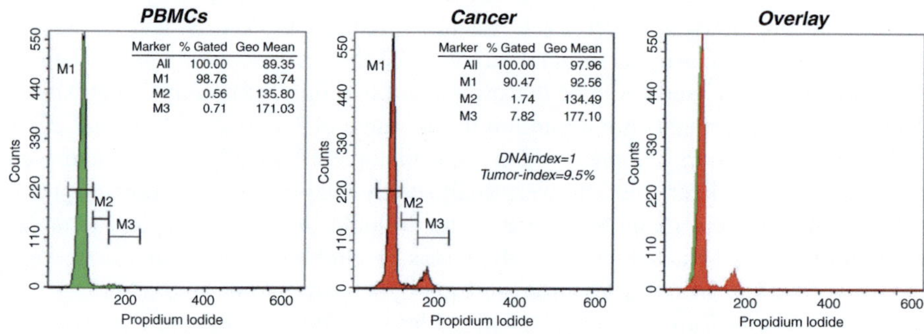

Fig. 10.2 Cell cycle distribution analysis using Intraoperative Flow cytometry (iFC) reveals a tumor of intermediate malignancy. Markers M1, M2, and M3 represent G0/G1, S, and G2/M cell cycle phases, respectively. On the left of each figure the cell cycle distribution of peripheral blood mononuclear cells (PBMCs) is presented as control. The presented case is diploi, with a DNA index of 1. In the overlay histogram the G0/G1 peak of cancer cells in red is discernible from that of normal cells in green. Tumor index (i.e., percentage of proliferative cells) was calculated at 9.5%. Pathology revealed the presence of an anaplastic ependymoma (WHO grade 3)

10.5 Immunophenotypic Analysis

Intraoperative immunophenotic analysis pave the way for multiple novel applications of flow cytometry and entails characterization of multiple cell surface markers on a per-cell basis. Apart for cell membrane markers, cytoplasmic and nuclear antigens can be detected by flow cytometry. In adults, central nervous system lymphoma can be diagnosed using intraoperative flow cytometry and analysis of specific cluster differentiation (CD) markers. The CD45, a glycoprotein expressed in all lymphohematopoietic cells, can be diagnostic for lymphoma and positivity for

CD19/CD20 (B-cell markers) or CD3 (T-cell marker) can be used for subclassification purposes [16]. Possible other tumor types can be diagnosed based on specific CD expression patterns or other specific markers. For example, glial fibrillary acidic protein (GFAP) is a glioma marker. Ependymomas show positivity for CD99 [17] (Fig. 10.3).

Neural cell adhesion molecule (NCAM/CD56) is expressed in brain tumors. In pediatric brain tumors CD56 immunopositivity was found to be inversely correlated with tumor grade [18]. Low-grade tumors exhibited significant higher CD56 expression than high-grade tumors and a negative linear correlation with Ki-67 index was reported. Furthermore, neoplastic tissue could be differentiated from normal brain based on CD56 expression. In a study of 46 pediatric brain tumor cases and 3 samples from epilepsy surgery cell cycle analysis was performed with propidium-iodine (PI) staining of CD56+ cells. Detection of neoplastic tissue compared to normal brain could be performed with 100% sensitivity and specificity using a threshold of 91% in G0/G1 phase fraction and G2/M fraction of 2%. There was a significant positive correlation between Ki-67 proliferation index and S + G2/M phase fraction and proliferation index (S + G2/M/G0/G1), suggesting excellent correlation with tumor's proliferation potentials [19].

Increased *CD24* gene expression has also been found in pediatric brain tumors being higher in medulloblastomas. Using intraoperative flow cytometry there was no CD24 expression in normal brain tissue, in low-grade astrocytomas and meningiomas. Both medulloblastomas and anaplastic ependymomas expressed CD24, whereas medulloblastomas had significant higher number of CD24 molecules/cell than ependymomas [6]. Apart from that, pediatric brain tumors have been found to express CD71. Previous studies have showed an increase in transferrin receptor (TfR1, CD71) in several cancers [20]. Therefore, monoclonal antibodies against TfR1 that have been conjugated to chemotherapeutic or cytotoxic agents have been

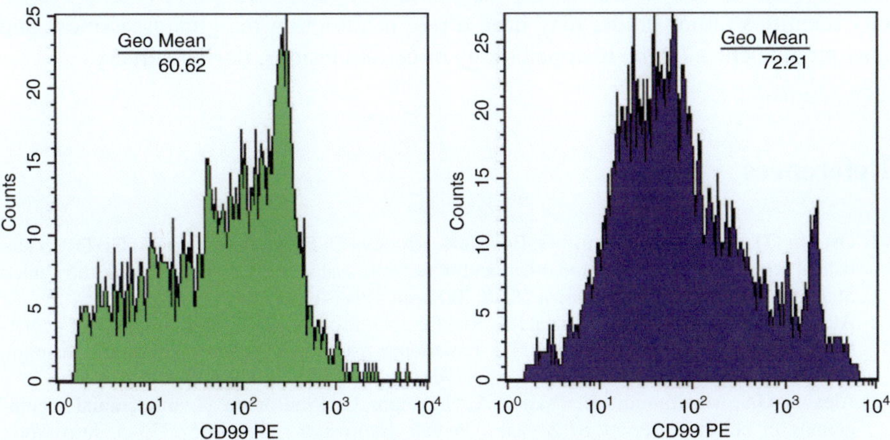

Fig. 10.3 CD99 expression in two ependymoma cases. The geometric mean of CD99 expression is presented in each histogram

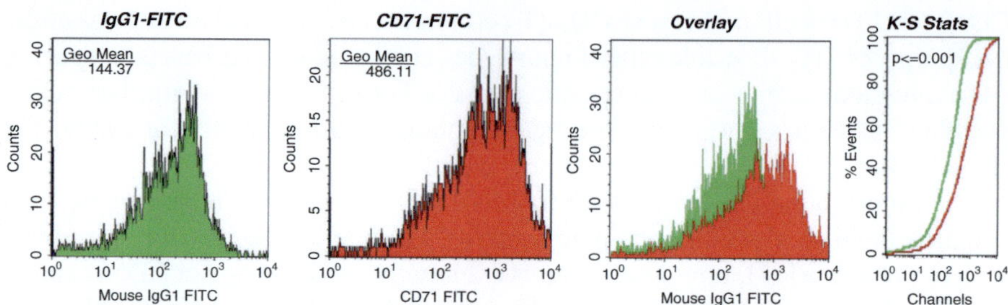

Fig. 10.4 CD71 expression in an aggressive primitive neuroectodermal tumor (red histogram). The overlay histogram revealed that this tumor exhibits significant CD71 expression, as verified by Kolmogorov–Smirnov analysis

developed and used in vitro and in vivo [21]. Moreover, functional nanoparticles to target TfR1 are currently developing and testing [22]. Regarding gliomas, Tf-CRM107, a protein that conjugated to diphtheria toxin, was administered stereotactically with catheter in patients with malignant brain tumors refractory to conventional therapy and a significant tumor response was observed [23]. In a series of 37 pediatric brain tumors there was CD71 expression in 26 (70%) cases. Atypical teratoid/rhabdoid tumors showed no CD71 expression, whereas almost half of medulloblastomas (58.3%) and nearly all ependymomas (90%) showed CD71 expression (Fig. 10.4).

10.6   Conclusion

Intraoperative flow cytometry is a promising novel technique with various applications in brain tumors. For pediatric brain tumor surgery, intraoperative flow cytometry identifies tumor grade, may have a role in resection margins assessment and may provide clues on the histopathology of certain lesions, during surgery.

References

1. Ostrom QT, Gittleman H, Truitt G, Boscia A, Kruchko C, Barnholtz-Sloan JS. CBTRUS statistical report: primary brain and other central nervous system tumors diagnosed in the United States in 2011–2015. Neuro Oncol. 2018;20(Suppl 4):iv1–iv86.
2. Alexiou GA, Moschovi M, Stefanaki K, Sfakianos G, Prodromou N. Epidemiology of pediatric brain tumors in Greece (1991-2008). Experience from the Agia Sofia Children's Hospital. Cent Eur Neurosurg. 2011;72(1):1–4. https://doi.org/10.1055/s-0030-1268495.
3. Alexiou GA, Mpairamidis E, Psarros A, Sfakianos G, Prodromou N. Intracranial meningiomas in children: report of 8 cases. Pediatr Neurosurg. 2008;44(5):373–5. https://doi.org/10.1159/000149903; Epub 2008 Aug 15.

4. Louis DN, Perry A, Wesseling P, Brat DJ, Cree IA, Figarella-Branger D, Hawkins C, Ng HK, Pfister SM, Reifenberger G, Soffietti R, von Deimling A, Ellison DW. The 2021 WHO classification of tumors of the central nervous system: a summary. Neuro-Oncology. 2021;23(8):1231–51. https://doi.org/10.1093/neuonc/noab106.
5. Vartholomatos E, Vartholomatos G, Alexiou GA, Markopoulos GS. The past, present and future of flow cytometry in central nervous system malignancies. Methods Protoc. 2021;4(1):11. https://doi.org/10.3390/mps4010011.
6. Alexiou G, Vartholomatos G. Intraoperative flow cytometry in pediatric brain tumors. In: Alexiou G, Prodromou N, editors. Pediatric neurosurgery for clinicians. Cham: Springer; 2022. https://doi.org/10.1007/978-3-030-80522-7_51.
7. Alexiou GA, Vartholomatos G, Goussia A, Batistatou A, Tsamis K, Voulgaris S, Kyritsis AP. Fast cell cycle analysis for intraoperative characterization of brain tumor margins and malignancy. J Clin Neurosci. 2015;22(1):129–32. https://doi.org/10.1016/j.jocn.2014.05.029.
8. Shioyama T, Muragaki Y, Maruyama T, Komori T, Iseki H. Intraoperative flow cytometry analysis of glioma tissue for rapid determination of tumor presence and its histopathological grade: clinical article. J Neurosurg. 2013;118(6):1232–8.
9. Jabarkheel R, Ho CS, Rodrigues AJ, Jin MC, Parker JJ, Mensah-Brown K, Yecies D, Grant GA. Rapid intraoperative diagnosis of pediatric brain tumors using Raman spectroscopy: a machine learning approach. Neurooncol Adv. 2022;4(1):vdac118. https://doi.org/10.1093/noajnl/vdac118.
10. Wach J, Banat M, Borger V, Vatter H, Haberl H, Sarikaya-Seiwert S. Intraoperative MRI-guided resection in pediatric brain tumor surgery: a meta-analysis of extent of resection and safety outcomes. J Neurol Surg A Cent Eur Neurosurg. 2021;82(1):64–74. https://doi.org/10.1055/s-0040-1714413.
11. Schwake M, Schipmann S, Müther M, Köchling M, Brentrup A, Stummer W. 5-ALA fluorescence-guided surgery in pediatric brain tumors-a systematic review. Acta Neurochir. 2019;161(6):1099–108. https://doi.org/10.1007/s00701-019-03898-1.
12. Bauer KD, Duque RE, Shankey TV. Clinical flow cytometry: principles and application. Baltimore: Williams and Wilkins; 1993.
13. Ben Arush MW, Linn S, Ben-Izhak O, Levy R, Nahum MP, Tsuk-Shina T, Guilbord JN, Elhasid R, Postovski S. Prognostic significance of DNA ploidy in childhood astrocytomas. Pediatr Hematol Oncol. 1999;16(5):387–96. https://doi.org/10.1080/088800199276930.
14. Kotylo PK, Robertson PB, Fineberg NS, Azzarelli B, Jakacki R. Flow cytometric DNA analysis of pediatric intracranial ependymomas. Arch Pathol Lab Med. 1997;121(12):1255–8.
15. Alexiou GA, Vartholomatos G, Stefanaki K, Lykoudis EG, Patereli A, Tseka G, Tzoufi M, Sfakianos G, Prodromou N. The role of fast cell cycle analysis in pediatric brain tumors. Pediatr Neurosurg. 2015;50(5):257–63. https://doi.org/10.1159/000439029.
16. Vartholomatos G, Alexiou GA, Voulgaris S, Kyritsis AP. Intraoperative immunophenotypic analysis for diagnosis and classification of primary central nervous system lymphomas. World Neurosurg. 2018;117:464–5. https://doi.org/10.1016/j.wneu.2018.03.022.
17. Choi YL, Chi JG, Suh YL. CD99 immunoreactivity in ependymoma. Appl Immunohistochem Mol Morphol. 2001;9(2):125–9. https://doi.org/10.1097/00129039-200106000-00004.
18. Vartholomatos G, Stefanaki K, Alexiou GA, Batistatou A, Markopoulos GS, Tzoufi M, Sfakianos G, Prodromou N. Pediatric brain tumor grading based on CD56 quantification. J Pediatr Neurosci. 2018;13(4):524–7.
19. Vartholomatos G, Alexiou GA, Stefanaki K, Lykoudis EG, Tseka G, Tzoufi M, Sfakianos G, Prodromou N. The value of cell cycle analysis by propidium-iodine staining of CD56+ cells in pediatric brain tumors. Clin Neurol Neurosurg. 2015;133:70–4. https://doi.org/10.1016/j.clineuro.2015.03.017.
20. Daniels TR, et al. The transferrin receptor and the targeted delivery of therapeutic agents against cancer. Biochim Biophys Acta. 2012;1820:291–317.

21. Ren WH, Chang J, Yan CH, Qian XM, Long LX, He B, Yuan XB, Kang CS, Betbeder D, Sheng J, Pu PY. Development of transferrin functionalized poly(ethylene glycol)/poly(lactic acid) amphiphilic block copolymeric micelles as a potential delivery system targeting brain glioma. J Mater Sci Mater Med. 2010;21:2673–81.
22. Ramalho MJ, Loureiro JA, Coelho MAN, Pereira MC. Transferrin receptor-targeted Nanocarriers: overcoming barriers to treat glioblastoma. Pharmaceutics. 2022;14(2):279. https://doi.org/10.3390/pharmaceutics14020279.
23. Weaver M, Laske DW. Transferrin receptor ligand-targeted toxin conjugate (Tf-CRM107) for therapy of malignant gliomas. J Neuro-Oncol. 2003;65(1):3–13.

Chapter 11
Intraoperative Flow Cytometry in Spine Tumors

Spyridon Voulgaris, Dimitrios Metaxas, and Georgios Alexiou

11.1   Introduction

Primary spinal cord tumors make up for 5–12% of all primary central nervous system (CNS) malignancies and 0.5% of newly diagnosed tumors [1]. The location within the spinal canal and cell of origin of these tumors are used to categorize them. Adults are more likely to have an intradural extramedullary neoplasm diagnosed (85%), and schwannomas and meningiomas make up between 55% and 60% of all tumors. Ependymomas and astrocytomas are the most prevalent types of the less common (10–12%) intramedullary tumors [1]. In contrast to adults, who experience in two-thirds extradural cancers, children experience intradural tumors at a similar or higher frequency than extradural tumors [2]. Uncommon are the intramedullary spinal cord metastases (ISCM) that typically result from a primary lung, breast, or melanoma tumor. ISCM affect between 0.5% and 2% of all patients with cancer and represent only 8.5% of all CNS metastases. Primary intramedullary spinal cord lymphoma (PISCL), a rare tumor that makes up just 1% of all CNS lymphomas, is another uncommon malignancy.

A vital tool in basic research, flow cytometry is a laser-based technology designed to identify and quantify physical and chemical cell characteristics. Flow cytometry is frequently used in clinical practice to diagnose and categorize patients with hematologic malignancies, as well as to identify rare events; nevertheless, its value as a research tool for solid tumors has been largely unexplored and underreported [3]. Flow cytometry permits the assessment of a tumor's ploidy which is associated with poor prognosis in several cancers. Cell cycle analysis is the one of the first applications of flow cytometry. Based on that, the cell cycle fractions, namely G0/G1, S,

S. Voulgaris · D. Metaxas · G. Alexiou (✉)
Department of Neurosurgery, University of Ioannina, Ioannina, Greece
e-mail: galexiou@uoi.gr

G. Alexiou, G. Vartholomatos (eds.), *Intraoperative Flow Cytometry*,
https://doi.org/10.1007/978-3-031-33517-4_11

and G2/M phase, can me estimated. Presence of aneuploidy can be also readily identified. In the past, cell cycle analysis required substantial time for preparation of tissue sample. Over the last years an innovative and rapid cell cycle analysis protocol (within 5–6 min) has been developed by our group (Ioannina protocol) which has the potential for intraoperative use [4]. This technique permits in brain tumor samples the detection of the grade of malignancy, histological type classification, and assessment of tumor margins [5, 6]. For the assessment of tumor margins this novel technique can identify tumor remnants thus permitting a complete excision. Herewith, we discuss the role of intraoperative flow cytometry for the assessment of spinal tumor grade, tumor type, and resection margins.

11.2 Challenges in Spinal Tumor Surgery

While the majority of primary extramedullary neoplasms are benign, intramedullary neoplasms are often malignant. In the majority, microsurgical resection is the established treatment in extramedullary spinal tumors. In meningiomas and schwannomas this is more or less easy to perform depending on the dural attachment and on adhesions to the spinal cord or the nerve rootlets. Maximum safe cytoreductive surgery is the gold standard in malignant intramedullary tumors. Nevertheless, clear visualization of solid tumor tissue, identification of tumor margins, and safe differentiation of normal neuronal tissue in extra- and intramedullary gliomas, recurrent or infiltrative meningiomas, and extra- and intramedullary ependymomas can be challenging [7].

To date, surgeons are using frozen section biopsy for the determination of exact tumor type, grade of malignancy, and tumor margins. However, low-quality sections, the reliance on the pathologist's expertise, the typical turnaround time of 20 minutes, and the rarity of discrepancies between the final diagnosis and the diagnostic of the frozen section biopsy are only a few of the disadvantages of frozen sections. The 5-aminolevulinc acid (5-ALA) has been also utilized to aid the resection of spine tumors [8]. Sodium fluorescein has been also evaluated and proved useful for preventing vascular injuries and in intradural lesions, fluorescence helps prior to the durotomy to distinguish the tumor from healthy tissue [9].

11.3 Intraoperative Flow Cytometry in Spine Tumors

Intraoperative flow cytometry for spinal cord tumors has a role in the discrimination of low from high-grade tumors, identification of exact tumor type, and assessment of tumor margins in infiltrative tumors. To date standard pathology report requires 2–3 weeks for completion. Furthermore, regarding tumor's margins visual delineation with standard surgical techniques is difficult. Frozen sections constitute the gold standard, however, analysis of multiple tissue samples is a difficult task and moreover spinal tumors are usually small in size, thus cancerous tissue might not be adequate. Intraoperative flow cytometry can be performed in very small tissue samples (usually 0.5–2 mm^3) thus this technique is ideal for spinal tumor's evaluation. Upon sample receipt cell cycle analysis and assessment of ploidy status can be performed within 6 minutes. High-grade tumors exhibit significant lower G0/G1 and significant higher S and G2/M phase fractions than low-grade tumors. Thus, using ROC curve analysis cut-off points can be calculated for the discrimination between the two entities (Fig. 11.1).

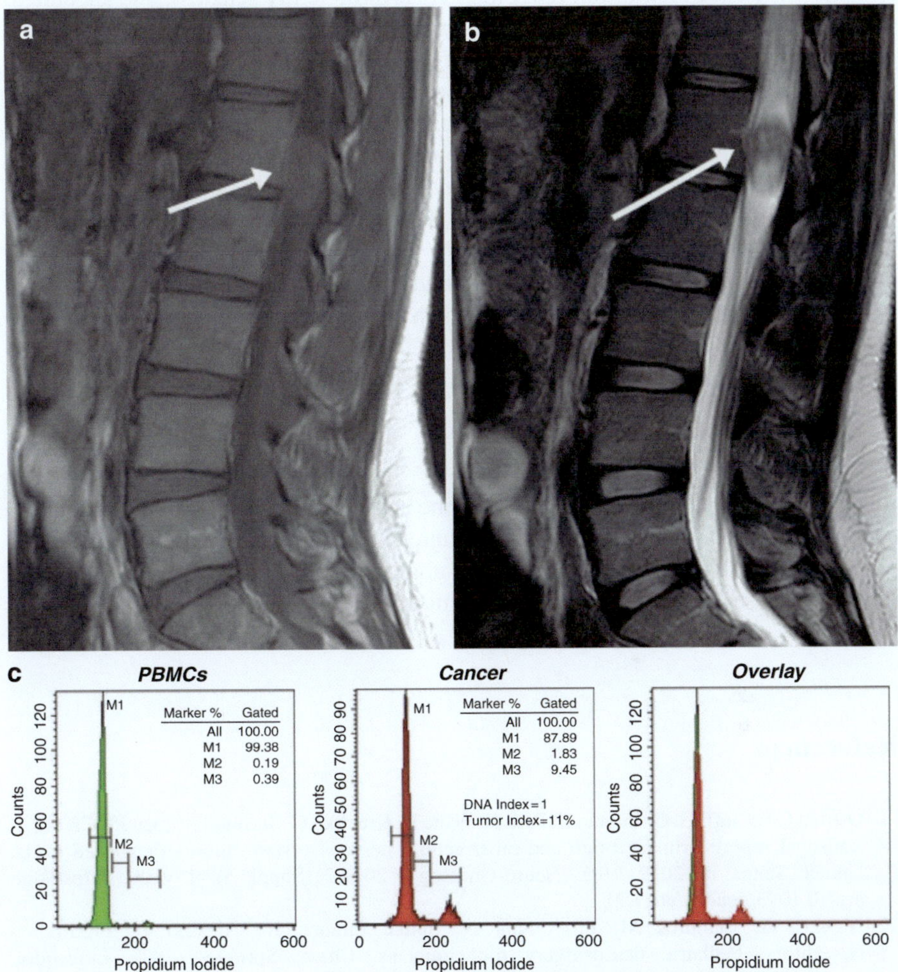

Fig. 11.1 (**a**) T1-weighted MRI revealing and intradural extramedullary tumor (arrow). (**b**) T2-weighted MRI. (**c**) Cell cycle distribution analysis using intraoperative flow cytometry in a spinal meningioma. Markers M1, M2, and M3 represent G0/G1, S, and G2/M cell cycle phases, respectively. On the left of each figure the cell cycle distribution of peripheral blood mononuclear cells (PBMCs) is presented as control. The presented case is diploid, with a DNA index = 1. In the overlay histogram the G0/G1 peak of cancer cells in red is discernible from that of normal cells in green. Tumor index (i.e., percentage of proliferative cells) was calculated at 11%. (Figure **c**, Courtesy by G. Vartholomatos)

Furthermore, ploidy status can be simultaneously established. High-grade tumors are usually aneuploids compared to low-grade tumors, which are usually diploids. When surgical margins are needed to be evaluated, several samples from tissue core and periphery can be analyses. Based on ploidy or malignancy index (S + G2/M phase fractions) normal tissue can be detected, verifying the presence of clear resection margins. Regarding the diagnosis of exact tumor type immunophenotypic characterization of spinal cord tumors can provide important clues. Evaluation of specific cluster differentiation (CD) markers is sufficiently sensitive and specific to confirm the histologic diagnosis in lymphoproliferative lesions. Similarly, by analyzing a brain tumor sample, diagnosis of the histological type might become possible using CD expression. Based on the previous studies intraoperative immunophenotypic analysis for the diagnosis of central nervous system lymphomas can be performed [10]. Furthermore, the neural cell adhesion molecule (NCAM, CD56) expression was associated with tumor's malignancy [11]. Other useful markers may progesterone (PR) and estrogen (ER) receptors and epithelial membrane antigen (EMA, MUC1, CD227) positivity for meningiomas. Gliomas may show glial fibrillary acidic protein (GFAP) positivity, whereas schwannomas on the SRY-related HMG-box 10 (SOX10) protein which is a transcription factor are positive.

11.4 Conclusion

Intraoperative flow cytometry might become a novel adjunct to standard pathology evaluation of spinal cord tumors. This technique might prove useful for the intraoperative discrimination of low from high-grade tumors, diagnosis of exact tumor type, and assessment of surgical resection margins in malignant intramedullary tumors.

References

1. Ostrom QT, Cioffi G, Gittleman H, Patil N, Waite K, Kruchko C, Barnholtz-Sloan JS. CBTRUS statistical report: primary brain and other central nervous system tumors diagnosed in the United States in 2012-2016. Neuro-Oncology. 2019;21(Suppl 5):v1–v100. https://doi.org/10.1093/neuonc/noz150.
2. Alexiou G, Lampros M, Prodromou N. Spinal tumors. In: Alexiou G, Prodromou N, editors. Pediatric neurosurgery for clinicians. Cham: Springer; 2022. https://doi.org/10.1007/978-3-030-80522-7_25.
3. Alexiou G, Vartholomatos G. Intraoperative flow cytometry in pediatric brain tumors. In: Alexiou G, Prodromou N, editors. Pediatric neurosurgery for clinicians. Cham: Springer; 2022. https://doi.org/10.1007/978-3-030-80522-7_51.
4. Alexiou GA, Vartholomatos G, Goussia A, et al. Fast cell cycle analysis for intraoperative characterization of brain tumor margins and malignancy. J Clin Neurosci. 2015;22(1):129–32.
5. Vartholomatos G, Alexiou G, Batistatou A, Kyritsis AP. Intraoperative cell-cycle analysis to guide brain tumor removal. Proc Natl Acad Sci U S A. 2014;111(36):E3755.

6. Vartholomatos G, Alexiou GA, Lianos GD, Harissis H, Voulgaris S, Kyritsis AP. Intraoperative cell cycle analysis for tumor margins evaluation: the future is now? Int J Surg. 2018;53:380–1.
7. Eicker SO, Floeth FW, Kamp M, Steiger HJ, Hänggi D. The impact of fluorescence guidance on spinal intradural tumour surgery. Eur Spine J. 2013;22(6):1394–401.
8. Wainwright JV, Endo T, Cooper JB, Tominaga T, Schmidt MH. The role of 5-aminolevulinic acid in spinal tumor surgery: a review. J Neuro-Oncol. 2019;141(3):575–84. https://doi.org/10.1007/s11060-018-03080-0.
9. Cardali SM, Ricciardo G, Garufi G, Raffa G, Messineo F, Scalia G, Conti A, Germanò A. Fluorescein-guided surgery for intradural spinal tumors: a single-center experience. Brain Spine. 2022;2:100908. https://doi.org/10.1016/j.bas.2022.100908.
10. Vartholomatos G, Alexiou GA, Voulgaris S, Kyritsis AP. Intraoperative immunophenotypic analysis for diagnosis and classification of primary central nervous system lymphomas. World Neurosurg. 2018;117:464–5. https://doi.org/10.1016/j.wneu.2018.03.022.
11. Vartholomatos G, Stefanaki K, Alexiou GA, Batistatou A, Markopoulos GS, Tzoufi M, Sfakianos G, Prodromou N. Pediatric brain tumor grading based on CD56 quantification. J Pediatr Neurosci. 2018;13(4):524–7. https://doi.org/10.4103/JPN.JPN_155_17.

Part IV
Intraoperative Flow Cytometry in Breast Malignancies

Chapter 12
Breast Cancer

Anna Batistatou and Sevasti Kamina

12.1 Introduction

Breast cancer is the most diagnosed cancer in women, and in the last decade there is a steady slow increase in incidence rates, by about 0.5% annually [1–3]. In a recent study by the American Cancer Society, it has been shown that 51% of all new cancer diagnoses for women comprise breast, lung, and colorectal cancer, with approximately one-third being breast cancer [1]. Breast cancer is the second cause of cancer death in women, after lung cancer and before colorectal cancer [1, 2]. Interestingly, although mortality rates for lung cancer are declining with accelerating rates, the decline is slowing for breast cancer [1]. This phenomenon provokes consideration for further actions needed to improve screening and treatment efficacies.

The great progress in breast cancer diagnosis and identification of prognostic and predictive markers, that has started about two decades ago—with estrogen receptors (ER), progesterone receptors (PR), and human epidermal growth factor receptor 2 (HER2)—is continuing in the present decade, with new markers but also with constant updating of the classic ones [4–8]. Besides estimation of Ki67, other predictive markers have emerged, i.e., germline BRCA mutation testing, PD-L1, PIK3CA mutation status, MSI/MMR, TMB, NTRK, etc. [9].

Pathology diagnosis remains the cornerstone for treatment. Classification of breast cancer has also evolved over the decades to reflect more accurately the

A. Batistatou (✉)
Department of Pathology, Faculty of Medicine, University of Ioannina, Ioannina, Greece
e-mail: abatista@uoi.gr

S. Kamina
Department of Pathology, University Hospital of Ioannina, Ioannina, Greece

G. Alexiou, G. Vartholomatos (eds.), *Intraoperative Flow Cytometry*,
https://doi.org/10.1007/978-3-031-33517-4_12

advances of basic and clinical research. Herein, we present the recent (5th Ed, 2019) World Health Organization (WHO) classification of breast carcinoma [10] with examples of the most common entities.

12.2   In Situ Breast Carcinoma [10, 11]

Under the term non-invasive lobular neoplasia, the entities of Lobular carcinoma in situ, not otherwise specified (LCIS NOS), Classic and Florid, and Pleomorphic Lobular Carcinoma are included. By definition, LCIS originates in the terminal duct lobular unit. An early pathogenetic event is the loss of E-cadherin (Fig. 12.1a, b).

The term ductal carcinoma in situ (DCIS) contains intraductal carcinoma, non-infiltrating, NOS, of low-, intermediate-, or high-nuclear grade (Fig. 12.1c). This carcinoma arises in the mammary-duct/lobular system and is heterogeneous. Solid,

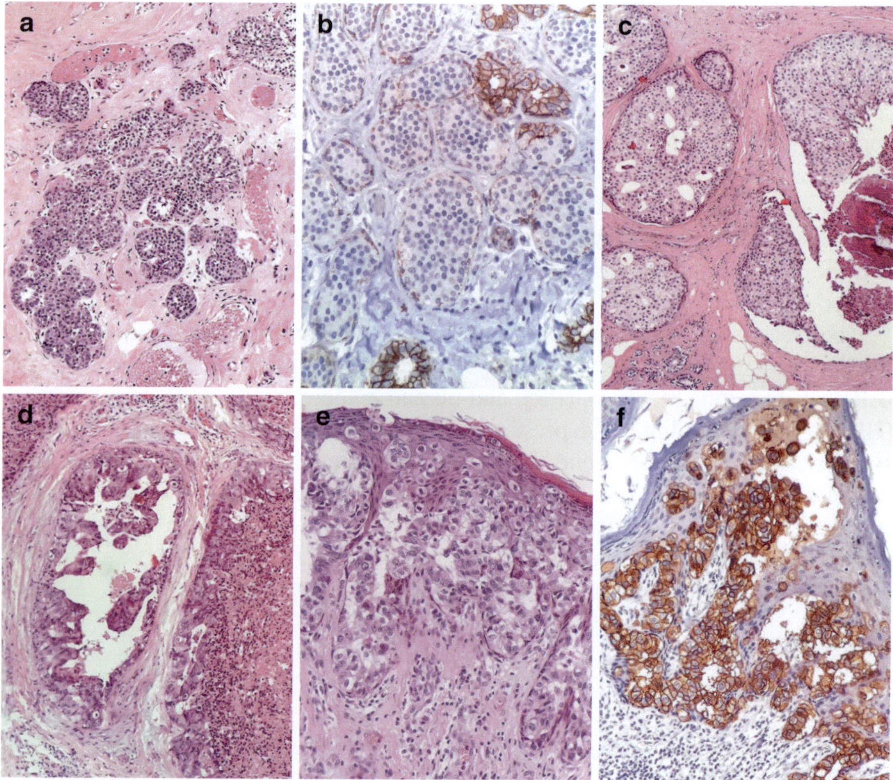

Fig. 12.1   (**a**) Classic lobular carcinoma in situ (Haematoxylin-eosinX100). (**b**) LCIS with the loss of immunohistochemical expression of E-cadherin (DABX200). (**c**) DCIS of high-nuclear grade (Haematoxylin-eosinX200). (**d**) Micropapillary DCIS (Haematoxylin-eosinX200). (**e**) Paget disease of the nipple (Haematoxylin-eosinX400). (**f**) HER-2 positive Paget disease (DABX400)

cribriform, papillary and micropapillary subtypes are well-recognised (Fig. 12.1d). It appears that pleomorphic lobular carcinoma in situ (LCIS) has overlapping features with DCIS [10, 11]. High-grade DCIS can also present as Paget disease of the nipple, where neoplastic cells are HER2 positive (Fig. 12.1e, f).

12.3 Infiltrating Breast Carcinoma [10, 11]

Invasive carcinoma of the breast includes carcinomas with invasion or microinvasion (micro-invasive carcinoma, less than or equal to 1 mm)(Fig. 12.2a). It includes infiltrating duct carcinoma NOS, lobular carcinoma NOS, invasive carcinoma with mixed ductal and lobular features, oncocytic carcinoma, lipid-rich carcinoma, glycogen-rich carcinoma, sebaceous carcinoma, tubular carcinoma, cribriform carcinoma NOS, mucinous adenocarcinoma, mucinous cystadenocarcinoma NOS, invasive micropapillary carcinoma, apocrine adenocarcinoma, metaplastic carcinoma, rare and salivary gland-type tumors, and neuroendocrine neoplasms. Classification is based on the architecture of the neoplasm, the cellular characteristics, and stromal features. The histological grade of the invasive cancer is based on a semiqualitative method (modified Nottingham score) taking in account the tubule/gland formation, the nuclear pleomorphism, and the mitotic count. The immunohistochemical expression of estrogen (ER) and progesterone (PR) receptors and the status of *ERBB2 (HER2)* gene amplification/overexpression of HER2 protein are important information to complement histological diagnosis. The Ki-67 proliferation index (assessed immunohistochemically) is important, as prognostic and predictive marker but also for identifying surrogate subtypes. The major subtypes are Luminal A-like, Luminal B-like (HER2 negative), Luminal B-like (HER2 positive), HER2 positive (non-luminal), and Triple negative.

Infiltrating duct carcinoma NOS is the most common type of the heterogeneous group of invasive breast carcinomas of no special type (IBC NST). Further subclassification is based on ER and HER2 status (Fig. 12.2b–d).

The hallmark of invasive lobular carcinoma is the presence of discohesive infiltrating neoplastic cells (Fig. 12.2e), which have the loss of E-cadherin expression and in the classic subtype express highly ER and are HER2 negative/non-amplified.

Neuroendocrine carcinoma is a specific entity with cells that have neuroendocrine morphology and express neuroendocrine immunohistochemical markers (Fig. 12.2f, g).

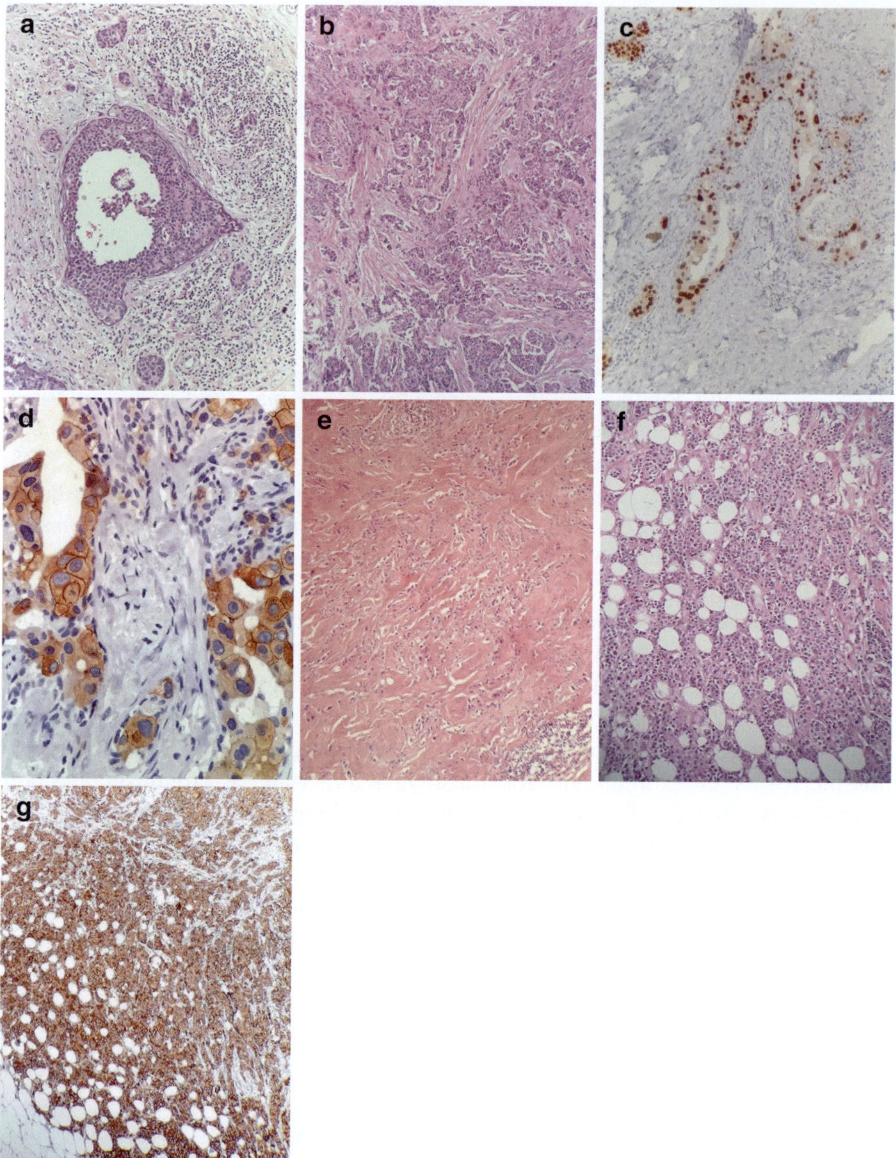

Fig. 12.2 (**a**) DCIS and Micro-invasive carcinoma (Haematoxylin-eosinX200). (**b**) Invasive breast carcinoma NST (Haematoxylin-eosinX100). (**c**) ER expression in invasive breast carcinoma NST (DABX200). (**d**) HER-2 positive invasive breast carcinoma NST (DABX400). (**e**) Invasive lobular carcinoma (Haematoxylin-eosinX100). (**f**) Invasive neuroendocrine carcinoma (Haematoxylin-eosinX200). (**g**) Immunohistochemical expression of synaptophysin in neuroendocrine carcinoma (DABX100)

References

1. Siegel RL, Miller KD, Fuchs HE, Jemal A. Cancer statistics, 2022. Cancer J Clin. 2022;72:7–33.
2. Torre LA, Siegel RL, Ward EM, Jemal A. Global cancer incidence and mortality rates and trends-an update. Cancer Epidemiol Biomark Prev. 2016;25:16–27. https://doi.org/10.1158/1055-9965.EPI-15-0578.
3. Pfeiffer RM, Webb-Vargas Y, Wheeler W, Gail MH. Proportion of US trends in breast cancer incidence attributable to long-term changes in risk factor distributions. Cancer Epidemiol Biomarkers Prev. 2018;27:1214–22.
4. Allison KH, Hammond MEH, Dowsett M, McKernin SE, Carey LA, Fitzgibbons PL, et al. Estrogen and progesterone receptor testing in breast cancer: ASCO/CAP guideline update. J Clin Oncol. 2020;38:1346–66.
5. Reis-Filho JS, Pusztai L. Gene expression profiling in breast cancer: classification, prognostication, and prediction. Lancet. 2011;378:1812–23. https://doi.org/10.1016/S0140-6736(11)61539-0.
6. Wolff AC, Hammond MEH, Allison KH, et al. Human epidermal growth factor receptor 2 testing in breast cancer: American Society of Clinical Oncology/College of American Pathologists clinical practice guideline focused update. J Clin Oncol. 2018;36:2105e22.
7. Krystel-Whittemore M, Wen HY. Update on HER2 expression in breast cancer. Diagn Histopathol. 2022;28(3):170–5.
8. Franchet C, Djerroudi L, Maran-Gonzalez A, Abramovici O, Antoine M, Becette V, et al. Ann Pathol. 2021;41(6):507–20. https://doi.org/10.1016/j.annpat.2021.07.014; Epub 2021 Aug 12.[2021 update of the GEFPICS' recommendations for HER2 status assessment in invasive breast cancer in France]
9. Najjar S, Allison KH. Updates on breast biomarkers. Virchows Arch. 2022;480(1):163–76. https://doi.org/10.1007/s00428-022-03267-x; Epub 2022 Jan 14
10. WHO Classification of Tumours Editorial Board. Breast tumours, WHO classification of tumours series, vol. 2. 5th ed. Lyon: International Agency for Research on Cancer; 2019.
11. https://www.cap.orgBreast.DCIS.

Chapter 13
Current Methods for Intraoperative Application

Maria Paraskevaidi

13.1 Introduction

Current technologies available for breast imaging can offer high diagnostic accuracy (sensitivity and specificity), but they have been mainly developed for breast cancer screening and presurgical planning. X-ray mammography, the most common clinical modality for breast imaging, has an estimated sensitivity and specificity ranging between 83–95% and 90–98%, respectively [1]. However, tools for the intraoperative assessment of margin clearance and sentinel lymph nodes that would enhance surgical outcomes and minimize tumour recurrence are much less developed.

As of today, staining of the excised tissue followed by histological assessment is considered the gold standard for margin classification and a final diagnosis. Although the diagnostic accuracy of this approach is high, the limitations coming with it are numerous, including laborious and time-consuming procedures beyond the operating theatre, lack of automation and the need for expert pathologists with significant inter-observer variability.

A recent prospective study from Sweden including almost 49,000 patients with breast cancer suggested that breast conserving surgery followed by radiotherapy offers better overall and breast cancer-specific survival when compared to total mastectomy with/without radiotherapy [2]. The authors highlighted that breast conservation should be given priority if both treatments are valid options for the respective patient [2].

M. Paraskevaidi (✉)
Department of Metabolism, Digestion and Reproduction, Faculty of Medicine, Institute of Reproductive and Developmental Biology, Imperial College London, London, UK
e-mail: m.paraskevaidi@imperial.ac.uk

G. Alexiou, G. Vartholomatos (eds.), *Intraoperative Flow Cytometry*,
https://doi.org/10.1007/978-3-031-33517-4_13

163

Given the high percentages of surgical margin positivity after breast conserving surgery (up to 20–40%) [3–9], which necessitates a second operation at a subsequent visit, novel technologies that would offer a rapid tool for diagnosis and margin assessment are highly sought after. Such a tool would allow immediate diagnosis and margin assessment but also minimize repeat visits and prolonged patient anxiety whilst improving prognosis.

Technological advancements during the last decades have allowed the introduction of other innovative techniques for near-real-time diagnosis and margin clearance assessment intraoperatively. Although this chapter is not an exhaustive systematic review of the literature, it will still cover key points and seminal studies around:

1. conventional intraoperative techniques employed for diagnosis and margin detection in breast cancer and
2. the performance of emerging technologies in the field of breast cancer surgery and their potential role in reducing positive margins and re-excision rates.

13.2 Intraoperative Techniques in Breast Cancer

13.2.1 Conventional Intraoperative Techniques

13.2.1.1 Frozen Sections

Frozen section analysis is the traditional choice for intraoperative diagnosis during breast conservation surgery. It includes collection of the resected tissue, embedding in an optical cutting temperature compound and freezing before sectioning the bulk sample into thin tissue sections. The sections need to, then, be deposited on glass slides and fixed for immunohistochemical staining with haematoxylin and eosin (H&E) for the histopathologist to make a final diagnosis and assess margin clearance. Morphological examination of the stained tissue can give information on whether the tissue consists of ductal carcinoma in situ, invasive ductal carcinoma, ductal hyperplasia, or normal breast gland. In a meta-analysis of different intraoperative techniques for margin assessment in breast cancer surgery [10], frozen sections achieved high diagnostic accuracy with a pooled sensitivity, specificity and area under the receiver operating characteristic curve (AUROC) of 85%, 96% and 96% after including nine different studies. Despite the high diagnostic performance that frozen sections can provide, this approach comes with a number of limitations, such as laborious sample preparation steps and prolonged operating times with the patient under anaesthesia as well as requirement of infrastructure and expert pathologists. Moreover, the method's accuracy can vary significantly since diagnosis is dependent on human interpretation which can introduce inter-observer variability. Reports have also indicated that frozen sections may cause artifacts in the fatty tissue as a result of the freezing and thawing process [8]. A previous survey enquiring lead pathologists ($n = 18$) about routine histopathological intraoperative margin assessment within major breast screening centres in the UK [10], confirmed that no institutions were using this approach routinely during breast cancer surgery. The survey's authors noted that only high-volume centres with suitable large pathology teams are able to provide a service like this to the required level, since interpretation of frozen specimens is more difficult that permanent section histology and as such a senior pathologist is required to produce confident reports [10].

13.2.1.2   Imprint Cytology

Because of the disadvantages of frozen sections mentioned above, imprint cytology has been suggested as an alternative, quicker, and more simple intraoperative method to analyse breast tissue excisions [8]. During imprint cytology, the excised mass is oriented and pressed onto glass slides which are then fixed and stained. It is based on the principle that only malignant cells will adhere to the slide (due to cellular surface characteristics) whilst adipose cells will not. In a meta-analysis of 11 different studies using imprint cytology as their method to assess surgical margins [10], the authors reported a pooled sensitivity, specificity and AUROC of 91%, 95% and 98%. However, this approach has variability in the sensitivity and is related to the size of the tumour and the cytological skills of the pathologist [11]. Skills in imprint cytology reporting have also been seen to decrease over the past years due to the decline in routine cytological assessment that makes analysis by experienced cytologists more troublesome [10]. Also the specimen's surface irregularity, dryness and presence of atypical cells can all lead to errors in the interpretation of the slide and final diagnosis [12].

13.2.1.3   Intraoperative Ultrasonography

Intraoperative ultrasonography can be used for visualising structural features and associated heterogeneity to assist with specimen margins in breast cancer. Surgeons locate the tumour in the breast using ultrasound and compare findings with preoperative digital images. After excision, the surgeon can use ultrasound to examine the specimen ex vivo to confirm that it resembles the candidate lesion targeted preoperatively [13]. Intraoperative ultrasound studies have also been meta-analysed to determine the diagnostic accuracy of this technology in breast cancer margin assessment [14]. Four studies were included and the pooled sensitivity, specificity and AUROC were reported as 59%, 81% and 78% respectively [10]. Apart from the low sensitivity of this approach, intraoperative ultrasound is operator-dependent and requires additional training and expertise.

13.2.2   Emerging Technologies for Intraoperative Applications

Given the limitations of conventional techniques used for intraoperative margin assessment, presented above, newly emerging technologies have been developed over the year to improve speed, cost, reliability and diagnostic accuracy. Herein, we describe a number of methods that have shown potential as tools for the intraoperative examination of breast cancers based on principles of flow cytometry, vibrational spectroscopy, mass spectrometry, bio-impedance spectroscopy, radiofrequency spectroscopy, optical coherence tomography, microcomputed tomography and other fluorescence-guided systems.

13.2.2.1   Intraoperative Flow Cytometry

Although flow cytometry has been used for decades for clinical diagnostic purposes, its use in intraoperative applications has been limited mostly due to time-consuming sample preparation steps. Recent developments have allowed the introduction of a rapid cell-cycle analysis protocol permitting the use of flow cytometry as an intraoperative tool for evaluating tumour margin status [15–17]. The diagnostic performance of intraoperative flow cytometry (iFC) was initially assessed in patients with brain tumours [15, 18, 19] as well as head and neck lesions [17], demonstrating promising results before the technique was used in breast cancer patients.

In a recent study conducted by Vatholomatos et al., iFC was employed for the first time for the rapid assessment of resection margins during breast conserving surgery [20]. The authors included 606 samples of margins ($n = 506$) and tumours ($n = 100$) from 99 patients with invasive ductal carcinoma of no special type and invasive lobular carcinoma. Using pathological examination as the gold standard, iFC achieved 92.5% diagnostic accuracy, 93.3% sensitivity and 92.4% specificity, whereas cytological assessment achieved 94.2% diagnostic accuracy and 94.6% specificity but a much lower sensitivity of 82.3%. The optimised, quick protocol used in this study achieved analysis of each sample between 3 and 5 min (Fig. 13.1). Considering the fast, objective, inexpensive and accurate manner of this approach, iFC shows great promise as a novel tool for the intraoperative evaluation of surgical margins in breast conserving surgery. Moreover, since flow cytometers are currently widely used in both clinical and research settings, their implementation in surgical theatres would be much easier, following large-scale multicentre clinical trials.

A more detailed description of the use of iFC in breast lumpectomy is given in the following chapter (Chap. 14).

13.2.2.2   Vibrational Spectroscopy

Vibrational spectroscopy techniques, such as Raman spectroscopy, study the interaction of light with biological matter after exposure to electromagnetic radiation to provide information about the biomolecules present within a sample. The

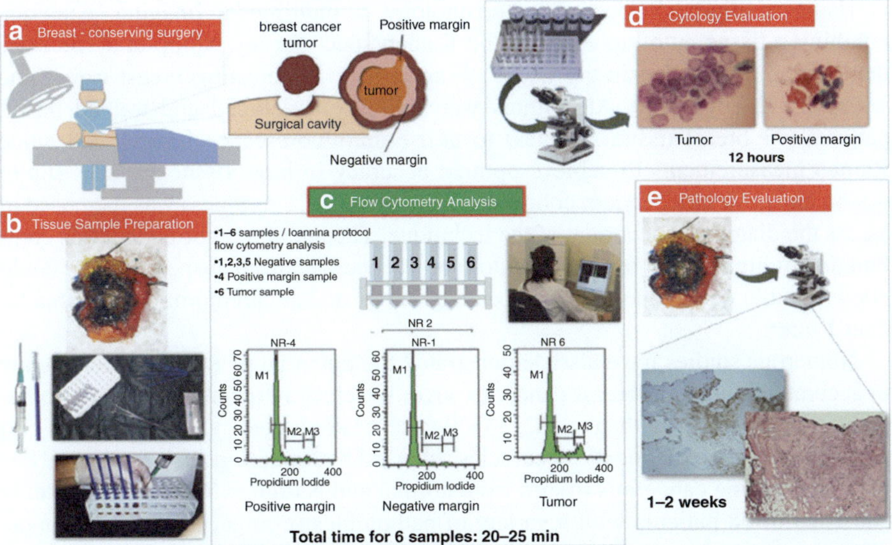

Fig. 13.1 Schematic representation of the experimental procedure to evaluate margins from excised breast cancer specimens using flow cytometry, cytology and pathology. (**a**), Breast - conserving surgery (**b**), Tissue Sample Preparation (**c**), Flow Cytology Analysis (**d**), Cytology Evaluation (**e**), Pathology Evaluation (Figure reproduced from Vartholomatos et al. [20])

vibrational movements caused by inelastic light scattering in Raman spectroscopy can reveal information about different biological molecules, such as lipids, carbohydrates, nucleic acids and proteins [21]. This simultaneously-derived information can be used to generate a holistic biochemical "fingerprint" of a sample, indicating the presence of absence of disease.

Raman spectroscopy has attracting great interest over the years for different clinical applications ranging from early detection and diagnosis to monitoring of human diseases including cancers, neurodegenerative diseases and infectious diseases [21]. Raman spectroscopy has been successfully employed in large- and smaller-cohort studies for the in vivo analysis and margin assessment of brain [22], gastric [23], head and neck [24], lung [25], oesophageal [26], skin [27–29] as well as breast [30] cancers.

In 2006 Haka et al. [31] presented the first demonstration of Raman spectroscopy in breast tissue in vivo in a study consisting of nine patients (30 Raman spectra were collected). Spectral information was generated in 1 s highlighting the potential real-time benefits of this technique as an in vivo tool for margin assessment during partial mastectomy breast surgery. Although the patient number was small with only one malignant sample, the sensitivity and specificity were 100%. More importantly, it is worth noting that the malignancy was only diagnosed after H&E histological assessment since it was grossly invisible during surgery and therefore patient had to undergo a second surgery. Had Raman spectroscopy been used in a real-time fashion during the initial surgery (since it had correctly classified the sample as malignant), the additional re-excision may have been avoided.

Using multimodal spectral histopathology, a multimodal imaging technique combining tissue autofluorescence and Raman spectroscopy, Shipp et al. recently demonstrated 95% sensitivity and 82% specificity in detecting breast carcinoma within 12–24 min [30]. Algorithms were initially developed and trained on 65 patients (91 breast tissue samples) to utilise autofluorescence images and guide Raman measurements to achieve optimal accuracy in large tissue surfaces (up to 4×65 cm^2). An independent cohort of 107 patients (121 samples) was then used to assess the diagnostic accuracy of the technique. The authors reported that this combination of high spatial resolution autofluorescence with Raman spectroscopy could allow reliable detection of invasive carcinoma or ductal carcinoma in situ smaller than 1 mm^2.

Numerous studies have also demonstrated the potential of Raman spectroscopy in accurately detecting breast cancer ex vivo, which is a crucial step before implementation into surgical theatre [32, 33]. Two separate studies by Haka et al. [34, 35] demonstrated high diagnostic accuracies achieved by Raman spectroscopic analysis in distinguishing cancerous tissues from normal and benign ex vivo. The first study consisted of 58 patients with a variety of pathologies (normal, fibrocystic change, fibroadenoma and infiltrating carcinoma) and had 94% sensitivity and 96% specificity [34] (Fig. 13.2), whereas the following study [24] was the first prospective application that closely mimicked the target patient population of an anticipated in vivo setting; this second study achieved a sensitivity of 83%, a specificity of 93%, a positive predictive value (PPV) of 36% and a negative predictive value (NPV) of 99% for distinguishing cancerous from normal and benign tissues [24]. Even though the authors concluded that the high NPV was the main clinically relevant outcome, the low PPV could still arise issues in a clinical setting since it would lead to unnecessary surgical excisions. However, the advantages of the latter study were that analysis time was ~30 min and was also performed adjacent to the operating theatre, which mimics the conditions for intraoperative use.

Talari et al. [32] used Raman spectroscopy to analyse 132 tissue microarray breast biopsies and demonstrated specificity of 70%, 100%, 90% and 97%, for identifying luminal A, luminal B, HER2 and triple negative subtypes, respectively. In a different study by Surmacki et al. [33], 82 tissue samples were studied, and the authors reported 86% sensitivity and 72% specificity in distinguishing normal and breast cancerous tissues.

Different experimental variants of Raman spectroscopy techniques have also shown promising results for breast cancer detection. Spatially offset Raman spectroscopy (SORS) enables acquisition of Raman spectra from regions spatially offset from the point of original laser incidence which allows biological investigation of deep layers of a sample [36–38]. This could be critical for the accurate detection of tumour margins since clear margin is ~2 mm for infiltrating carcinoma. Using SORS in an ex vivo setting to analyse 35 breast tissue samples, Keller et al. [37] achieved a sensitivity of 95% and specificity of 100% after comparison with the histopathological assessment as the gold standard. Surface-enhanced Raman spectroscopy (SERS) is another variant of Raman that uses colloidal suspensions or substrates to enhance the Raman signal 10^3–10^{10} times. Wang et al. [38] used SERS

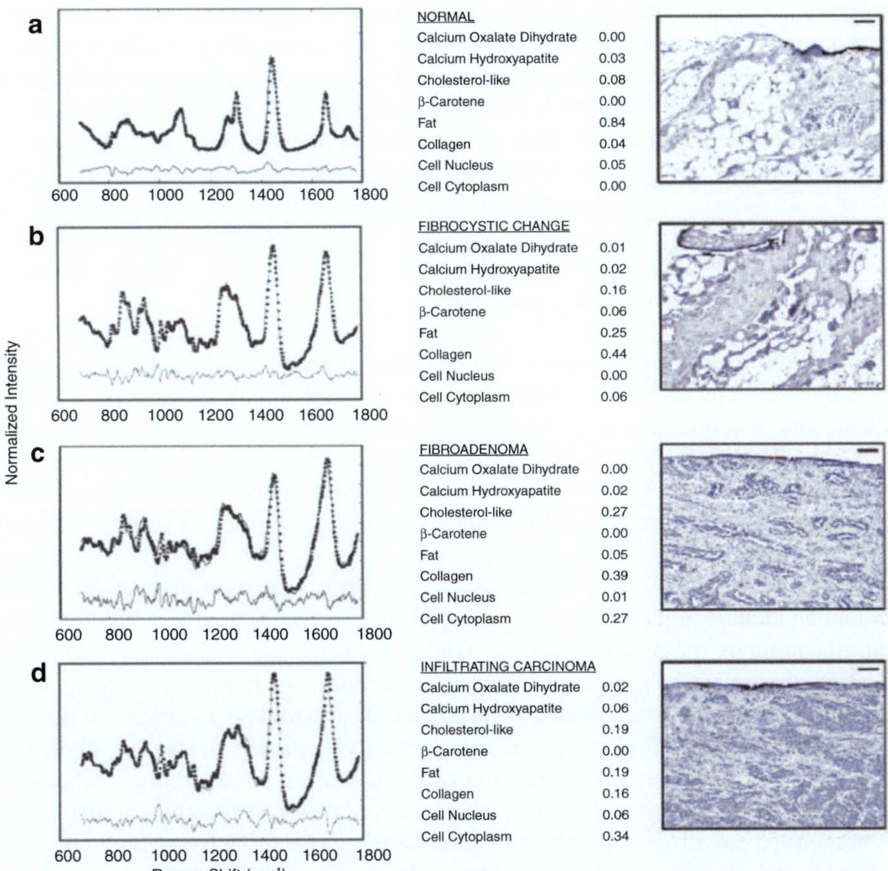

Fig. 13.2 Raman spectroscopy of ex vivo breast tissues. Raman spectra acquired from normal, benign and malignant samples of breast tissue with corresponding images from haematoxylin & eosin(H&E)-stained sections used to make the histopathologic diagnosis for normal breast tissue (**a**), fibrocystic change (**b**), fibroadenoma (**c**) and infiltrating carcinoma (**d**). (Figure reproduced from Haka et al. [34])

to detect tumour at the excision surface with 89% sensitivity and 92% specificity. In this study, nanoparticles were topically applied on excised fresh tissues ($n = 57$) to enable rapid visualisation of a multiplexed panel of cell surface biomarkers to simultaneously quantify their expression (HER2, ER, EGFR and CD44).

Even though the majority of Raman studies in breast cancer so far have been performed in ex vivo settings, technological advancements in Raman spectrometers have permitted the advent of portable, handheld devices for point-of-care testing. The introduction of fibre laser probes in Raman spectroscopy is now also expediting the use in in vivo settings for disease diagnostics and evaluation of surgical intraoperatively [39], however, large-scale trials are still needed. A noteworthy study of Raman spectroscopy for in vivo cancer detection and margin assessment using a laser fibre handheld instrument is this by Jermyn et al [22]. In this study, a handheld Raman probe was used for the local detection of cancer cells in the human brain. The authors were able to differentiate normal brain from dense cancer and normal brain invaded by cancer with a sensitivity of 93% and specificity of 91%. With analysis time being ~0.2 s per scan, such an intraoperative technology could classify cell populations in real time, rendering it ideal for accurate surgical resection and immediate decision-making in many malignancies, including breast.

13.2.2.3   Mass Spectrometry Techniques

Mass spectrometry analyses molecules by measuring the mass-to-charge ratio (m/z) of molecular ions and their charged fragments. Such technologies are valuable for identifying and quantifying tissue-specific ionic content linked to cellular metabolism. In clinical medicine, different variations of mass spectrometry techniques exist serving different medical applications, such as detection of disease biomarkers in biological fluids, imaging diagnostics or monitoring of disease progression and response to treatment.

Some examples of mass spectrometry platforms that have shown diagnostic potential include liquid chromatography-mass spectrometry (LC-MS) [40], gas chromatography-mass spectrometry (GC-MS) [41] and matrix-assisted laser desorption ionisation (MALDI) [42]. For decades, such platforms have been employed to study cancer metabolism and identify biomarkers indicative of disease states and underlying aetiology. However, these methods tend to be laborious, requiring extensive sample preparation or the use of chromatographic techniques prior to mass spectrometry analysis, which prevent their use as intraoperative tools. The more recent advent of ambient ionisation mass spectrometry technologies has allowed analysis of samples without the need for prior sample preparation steps and therefore has permitted real-time analysis and opening avenues for their use as intraoperative cancer diagnostic tools. Over the years, a number of studies have employed ambient ionisation mass spectrometry to detect different malignancies, such as brain [43], cervical [44, 45], ovarian [46, 47], colorectal [48] and breast [49, 50] cancers, among others [43].

In the field of breast cancer, St John et al. [49] used rapid evaporative ionisation mass spectrometry (REIMS) which utilises commonly-used surgical methods, such as surgical diathermy or laser surgery, to cause sample evaporation and generation gas-phase ions; the tissue-derived "smoke" includes important biological information to characterise key lipid species present in and cancerous tissues [43]. This study used REIMS coupled to diathermy, also known as the intelligent knife – iKnife, and reported that the differential metabolic profiles of breast cancer and normal tissues could detect cancer with 93.4% sensitivity and 94.9% specificity (Fig. 13.3). The analysis was performed by analysing 359 individual specimens; 253 normal (932 sampling points) and 106 tumour specimens (226 sampling points) from 113 patients. Using a validation set of 260 newly acquired tissues (normal $n = 161$, tumour $n = 99$), the iKnife achieved a sensitivity and specificity of 90.0%

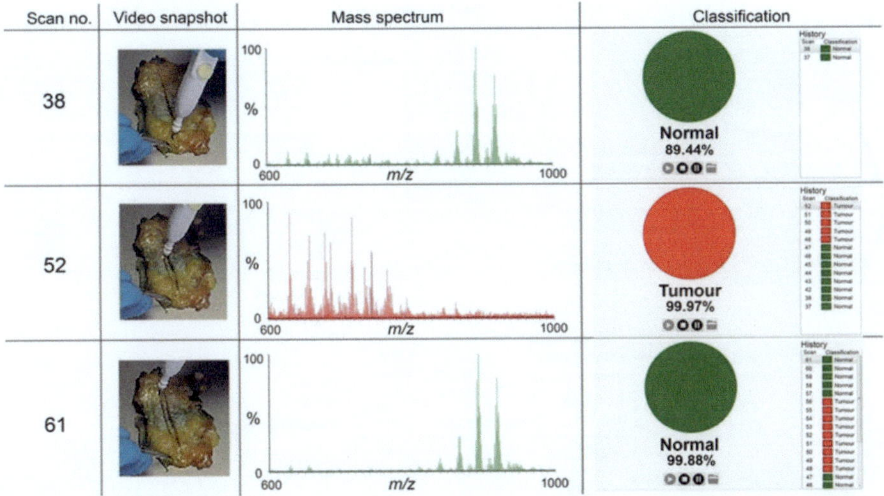

Fig. 13.3 The iKnife used in a mastectomy specimen as an ex vivo validation case study. The electrosurgical hand-piece was moved through the mastectomy specimen from normal breast tissue, into tumour and out through normal tissue. A simultaneous video recording reveals the position of the hand-piece in relation to the specimen and the generated spectra and demonstrates good correlation with the recognition software compared to macroscopic findings. (Reproduced from St John et al. [49])

and 98.8%, respectively. To demonstrate the technique's potential in an intraoperative setting, the authors also conducted a proof-of-concept study in six case studies showing that 99.27% (n = 5422/5462) were interpretable by the ex vivo model whilst only 0.73% (n = 40/5462) of spectra were classified as outliers. The authors concluded that this system could allow real-time analysis of both ex vivo and in vivo breast tissue, highlighting its potential as an intraoperative tool for the classification of resection margins (Fig. 13.4).

A different handheld device, named MasSpec Pen, was developed by Zhang et al. [51] and assessed as a tool to detect cancerous tissues and achieve negative margins. MasSpec Pen brings a small volume water droplet in physical contact with a tissue surface and after 3 s the water is transported to a mass spectrometer extracting diagnostic information about proteins, lipids and metabolites. In the specific study, the MassSpec was employed to analyse 20 human cancer thin tissue sections and 253 human patient tissue samples including normal and cancerous tissues from breast, lung, thyroid and ovary. After comparison with histological findings, the device allowed overall cancer prediction with high sensitivity (96.4%), specificity (96.2%) and overall accuracy of 96.3%. For breast cancer (n = 45), 87.5% sensitivity, 100% specificity (AUC = 1.0) and an overall accuracy of 95.6% were achieved. The authors also tested the suitability of this technology in vivo during the surgery of tumour-bearing mouse models, without causing any observable tissue damage, demonstrating its potential for intraoperative applications.

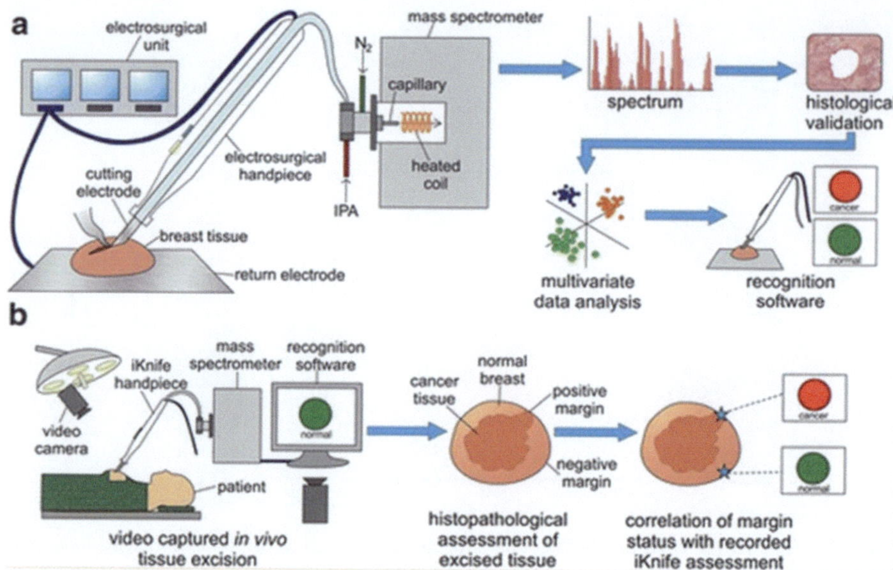

Fig. 13.4 Ex vivo and intraoperative workflows of the iKnife (Rapid Evaporative Ionisation Mass Spectrometry (REIMS) coupled to surgical diathermy) in breast cancer. (**a**) Ex vivo workflow from generation of spectra by mass spectrometry (MS) analysis of surgical aerosol through to model building by multivariate statistics leading to ex vivo recognition of tissue in real time. (**b**) Intraoperative workflow from generation of spectra in real time by on-line MS analysis, through to determination of margin status by histopathological assessment and correlation to iKnife results. (Reproduced from St John et al. [49])

Desorption electrospray ionisation (DESI) is another mass spectrometry technique falling under the umbrella of ambient ionisation techniques. DESI directs electrically-charged solvent droplets onto the surface of a sample, causing desorption of the sample's surface and generating secondary gas-phase ions, which are then imported and analysed with a mass spectrometer [52]. DESI mass spectrometry imaging (DESI-MSI) allows simultaneous spatial and molecular information for a biological sample, therefore providing the distribution and identity of biomolecules [53] and it is becoming increasingly used in cancer studies as it allows fast surface sampling without the need for laborious sample preparation [54]. The first application of DESI-MSI in a small set of breast tissue samples (benign ductal carcinoma and invasive ductal carcinoma) was performed by Dill et al. [55] in 2009, showing differences in the relative intensities and spatial distributions of various lipids (Fig. 13.5).

In a different study, Calligaris et al. [50] used DESI-MSI to image breast tissue samples from 14 patients showing that tumour margins could be identified using the spatial distributions and intensities of different lipids, which were more abundant in the cancerous tissues. The cancer margins delineated by the molecular images from DESI-MSI were consistent with margins obtained from histological staining

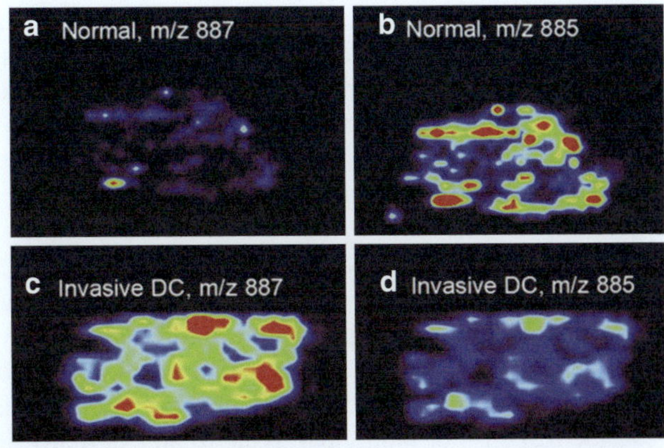

Fig. 13.5 Images from human breast tissue section after DESI-MSI analysis. Distributions of *m/z* 887 and *m/z* 885 ions in normal and invasive ductal carcinoma specimens. (**a**) Normal, m/z 887 (**b**) Normal, m/z 885 (**c**) Invasive Ductal Carcinoma, m/z 887 (**d**) Invasive Ductal Carcinoma, m/z 885. (Reproduced from Dill et al. [55]).

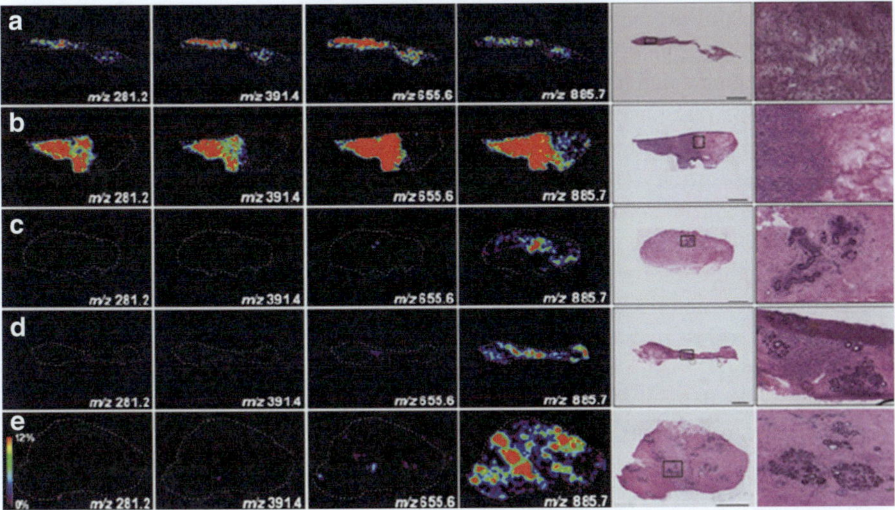

Fig. 13.6 DESI mass spectrometry images from specimens of one patient. Images were acquired from the tumour centre (**a**), the tumour edge (**b**), 2 cm away from the tumour (**c**), 5 cm away from the tumour (**d**) and contralateral side (**e**) tissue sections showing the distributions of ions at *m/z* 281.2, *m/z* 391.4, *m/z* 655.6 and *m/z* 885.7. (Right) Light microscopy images of the H&E-stained sections are shown. (Scale bars, 2 mm). (Reproduced from Calligaris et al. [50])

(Fig. 13.6). The authors concluded that such an approach could be useful as a rapid intraoperative detection tool of remaining cancerous tissue during breast conserving surgery.

DESI-MSI was also assessed in a following study by Guenther et al. [56] using 126 tissue biopsies from 50 patients undergoing surgical resections for breast cancer. Data extracted from DESI-MSI measurements were separated in two groups (tumour from 28 patients and "tumour bed" from 22 patients) and subjected to multivariate statistical analysis. "Tumour bed" samples were used as the normal control group and were confirmed as morphologically normal tissue by histologic examination. Diagnosis of breast cancer was achieved with an accuracy of 98.2% based on DESI-MSI data (PPV 96%, NVP 100%, specificity 96%, sensitivity 100%).

13.2.2.4 ClearEdge (Bio-impedance Spectroscopy)

The ClearEdge system, developed by LS BioPath, is a mobile, battery operated handheld imaging device intended for intraoperative use during breast cancer surgery. This system is equipped with a single-use prove which can guide surgeons in deciding margin clearance and enable immediate and accurate removal of diseased tissue (Fig. 13.7). This technology employs bio-impedance spectroscopy to measure the response of biological tissue to an externally applied electrical current. In the first intraoperative study of ClearEdge by Dixon et al. [57], the imaging device was used to examine margins of excised tissue intraoperatively in patients undergoing breast conserving surgery in two phases of independent cohorts. Phase 1 consisted of 58 patients and had 334 margins assessed, whereas Phase 2 consisted of 63 patients and 335 margins were assessed. The margin assessment accuracies in Phase 1 and Phase 2 compared to pathology results were very similar: sensitivity (84.3% and 87.3%), specificity (81.9% and 75.6%), positive predictive value (67.2% and 63.6%) and negative predictive value (92.2% and 92.4%). The false positive rate (18.1% and 24.4%) and false negative rate (15.7% and 12.7%) were low in both phases. The imaging information was collected in <5 min with each image requiring 3 s acquisition time. The authors also reported that the ClearEdge has the ability to automatically adjust its baseline every time based on the individual patient's breast tissue by an initial reading taken on normal tissue distant from the tumour site; this may enhance its detection sensitivity in each patient.

Starting in August 2022, the intraoperative performance of ClearEdge device in breast conserving surgery will be assessed in a 26 month, multicentre randomised controlled clinical (RCT) trial. This RCT will include 288 participants and conclude on whether there is an improvement in the detection of ductal carcinoma in situ or invasive cancer involved margins. This will be determined by measuring whether

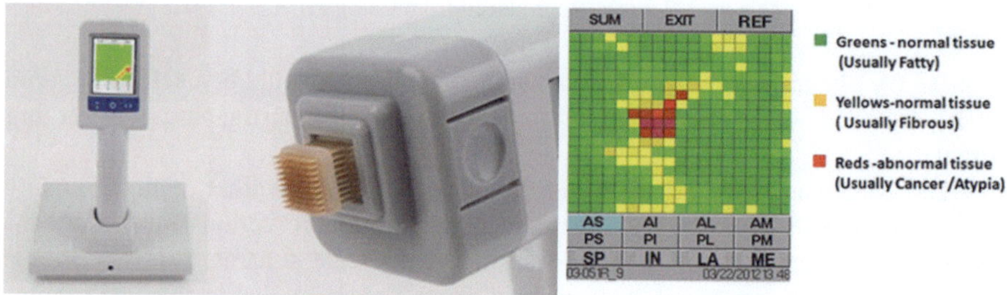

Fig. 13.7 ClearEdge device (left), disposable head (middle) and colour coded image display (right). (Reproduced from Dixon et al. [57])

removal at the time of primary surgical treatment can reduce the need for repeat surgeries as compared to the Standard of Care procedures, which does not use the device.

13.2.2.5   MarginProbe (Radiofrequency Spectroscopy)

MarginProbe (Dilon Technologies, USA), is used as a real-time, intraoperative detection tool of cancerous tissue at the edges of excised breast tissue to enable surgeons to immediately resect additional diseased tissue. MarginProbe uses radio frequency fields to measure changes in the electrical properties of biological tissues that occur in the presence of cancerous lesions (Fig. 13.8) and to provide an immediate result within the operating room. The system is comprised of two components: a detachable, sterile, single-use probe and a console with a user interface system showing the result (Fig. 13.9a).

Numerous studies and randomised controlled trials (RCTs) have tested the potential of MarginProbe in assessing margin status in breast conservation surgery [14, 59–72]. Clinical studies, including four RCTs, that have assessed the performance of MarginProbe are summarised in Table 13.1. Although it has been reported that the device can provide quick results (~5–7 min) and achieve ~50% reduction in the need for excisions, diagnostic sensitivity and specificity values vary between different studies and are modest (~70%).

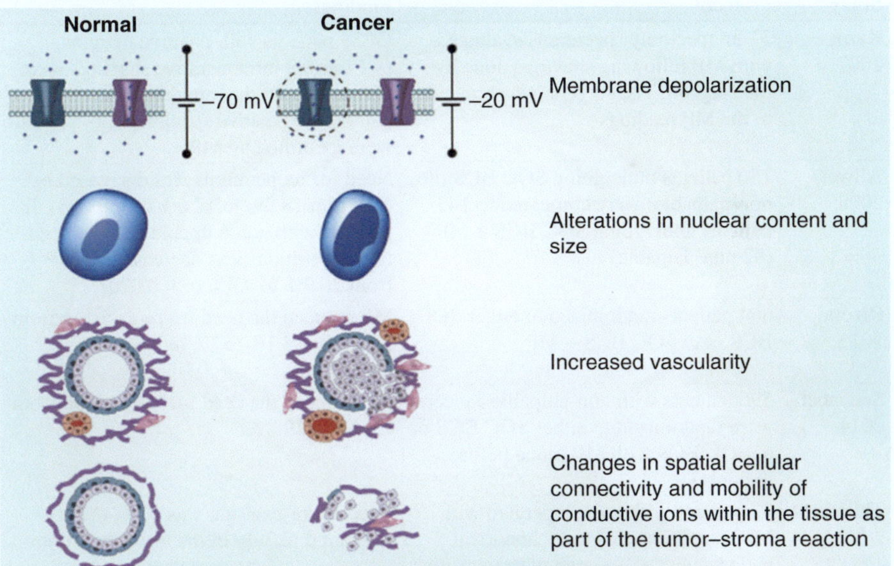

Fig. 13.8 Reasons for bioelectric differences in normal versus cancerous samples. The electrical properties of cells are affected when tissue becomes malignant. Changes in membrane properties, cells becoming larger as does the volume of their core (nucleus), changes in bonding of cells to each other, less order is observed among cells and growing tumours inducing generation of blood vessels in their vicinity (angiogenesis). (Reproduced from Thill et al. [58])

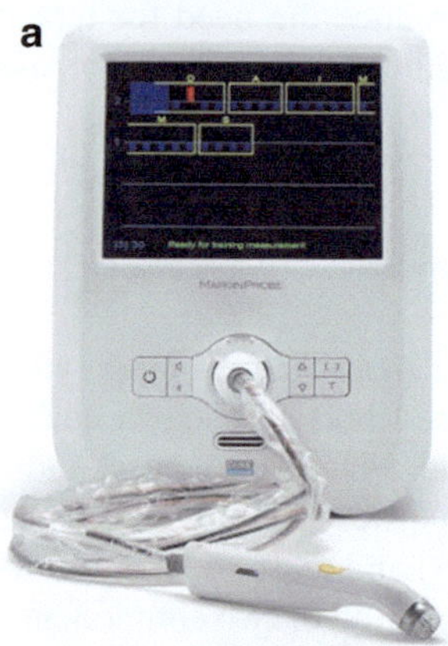
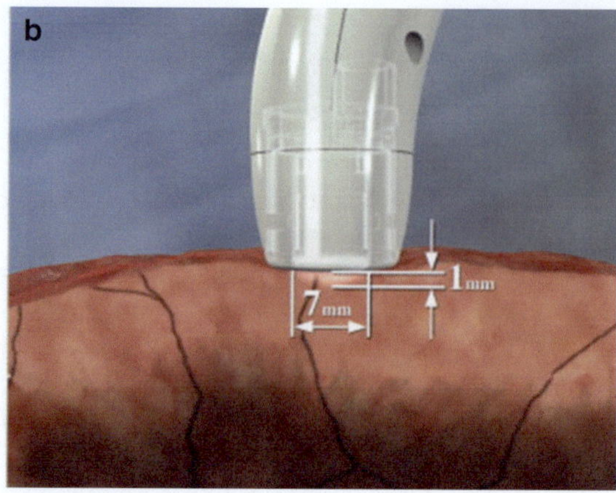

Fig. 13.9 (**a**) The MarginProbe system with the probe and device output display. Data accumulate on the screen from left to right and from top to bottom. Blue and red bars are negative and positive readings, respectively. Yellow frames and labels mark the margins from which readings were obtained. (**b**) The effective detection volume of the probe is 0.7 cm in diameter and 0.1 cm deep. (Reproduced from Dilon Medical Technologies, Inc. (https://dilon.com/marginprobe/) and from Karni et al. [59])

Table 13.1 Clinical studies and Randomised Controlled Trials (RCTs) of MarginProbe. Reproduced from Hoffman and Ashkenazi [72]

Study	Protocol	Findings
Karni 2007	57 lumpectomy specimens evaluated with MP following shavings done by the surgeon. The surgeon was blinded to the MP readings	Of 31 patients with positive margins ($\leq$1 mm), 9 intraoperative shavings were performed. Of the remaining 22 pathology- positive specimens, 19 patients were identified by MP
Allweis 2008	150 patients undergoing SOC BCS (86 non-palpable) were compared to 143 patients undergoing SOC BCS + MP (82 non-palpable)	Need for reoperations was decreased by MP from 18.6% to 12.6% ($p = 0.098$). In patients with non-palpable tumors, need for reoperations was decreased by MP from 20.9% to 9.8% ($p = 0.020$)
Rivera 2012	664 patients randomized to either SOC BCS or to SOC BCS + MP	MP reduced the need for re-excision from 29.9% to 14.1% (57% reduction; $p < 0.001$)
Schnabel 2014	596 patients with non-palpable cancers were randomized to either SOC BCS or to SOC BCS with MP (done before imaging)	MP reduced the need for re-excision from 25.8% to 19.8%
Thill 2014	42 patients with DCIS operated with MP were compared to 67 historical patients with a 39% rate of re-excision	Need for re-excision was 17%, lower compared to 39% in the historical controls
Sebastian 2015	Patients operated by 4 surgeons with MP compared to historical controls operated by the same surgeons	Re-excision rates reduced from 25.8% to 9.7%

Table 13.1 (continued)

Study	Protocol	Findings
Blohmer 2016	150 patients operated with MP were compared to 172 historical controls	MP decreased the need for re-excision in patients with invasive cancer (14.6% from 29.7%), invasive lobular subtype (19.0% from 37.0%) and DCIS (23.1% from 61.1%)
Coble 2017	Retrospective study of 137 patients operated with MP and 119 patients who received full cavity shaving	The need for re-excision was less in patients operated with MP (6.6% vs. 15.1%, $p = 0.026$). The breast volume resected was also less in patients operated with MP (78 ml vs. 116 ml; $p = 0.002$)
Kupstas 2018	240 consecutive patients; 120 operated without MP (SOC) between 10/2014 and 9/2015 were compared to 120 patients operated with MP between 10/2015 and 10/2016	Total re-excision rate was 18.2% in the SOC group and 9.2% in the MP group ($p = 0.039$). The conversion to mastectomy was the same in both groups (3.3%)
Gooch 2019	Cohort study of 341 patients undergoing BCS with use of the MP	Of 341 patients, 135 (39.6%) had a lumpectomy with positive margins. MP identified 101 (75%) of these margins. Additional shaving from negative margins resulted in positive final margins in 17 patients
Geha 2020	46 patients randomized to either SOC BCS or to SOC BCS with MP	8 (34.8%) were in need of re-excision in the control group compared to 1 (4.3%) in the MP group ($p = 0.022$)
LeeVan 2020	MP evaluated as adjunct to SOC BCS	MP demonstrated a sensitivity of 67%, specificity of 60%, positive predictive value of 16% and negative predictive value of 94%, results similar to specimen radiography and gross pathologic evaluation
Cen 2021	42 patients without complete response following neoadjuvant chemotherapy who underwent BCS, 16 were operated with the aid of MP and 26 were operated without the aid of MP	One of 16 operated with the aid of MP had involved/close margins, lower when compared to 8 with involved/closed margins of 26 who were operated without the aid of MP

MP Margin Probe©, *BCS* breast conserving surgery, *SOC* standard of care (refers to lumpectomy with re-excision of questionable margins guided by palpation or specimen radiography)

More specifically, Karni et al. [59] used MarginProbe to analyse 57 lumpectomy specimens and compared the diagnostic accuracy of the probe and histological results. Nineteen out of 22 (86%) pathology-positive patients were detected with the device. Sensitivity and specificity per margin were 71% and 68%, respectively, within a range of positive margin definitions (0–0.4 cm) (Fig. 13.9B).

In a different prospective, randomised trial by Allweis et al. [60], 300 patients were enrolled and, after exclusion of 7 patients that did not fit the inclusion criteria, 293 were analysed with the probe (143 and 150 in the "device" and "control" arms). Final diagnosis was confirmed using histology as the gold standard. Reoperation rate including mastectomy in the entire cohort was lower in the "device" arm when compared to the "control" arm, 12.6% (18/143) versus 18.6% (28/150), respectively; however, this difference did not achieve statistical significance ($p = 0.098$). When restricting to patients with non-palpable tumours only, the need for reoperations including mastectomy was decreased by the device from 20.9% (18/86) to 9.8% (8/82) ($p = 0.020$). The authors also showed that repeat lumpectomy rate was significantly reduced by 56% in the device arm: 5.6% (8/143) versus 12.7% (19/150) ($p = 0.0027$) in the control arm and therefore suggested that MarginProbe shows potential in decreasing the rate of repeat re-excisions.

The diagnostic performance of MarginProbe was also evaluated after analysis of freshly excised lumpectomy and mastectomy specimens from 76 patients [61]. Overall a total of 869 tissue measurement sited were obtained and 753 were analysed with 165 being cancerous and 588 being nonmalignant. The probe performed well on relatively homogeneous sites achieving 100% sensitivity (95% CI: 0.85–1) and 87% specificity (95% CI: 0.83–0.90), however, for the full dataset sensitivity was 70% (95% CI: 0.63–0.77) and specificity 70% (95% CI: 0.67–0.74). Device sensitivity was estimated to range between 56% and 97% as the cancer feature size increased from 0.7 to 6.6 mm.

In a multicentre randomised prospective study including 596 patients, Schnabel et al. [63] were able to resect all positive margins on positive main specimens in 62% (101 of 163) of cases in the device arm, versus 22% (33 of 147) in the control arm ($p < 0.001$). A total of 19.8% (59 of 298) of patients in the device arm underwent a re-excision procedure compared with 25.8% (77 of 298) in the control arm (6% absolute, 23% relative reduction). The margin-level sensitivity of the device was 75.2% (95% CI: 69.4–81.0) with that of the control arm being 33.9% (95% CI: 27.6–40.2), whilst margin-level specificity was only 46.4% (95% CI: 42.9–49.9) versus 83.4% of the control arm (95% CI: 81.0–85.8). False negative rates were 24.8 and 66.1% in the device and control arms, respectively, whereas false positive rates were 53.6 and 16.6%, in device and control arms, respectively.

Thill et al. [14] employed the MarginProbe to assess margins during breast conserving surgery of ductal carcinoma in situ in 42 patients enrolled in three different institutions. The device was used as an adjunctive tool to standard of care and was associated with a reduction in re-excision rates by 56%, from 39% to 17% ($p = 0.018$). Sensitivity was 57% (95% CI 48–66) and specificity 50% (95% CI 42–58). When using a clear margin threshold of 1 mm, sensitivity was slightly improved to 65% (95% CI 51–76) whereas specificity remained at 50% (95% CI 43–57).

Another study included 214 patients who received neoadjuvant chemotherapy (NAC) and 61 patients (28.5%) who had both NAC and breast conservation surgery [71]. Out of 61 patients that had surgery after NAC, 19 had pathologic complete response and were excluded from the analysis. Of the remaining 42 patients, 9 had close or positive margins that required re-excision. The authors demonstrated that MarginProbe use was associated with a lower-re-excision rate for patients who had NAC and surgery (6% versus 31%), supporting the use of this technique as an intraoperative tool in breast conservative surgery after NAC.

A more recent study by Hoffman and Ashkenazi [72] critically assessed the value of MarginProbe in detecting positive resection margins. The authors used MarginProbe in 48 patients with 51 tumour samples. Thirteen of the 51 lumpectomies had pathological close or involved margins. The probe was able to correctly identify only 3/13 positive margins with 97/287 margins being recorded as false positive readings. The achieved sensitivity, specificity, positive predictive value and negative predictive value were 23.1% (95%CI 5.0% 53.8%), 66.4% (95%CI 60.7%–71.9%), 3% (95%CI 0.6%–8.5%) and 95.1% (95%CI 91.1%–97.6%), respectively. Reviewing findings of previous studies on the probe device (Table 13.1), the authors noted that these were confounded by the fact that re-excision rates were at times calculated taking into consideration further shavings taken by the surgeons. Thus, lumpectomy margins shaving guided by intraoperative specimen mammography or by "surgeons' discretion" were not distinguished from MarginProbe-guided shavings. Based on their results, the authors of this study concluded that MarginProbe's ability to detect breast cancerous tissue within 1 mm of resection margins is low and its high false positive rate results in unacceptable unnecessary shavings. Going forward, further evaluation of the probe should be based on comparing the probe's result to pathology report.

13.2.2.6 Optical Coherence Tomography

Optical coherence tomography (OCT) is a high-resolution microscopic optical imaging technique that can provide real-time multidimensional images of subsurface tissue structures [73, 74] (penetration depth in breast tissues is ~1–2 mm), which renders it an ideal candidate for intraoperative tumour margin assessment. In 2009, Nguyen et al. [75] employed OCT for the intraoperative evaluation of breast tumour margins in a study of 37 patients that were split into a training ($n = 17$ patients) and a study group ($n = 20$). The training group was initially used to establish and optimise standard imaging protocols and OCT evaluation showed that areas of higher scattering tissue with a heterogeneous pattern were indicative of cancerous tissue in contrast to lower scattering adipocytes found in normal breast tissue. The study group was then used for the feasibility study. Out of these 20 lumpectomy specimens, 11 were identified with a positive or close surgical margin and 9 were identified with a negative margin under OCT. Based on histologic findings, 9 true positives, 9 true negatives, 2 false positives and 0 false negatives were found, yielding a sensitivity of 100% and specificity of 82%.

In a more recent study by Erickson-Batt et al. [76], a handheld surgical OCT imaging probe was developed for the in vivo analysis of 35 patients to assess margins both in the resection bed and on excised specimens. The OCT images showed structural differences between normal and cancerous tissue within the resection bed following wide local excision of the human breast. The ex vivo images were compared with standard postoperative histopathology and yield sensitivity of 91.7% (95% CI, 62.5%–100%) and specificity of 92.1% (95% CI, 78.4%–98%).

A different study using novel imaging techniques including high-resolution full-field optical coherence tomography (FFOCT) and dynamic cell imaging (DCI), reported high accuracy in detecting breast cancer and nodal metastasis [77]. A total of 314 specimens, including 173 breast biopsies (malignant, 132; benign/normal, 41) and 141 resected lymph nodes (tumour-positive, 48; tumour-negative, 93), were obtained from 158 patients during breast surgery for prospective imaging evaluations. In breast cancer diagnosis, the minimum sensitivities (FFOCT, 85.6%; DCI, 88.6%) and specificities of optical imaging (FFOCT, 85.4%; DCI, 95.1%) were high, although they diverged somewhat in nodal assessments (FFOCT sensitivity, 66.7%; FFOCT specificity, 79.6%; DCI sensitivity, 83.3%; DCI specificity, 98.9%). The potential use of FFOCT or DCI for margin assessment was preliminarily explored in a patient showing that margin distances determined by FFOCT, DCI and H&E staining were well matched.

13.2.2.7   Microcomputed Tomography

Microcomputed tomography (micro-CT) is a relatively new technology for breast tissue evaluation [78, 79], providing three-dimensional (3D) imaging of specimens with remarkable spatial resolution down to <1 μm [80]. Using micro-CT Tang et al. [81] performed a pilot study to evaluate shaved cavity margins (SCM) and develop this method for lumpectomy margin status prediction intraoperatively to enable rapid identification of tumour margins and reduce re-excision rates. Twenty-five SCM from six lumpectomies were evaluated with this method and results were compared to histopathological results. SCM were found negative by micro-CT in 19/25 (76%) which agreed with the negative reports (≥2 mm) by histopathology in 19/25 (76%). Margin status by micro-CT was concordant with histopathology in 23/25 (92%). Overall, the authors reported that micro-CT had an 83.3% positive predictive value, a 94.7% negative predictive value, 83.3% sensitivity and 94.7% specificity for evaluation of SCM.

In a more recent larger-cohort study by DiCorpo et al. [82], micro-CT was used to image 173 partial mastectomies (129 ductal carcinomas, 14 lobular carcinomas, 28 DCIS). Micro-CT revealed cancer touching the specimen edge for 93% of the 114 cases that had positive margins after histology, and 28 of the cases not seen as margin positive on pathological analysis; cancer occupied 1.55% of surface area when both the pathologist and Micro-CT suggested cancer at the edge, but only 0.45% of surface area for the "Micro-CT-Only-Positive Cases". The authors highlighted that micro-CT could, therefore, detect cancers that touch a very small region of the specimen surface, which is likely to be missed on sectioning.

13.2.2.8   Novel Pegulicianine Fluorescence-Guided System

A novel fluorescence-guided system (FGS) has been recently developed to accurately identify the microscopic extent of breast tumours and complete tumour excision during breast conservation surgery. The innovative system, developed by

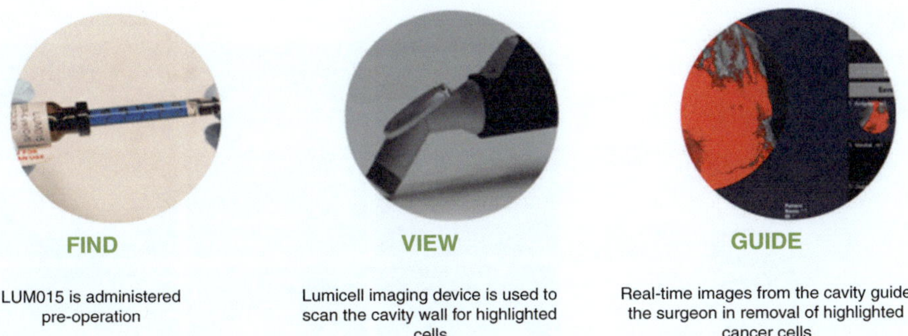

Fig. 13.10 Overview of a fluorescence-guided system (FGS) designed by Lumicell for real-time analysis of breast tissues during surgery. LUM015 is an investigational onco-fluorescent agent that targets the tumour microenvironment and is designed to fluoresce near cancer cells at the tumour margin when activated by proteases (left). A handheld, single-cell resolution imaging device is designed to fit into the lumpectomy cavity to scan for residual cancer at the margins (middle). Proprietary decision software produces real-time images indicating the potential location of residual cancer (right). (Reproduced from Lumicell, Inc. (http://www.lumicell.com/about/contact.php))

Lumicell, Wellesley, MA, is comprised of an activatable fluorescent agent, a handheld device and a patient-specific tumour detection algorithm (Fig. 13.10). Previous studies of pegulicianine FGS (pFGS) in 55 patients from one clinical centre showed that the technology could identify residual breast cancer in real time by directly analysing the lumpectomy cavity [83, 84].

In an interesting study published in 2022, Hwang et al. [85] *used* a novel pegulicianine fluorescence-guided system (pFGS) to assess its clinical impact for the intraoperative margin assessment during breast conserving surgery (BCS) (Fig. 13.11). This was a prospective single arm study conducted as a nonrandomised multicentre controlled trial performed within 16 breast centres in the USA. Female patients 18 years and older with newly diagnosed primary invasive breast cancer or ductal carcinoma in situ (DCIS) undergoing BCS were included; patients with previous breast cancer surgery and a history of dye allergies were excluded from this trial. Of 283 eligible patients recruited, 234 received a pegulicianine injection and were included in the safety analysis; of these, 230 were included in the efficacy analysis with all patients being monitored for a 30-day follow-up period. Participants received an injection of a novel imaging agent (pegulicianine) ~3.2 h prior to surgery at a dose of 1 mg/kg. After completing standard of care (SOC) excision, pFGS was used to scan the lumpectomy cavity to guide the removal of additional shave margins. Correlation of pFGS with final margin status on a per-margin analysis showed a marked improvement in sensitivity over standard pathology assessment of the main lumpectomy specimen (69.4% vs. 38.2%, respectively), whereas specificity was lower in comparison to pathology (70.4% vs. 91.2%). On a per-patient level, the false negative rate of pFGS was 23.7% (9 of 38) and sensitivity was 76.3% (29 of 38). Among 32 patients who underwent excision of pFGS-guided shaves, pFGS prevented the need for re-excision in 6 (19%). The authors confirmed the clinical

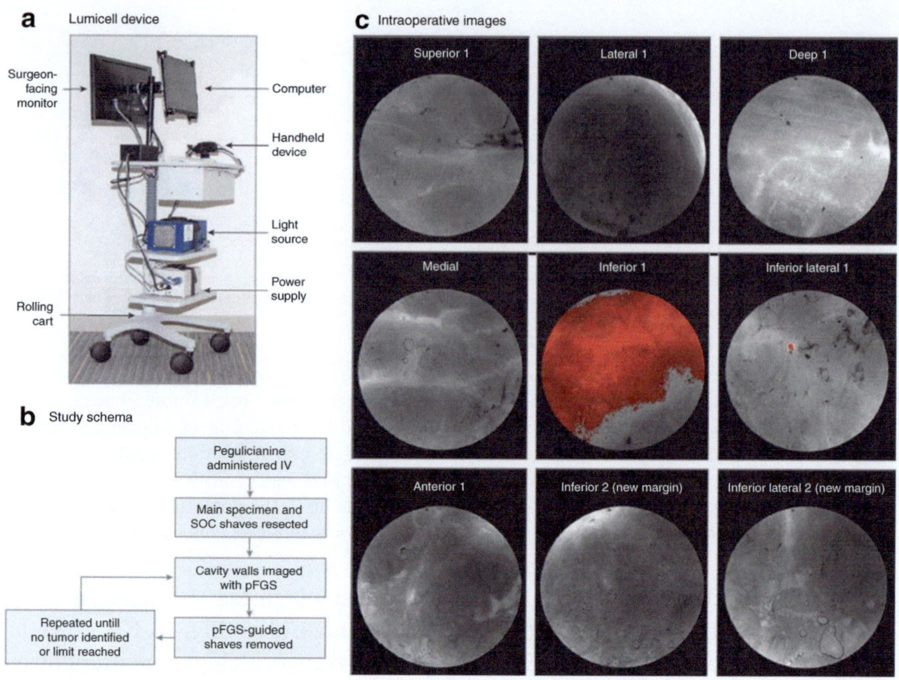

Fig. 13.11 The pegulicianine fluorescence-guided system (pFGS), study design for intraoperative use and intraoperative images. (**a**) The Lumicell study monitor was present either in person or virtually for each procedure to oversee device use and data collection. (**b**) Study schema for intraoperative use of the Lumicell device. Up to 2 additional shave margins were allowed per margin orientation. (**c**) Intraoperative images demonstrating a red signal indicating pFGS uptake. Additional shave margins were excised in the inferior and inferior lateral orientations with resultant elimination of signal. IV indicates intravenously. (Reproduced from Hwang et al. [85])

safety of the dye and concluded that pFGS reduced the need for second surgery in those who underwent additional pFGS-guided excisions and highlighted the need for follow-up on prospective randomised clinical trials.

13.3 Conclusions

Although there has been a significant progress over the last decades, it is evident that there is still a significant unmet need for a better, more accurate detection method to be intraoperatively used in patients undergoing breast conserving surgery to prevent local recurrence and additional surgery in the case of positive margins. A number of methods, such as frozen sections and imprint cytology, are currently used in clinical routine, however, these have significant clinical and technical limitations, including time-consuming sample preparation and analysis steps, manpower requirements and the potential for false positive interpretation. Moreover, current intraoperative examinations do not accurately identify the microscopic extent of tumour leading to incomplete surgical treatment in which case patients require re-excision; surgical margins determined by histopathology several days after initial lumpectomy can be found positive in up to 20–40% of patients [5–9]. Specimen radiology and intraoperative ultrasound can alternatively be used for margin status assessment within the operating theatre, however, compared to traditional pathological results they still have inferior accuracy [10] and have not translated to reductions in reoperation rates [86].

A number of emerging technologies with potential for intraoperatively detecting breast tumour margins have been described and discussed in this chapter. Such techniques could reduce positive margins, prevent breast cancer recurrence and further systemic therapy and lead to better cosmetic outcomes. Extra consideration should be taken for the analysis of human breast cancer tissues since they consist of multiple histopathological features and heterogenous borderline lesions, which comes in contrast with other cancers such as gastric, colorectal or pancreatic that mostly comprise of adenocarcinomas. Importantly, technologies that have shown promising data in intraoperative ex vivo settings should also be evaluated in in vivo settings if their intended application is real-time margin assessment within the surgical theatre.

References

1. Mushlin AI, Kouides RW, Shapiro DE. Estimating the accuracy of screening mammography: a meta-analysis. Am J Prev Med. 1998;14:143–53.
2. de Boniface J, Szulkin R, Johansson AL. Survival after breast conservation vs mastectomy adjusted for comorbidity and socioeconomic status: a Swedish national 6-year follow-up of 48 986 women. JAMA Surg. 2021;156:628–37.
3. de Koning SGB, Peeters M-JTV, Jóźwiak K, Bhairosing PA, Ruers TJ. Tumor resection margin definitions in breast-conserving surgery: systematic review and meta-analysis of the current literature. Clin Breast Cancer. 2018;18:e595–600.
4. Wj H, As E, Js R, Parker C, Dh B. Rates of margin positive resection with breast conservation for invasive breast cancer using the NCDB. Breast. 2021;60:86–9. https://doi.org/10.1016/j.breast.2021.08.012.
5. Chagpar AB, et al. A randomized, controlled trial of cavity shave margins in breast cancer. N Engl J Med. 2015;373:503–10. https://doi.org/10.1056/NEJMoa1504473.
6. Coopey S, et al. The safety of multiple re-excisions after lumpectomy for breast cancer. Ann Surg Oncol. 2011;18:3797–801. https://doi.org/10.1245/s10434-011-1802-4.
7. Coopey SB, et al. Lumpectomy cavity shaved margins do not impact re-excision rates in breast cancer patients. Ann Surg Oncol. 2011;18:3036. https://doi.org/10.1245/s10434-011-1909-7.
8. Esbona K, Li Z, Wilke LG. Intraoperative imprint cytology and frozen section pathology for margin assessment in breast conservation surgery: a systematic review. Ann Surg Oncol. 2012;19:3236–45. https://doi.org/10.1245/s10434-012-2492-2.
9. McCahill LE, et al. Variability in reexcision following breast conservation surgery. JAMA. 2012;307:467–75. https://doi.org/10.1001/jama.2012.43.
10. St John ER, et al. Diagnostic accuracy of intraoperative techniques for margin assessment in breast cancer surgery. Ann Surg. 2017;265:300–10.

11. Laucirica R. Intraoperative assessment of the breast: guidelines and potential pitfalls. Arch Pathol Lab Med. 2005;129:1565–74.

12. Weinberg E, et al. Local recurrence in lumpectomy patients after imprint cytology margin evaluation. Am J Surg. 2004;188:349–54.

13. Pradipta AR, et al. Emerging technologies for real-time intraoperative margin assessment in future breast-conserving surgery. Adv Sci. 2020;7:1901519.

14. Thill M, Dittmer C, Baumann K, Friedrichs K, Blohmer J-U. MarginProbe® – final results of the German post-market study in breast conserving surgery of ductal carcinoma in situ. Breast. 2014;23:94–6. https://doi.org/10.1016/j.breast.2013.11.002.

15. Alexiou GA, et al. Fast cell cycle analysis for intraoperative characterization of brain tumor margins and malignancy. J Clin Neurosci. 2015;22:129–32. https://doi.org/10.1016/j.jocn.2014.05.029.

16. Vartholomatos G, et al. Intraoperative cell cycle analysis for tumor margins evaluation: the future is now? Int J Surg. 2018;53:380–1. https://doi.org/10.1016/j.ijsu.2018.03.046.

17. Vartholomatos G, et al. Intraoperative flow cytometry for head and neck lesions. Assessment of malignancy and tumour-free resection margins. Oral Oncol. 2019;99:104344. https://doi.org/10.1016/j.oraloncology.2019.06.025.

18. Shioyama T, Muragaki Y, Maruyama T, Komori T, Iseki H. Intraoperative flow cytometry analysis of glioma tissue for rapid determination of tumor presence and its histopathological grade. J Neurosurg. 2013;118:1232–8.

19. Alexiou GA, et al. The role of fast cell cycle analysis in pediatric brain tumors. Pediatr Neurosurg. 2015;50:257–63.

20. Vartholomatos G, et al. Rapid assessment of resection margins during breast conserving surgery using intraoperative flow cytometry. Clin Breast Cancer. 2021;21:e602–10.

21. Paraskevaidi M, et al. Clinical applications of infrared and Raman spectroscopy in the fields of cancer and infectious diseases. Appl Spectrosc Rev. 2021;56:804–68.

22. Jermyn M, et al. Intraoperative brain cancer detection with Raman spectroscopy in humans. Sci Transl Med. 2015;7:274ra219. https://doi.org/10.1126/scitranslmed.aaa2384.

23. Lin K, et al. Rapid fiber-optic Raman spectroscopy for real-time in vivo detection of gastric intestinal metaplasia during clinical gastroscopy. Cancer Prev Res. 2016;9:476–83.

24. Malik A, et al. In vivo Raman spectroscopy–assisted early identification of potential second primary/recurrences in oral cancers: an exploratory study. Head Neck. 2017;39:2216–23.

25. McGregor HC, et al. Real-time endoscopic Raman spectroscopy for in vivo early lung cancer detection. J Biophotonics. 2017;10:98–110.

26. Wang J, et al. Simultaneous fingerprint and high-wavenumber fiber-optic Raman spectroscopy improves in vivo diagnosis of esophageal squamous cell carcinoma at endoscopy. Sci Rep. 2015;5:1–10.

27. Zhao J, Lui H, Kalia S, Zeng H. Real-time Raman spectroscopy for automatic in vivo skin cancer detection: an independent validation. Anal Bioanal Chem. 2015;407:8373–9.

28. Zhao J, Zeng H, Kalia S, Lui H. Wavenumber selection based analysis in Raman spectroscopy improves skin cancer diagnostic specificity. Analyst. 2016;141:1034–43.

29. Schleusener J, et al. In vivo study for the discrimination of cancerous and normal skin using fibre probe-based Raman spectroscopy. Exp Dermatol. 2015;24:767–72.

30. Shipp DW, et al. Intra-operative spectroscopic assessment of surgical margins during breast conserving surgery. Breast Cancer Res. 2018;20:69. https://doi.org/10.1186/s13058-018-1002-2.

31. Haka AS, et al. In vivo margin assessment during partial mastectomy breast surgery using Raman spectroscopy. Cancer Res. 2006;66:3317–22.

32. Talari AC, Rehman S, Rehman IU. Advancing cancer diagnostics with artificial intelligence and spectroscopy: identifying chemical changes associated with breast cancer. Expert Rev Mol Diagn. 2019;19:929–40.

33. Surmacki J, Brozek-Pluska B, Kordek R, Abramczyk H. The lipid-reactive oxygen species phenotype of breast cancer. Raman spectroscopy and mapping, PCA and PLSDA for invasive ductal carcinoma and invasive lobular carcinoma. Molecular tumorigenic mechanisms beyond Warburg effect. Analyst. 2015;140:2121–33.

34. Haka AS, et al. Diagnosing breast cancer by using Raman spectroscopy. Proc Natl Acad Sci. 2005;102:12371–6.
35. Haka AS, et al. Diagnosing breast cancer using Raman spectroscopy: prospective analysis. J Biomed Opt. 2009;14:054023.
36. Stone N, Baker R, Rogers K, Parker AW, Matousek P. Subsurface probing of calcifications with spatially offset Raman spectroscopy (SORS): future possibilities for the diagnosis of breast cancer. Analyst. 2007;132:899–905.
37. Keller MD, et al. Development of a spatially offset Raman spectroscopy probe for breast tumor surgical margin evaluation. J Biomed Opt. 2011;16:077006.
38. Wang Y, et al. Raman-encoded molecular imaging with topically applied SERS nanoparticles for intraoperative guidance of Lumpectomy. Cancer Res. 2017;77:4506–16.
39. Stevens O, Petterson IEI, Day JC, Stone N. Developing fibre optic Raman probes for applications in clinical spectroscopy. Chem Soc Rev. 2016;45:1919–34.
40. Yang N, et al. Urinary glycoprotein biomarker discovery for bladder cancer detection using LC/MS-MS and label-free quantification. Clin Cancer Res. 2011;17:3349–59.
41. Lubes G, Goodarzi M. GC–MS based metabolomics used for the identification of cancer volatile organic compounds as biomarkers. J Pharm Biomed Anal. 2018;147:313–22.
42. Rodrigo MAM, et al. MALDI-TOF MS as evolving cancer diagnostic tool: a review. J Pharm Biomed Anal. 2014;95:245–55.
43. Balog J, et al. Intraoperative tissue identification using rapid evaporative ionization mass spectrometry. Sci Transl Med. 2013;5:194ra193.
44. Paraskevaidi M, et al. Laser-assisted rapid evaporative ionisation mass spectrometry (LA-REIMS) as a metabolomics platform in cervical cancer screening. EBioMedicine. 2020;60:103017.
45. Tzafetas M, et al. The intelligent-knife (i-knife) and its intraoperative diagnostic advantage for the treatment of cervical disease. Proc Natl Acad Sci U S A. 2020;117:7338–46.
46. Phelps DL, et al. The surgical intelligent knife distinguishes normal, borderline and malignant gynaecological tissues using rapid evaporative ionisation mass spectrometry (REIMS). Br J Cancer. 2018;118:1349–58. https://doi.org/10.1038/s41416-018-0048-3.
47. Dória ML, et al. Epithelial ovarian carcinoma diagnosis by desorption electrospray ionization mass spectrometry imaging. Sci Rep. 2016;6:39219.
48. Alexander J, et al. A novel methodology for in vivo endoscopic phenotyping of colorectal cancer based on real-time analysis of the mucosal lipidome: a prospective observational study of the iKnife. Surg Endosc. 2017;31:1361–70. https://doi.org/10.1007/s00464-016-5121-5.
49. St John ER, et al. Rapid evaporative ionisation mass spectrometry of electrosurgical vapours for the identification of breast pathology: towards an intelligent knife for breast cancer surgery. Breast Cancer Res. 2017;19:59.
50. Calligaris D, et al. Application of desorption electrospray ionization mass spectrometry imaging in breast cancer margin analysis. Proc Natl Acad Sci U S A. 2014;111:15184–9. https://doi.org/10.1073/pnas.1408129111.
51. Zhang J, et al. Nondestructive tissue analysis for ex vivo and in vivo cancer diagnosis using a handheld mass spectrometry system. Sci Transl Med. 2017;9:eaan3968.
52. Takáts Z, Wiseman JM, Gologan B, Cooks RG. Mass spectrometry sampling under ambient conditions with desorption electrospray ionization. Science. 2004;306:471–3.
53. Buchberger AR, DeLaney K, Johnson J, Li L. Mass spectrometry imaging: a review of emerging advancements and future insights. Anal Chem. 2018;90:240–65. https://doi.org/10.1021/acs.analchem.7b04733.
54. Ifa DR, Eberlin LS. Ambient ionization mass spectrometry for cancer diagnosis and surgical margin evaluation. Clin Chem. 2016;62:111–23.
55. Dill AL, Ifa DR, Manicke NE, Ouyang Z, Cooks RG. Mass spectrometric imaging of lipids using desorption electrospray ionization. J Chromatogr B. 2009;877:2883–9.
56. Guenther S, et al. Spatially resolved metabolic phenotyping of breast cancer by desorption electrospray ionization mass spectrometry. Cancer Res. 2015;75:1828–37. https://doi.org/10.1158/0008-5472.Can-14-2258.

57. Dixon JM, et al. Intra-operative assessment of excised breast tumour margins using ClearEdge imaging device. Eur J Surg Oncol. 2016;42:1834–40. https://doi.org/10.1016/j. ejso.2016.07.141.
58. Thill M. MarginProbe®: intraoperative margin assessment during breast conserving surgery by using radiofrequency spectroscopy. Expert Rev Med Devices. 2013;10:301–15.
59. Karni T, et al. A device for real-time, intraoperative margin assessment in breast-conservation surgery. Am J Surg. 2007;194:467–73.
60. Allweis TM, et al. A prospective, randomized, controlled, multicenter study of a real-time, intraoperative probe for positive margin detection in breast-conserving surgery. Am J Surg. 2008;196:483–9. https://doi.org/10.1016/j.amjsurg.2008.06.024.
61. Pappo I, et al. Diagnostic performance of a novel device for real-time margin assessment in lumpectomy specimens. J Surg Res. 2010;160:277–81. https://doi.org/10.1016/j. jss.2009.02.025.
62. Rivera RJ, Holmes DR, Tafra L. Analysis of the impact of intraoperative margin assessment with adjunctive use of MarginProbe versus standard of care on tissue volume removed. Int J Surg Oncol. 2012;2012:868623.
63. Schnabel F, et al. A randomized prospective study of lumpectomy margin assessment with use of MarginProbe in patients with nonpalpable breast malignancies. Ann Surg Oncol. 2014;21:1589–95. https://doi.org/10.1245/s10434-014-3602-0.
64. Sebastian M, Akbari S, Anglin B, Lin EH, Police AM. The impact of use of an intraoperative margin assessment device on re-excision rates. Springerplus. 2015;4:1–6.
65. Blohmer J-U, et al. MarginProbe© reduces the rate of re-excision following breast conserving surgery for breast cancer. Arch Gynecol Obstet. 2016;294:361–7.
66. Coble J, Reid V. Achieving clear margins. Directed shaving using MarginProbe, as compared to a full cavity shave approach. Am J Surg. 2017;213:627–30.
67. Kupstas A, et al. A novel modality for intraoperative margin assessment and its impact on re-excision rates in breast conserving surgery. Am J Surg. 2018;215:400–3.
68. Gooch JC, et al. The relationship of breast density and positive lumpectomy margins. Ann Surg Oncol. 2019;26:1729–36.
69. Geha RC, Taback B, Cadena L, Borden B, Feldman S. A single institution's randomized double-armed prospective study of lumpectomy margins with adjunctive use of the MarginProbe in nonpalpable breast cancers. Breast J. 2020;26:2157–62.
70. LeeVan E, Ho BT, Seto S, Shen J. Use of MarginProbe as an adjunct to standard operating procedure does not significantly reduce re-excision rates in breast conserving surgery. Breast Cancer Res Treat. 2020;183:145–51. https://doi.org/10.1007/s10549-020-05773-5.
71. Cen C, et al. Margin assessment and re-excision rates for patients who have neoadjuvant chemotherapy and breast-conserving surgery. Ann Surg Oncol. 2021;28:5142–8.
72. Hoffman A, Ashkenazi I. The efficiency of MarginProbe in detecting positive resection margins in epithelial breast cancer following breast conserving surgery. Eur J Surg Oncol. 2022;48:1498–502. https://doi.org/10.1016/j.ejso.2022.02.021.
73. Boppart SA, et al. In vivo cellular optical coherence tomography imaging. Nat Med. 1998;4:861–5.
74. Huang D, et al. Optical coherence tomography. Science. 1991;254:1178–81.
75. Nguyen FT, et al. Intraoperative evaluation of breast tumor margins with optical coherence tomography. Cancer Res. 2009;69:8790–6. https://doi.org/10.1158/0008-5472.Can-08-4340.
76. Erickson-Bhatt SJ, et al. Real-time imaging of the resection bed using a handheld probe to reduce incidence of microscopic positive margins in cancer surgery. Cancer Res. 2015;75:3706–12. https://doi.org/10.1158/0008-5472.Can-15-0464.
77. Yang H, et al. Use of high-resolution full-field optical coherence tomography and dynamic cell imaging for rapid intraoperative diagnosis during breast cancer surgery. Cancer. 2020;126:3847–56. https://doi.org/10.1002/cncr.32838.
78. Gufler H, Franke FE, Wagner S, Rau WS. Fine structure of breast tissue on micro computed tomography: a feasibility study. Acad Radiol. 2011;18:230–4.

79. Gufler H, Wagner S, Franke FE. The interior structure of breast microcalcifications assessed with micro computed tomography. Acta Radiol. 2011;52:592–6.
80. Ritman EL. Current status of developments and applications of micro-CT. Annu Rev Biomed Eng. 2011;13:531–52.
81. Tang R, et al. A pilot study evaluating shaved cavity margins with micro-computed tomography: a novel method for predicting lumpectomy margin status intraoperatively. Breast J. 2013;19:485–9. https://doi.org/10.1111/tbj.12146.
82. DiCorpo D, et al. The role of micro-CT in imaging breast cancer specimens. Breast Cancer Res Treat. 2020;180:343–57. https://doi.org/10.1007/s10549-020-05547-z.
83. Smith BL, et al. Real-time, intraoperative detection of residual breast cancer in lumpectomy cavity walls using a novel cathepsin-activated fluorescent imaging system. Breast Cancer Res Treat. 2018;171:413–20.
84. Smith BL, et al. Feasibility study of a novel protease-activated fluorescent imaging system for real-time, intraoperative detection of residual breast cancer in breast conserving surgery. Ann Surg Oncol. 2020;27:1854–61.
85. Hwang ES, et al. Clinical impact of intraoperative margin assessment in breast-conserving surgery with a novel pegulicianine fluorescence–guided system: a nonrandomized controlled trial. JAMA Surg. 2022;157:573.
86. Weber WP, et al. Accuracy of frozen section analysis versus specimen radiography during breast-conserving surgery for nonpalpable lesions. World J Surg. 2008;32:2599–606.

Chapter 14
Intraoperative Flow Cytometry in Lumpectomy

Angelos Pazidis and Haralampos V. Harissis

14.1 Introduction

It is estimated that more than 400,000 women are diagnosed with breast cancer every year in the European Union and a little less than 100,000 die of the disease in the same period of time. The improved therapies, both surgical and non-surgical, and also the early-stage diagnosis has led to a general improvement in the survival figures but the incidence keeps rising [1].

New therapies and new approaches always emerge in the field of breast cancer but surgery has always been the core of every therapeutic approach in the vast majority of the cases.

14.2 The Evolution of Breast Conserving Therapy (BCT)

Mastectomy used to be the classical surgical treatment for breast cancer. More limited excisions, like quadrantectomies and lumpectomies, were initially considered for patients with smaller tumours and were offered very cautiously. The picture in the surgical field started to change with the first studies published in the 1980s which revealed that the survival rates between the patients who had a radical mastectomy and those who underwent less radical operations with breast

A. Pazidis
Clinical Fellow in Pelvic Floor Surgery at NHS Tayside, Dundee, Scotland, UK

H. V. Harissis (✉)
Breast Unit, University Hospital of Ioannina, Ioannina, Greece

G. Alexiou, G. Vartholomatos (eds.), *Intraoperative Flow Cytometry*,
https://doi.org/10.1007/978-3-031-33517-4_14

conservation were not significantly different [2–5]. For some of the studies there was no difference in overall survival, disease free survival and distant-disease free survival [6]. Even then, the definition of a small or early-stage tumour varied amongst different studies, with some considering tumours <2 cm suitable for BCT while others included tumours of up to 4 cm [4, 5], thus making those first results difficult to combine and, more importantly, to translate to clinical practice.

More coherent evidence regarding the similar outcomes between and BCT and mastectomy with a clear cut-off for the tumour size amenable to local excision (set at 5 cm) was given by the 10,801 trial, a multi-centre, randomised prospective trial carried out by the European Organization for Research and Treatment of Cancer. The study found no statistically significant difference in the overall survival rate and in the distant metastasis free survival between the patients who had a modified radical mastectomy and those who had lumpectomy and radiotherapy. It did sow though a higher rate of locoregional recurrence in the BCT group [6]. The same or similar results have been reproduced by more other trials with long follow-up data which have not shown any significant differences in any of the survival parameters [7, 8].

After the safety of BCT and the good results published, the approach gained greater acceptance by breast surgeons and was widely adopted. Newer studies that were published in 2010s not only confirmed the results of the previous studies but also found that BCT might actually be superior to the traditional modified radical mastectomy, at least in certain patient subgroups. The biggest studies published come from big databases of prospectively collected data, such as registries, and incorporate a sizeable population of patients and as such give real-life information. The results from a Norwegian registry study showed that BCT patients had a better or at least equal overall and breast-cancer-specific survival compared to mastectomy patients, a benefit that applied to patients with up to cT2N1M0 tumours [9]. Almost identical results were published in a study based on data from Surveillance, Epidemiology and End Results-SEER database. The study also referred to patients with the up to cT2N1M0 cancers and showed a clear survival benefit for the BCT group (lumpectomy and radiotherapy) compared to mastectomy with or without radiotherapy. The results seem to clearly favour BCT as far as the 5- and 10-year breast cancer-specific survival is concerned and the difference is not affected by the patients' age or nodal status [10]. Similar impressive and encouraging results were also published elsewhere, showing that the benefit is maintained and is independent of the tumour characteristics and other prognostic factors [11] although other studies have suggested that the overall survival is similar between the two groups in more advanced nodal stages (N2-N3) and that possibly the benefit in survival seen in the BCT groups might be more pronounced in patients older than 50 years [12] or might depend on the receptor status of the tumours, with better survival figures in HR-negative patients [13].

14.3 The Surgical Margins

Early on in the course of BCT the question of the adequate resection margins was raised and with it came the question of the significance of the clear margins and the impact of the involved (or not clear) margins on the long-term therapy outcomes. Many factors have been studied and found to be associated with an increased risk of local recurrence and/or lower survival rates, amongst which the patient's age, the tumour characteristics or the use of hormone therapy.

14.3.1 The Significance of the Resection Margin

The involved margin in a lumpectomy seems to be, according to some studies at least, the single, most important predictor of local recurrence as far as the surgical management is concerned [14, 15], with the risk being more than twofold in patients with inadequate margins [16].

Published data suggested that there might be a correlation between involved margins and distant metastasis, and the time-to-distant disease, especially in younger women, and this is perceived to contribute significantly to the decreased survival rates and higher risk of death in those patients [17]. The link between local recurrence and distant metastasis has been described in many studies but whether there is a causative relationship or just a correlation could not be established [18], but the connection is certainly very strong with the risk for distant metastases being almost 2.5 times higher in patients with a local recurrence [19]. Of course it has to be said that this higher risk might not apply universally to all cases with involved margins; for example, a study form the Netherlands has shown that margin involvement over a length of less than 4 mm does not seem to adversely affect the locoregional control of the disease compared to "no ink on tumour" cases [20].

14.3.2 Defining the Negative Resection Margin

It has now been established that the negative margin is of utmost importance for the locoregional control of the disease while it also plays a pivotal role in the distant recurrences and the survival rates of the patients managed with BCT. The definition of the negative margin though has not been clear and unequivocal in the history of BCT. In the beginning, clear margins of 10 mm, or occasionally more, were required for a local excision to be considered adequate. The lack of robust data and general consensus meant that even the big randomised controlled studies that more or less lead to the wider adoption of BCT used different definitions of a negative margin, ranging between the currently accepted "no ink on tumour" (namely no cancer cells detected on the resection margins of the specimen the surface of which are dyed with ink before the specimen is sectioned for histopathological examination) on one side of the spectrum, all the way up to requiring a rim of 2–3 cm of normal breast tissue around the tumour on the other extreme [21, 22]. Of course, this created significant heterogeneity between the studies thus making data synthesis and the interpretation of the results more difficult and uncertain.

The debate about the margins continued for a long time, and the definition of the negative margin differed so much so amongst researchers as amongst clinical specialists. Very indicative of this lack of agreement was the fact that in the early 2000s in the fifth International consensus conference of the Breast health institute in Milan everyone agreed the "no ink on tumour" is absolutely essential but many specialists expressed the view that wider margins might be more appropriate [23]. Roughly at the same period, in 2005, a big survey in which more than 1000 radiotherapy oncologists from the USA and Europe were involved was published. The survey revealed that less than half of the responders would consider "no tumour on ink" as a negative margin while the rest would require a clear margin of 1 mm, 2 mm or even 5 mm from the edge of the tumour [24]. A few years later, in 2010, a big systematic review and meta-analysis that in total involved more than 14,500 patients added, according to some interpretations, to the uncertainty by revealing a weak trend towards better locoregional control of the disease with wider margins (but no added benefit for more than 2 mm). Factoring out, though, the patients who received any sort of adjuvant therapy there was no difference between the various margin groups and the researchers concluded that no actual benefit could be expected by wider than "no ink on tumour" margins [25].

A further, crucial step was taken a few years later, when the Society of Surgical Oncology and the American Society for Radiation Oncology jointly concluded in a consensus that effectively stated that margins wider than "no ink on tumour" are unlikely to offer any benefit in the locoregional control of the disease [26]. The consensus statement was based on a carefully organised and conducted systematic review and meta-analysis of 33 studies that collectively included more than 28,000 patients and found that the odds for local recurrence truly increased with the actual status of the margins, namely the presence or absence of tumour cells on the resection margin, but not with the distance of the tumour from the margin [27]. After the consensus guideline was published, and widely accepted in clinical practice, the re-excision rates for positive margins almost halved, dropping from 22% (when a variable margin of 1 or 2 mm was considered necessary in many cases) to 14% with the new definition, a meta-analysis found [28]. The exact same trend was observed in a retrospective analysis of data from the American society of Breast Surgeons Mastery database aiming to identify the reasons for re-excision. The overall excision rate amongst 6725 patients was found to be 21.6% but only half of them (49.7%) had tumour on the inked margin and the rest underwent a re-excision in order to ensure a clear margin of 1 mm or 2 mm [29].

14.3.2.1 Special Considerations-BCT and Margins in DCIS

BCT is feasible and safe for patients with DCIS given that the disease can be completely resected with good cosmetic outcome. The completeness of the resection brings the resection margins in the discussion again. It has been shown and is more or less widely accepted that wider margins are more appropriate in DCIS than in invasive cancer cases. A big meta-analysis followed by a consensus guideline, found that patients with DCIS treated with local excisions had a two-fold greater risk of local recurrence if the initial resection margins were narrower than 2 mm, which is now the accepted cut-off [30, 31]. Whether all the patients with narrower margins will definitely require re-excision though still remains in question as does the long-term survival benefit of a re-excision in these cases [32].

14.4 Trying to Ensure Negative Margins; Techniques and Different Approaches

Ensuring a pathologically negative margin is very important and positive margins can adversely affect the patients' oncological outcome. Of course re-excision, either local or with a mastectomy, can many cases mitigate the effects of an initially positive margin, as discussed above. This comes at a price though. The patients will require a second operation, with the additional financial cost for the system but, more importantly, the added psychological burden for the patient. A second operation also means a worse cosmetic outcome in at least some of the cases and, depending on the particular circumstances, might even necessitate a formal mastectomy [33]. Several techniques or approaches to minimise the margin positivity in the initial operation have been described in the literature.

The first step should of course always be a detailed preoperative assessment of the tumour with the appropriate imaging modalities in order to establish the feasibility of the BCT approach and then to plan, preoperatively, the margins of the excision. These methods have been extensively reviewed in the literature and their description here goes beyond the scope if this chapter.

Focusing on the intraoperative assessment of the resection margins, different centres tried to solve the problem in different ways. One of the first and most logical approaches, also utilised in other fields of surgery, was the use of frozen section of the margins and the imprint cytology. A recent meta-analysis collected and analysed data from 35 studies exploring different techniques of intraoperative margin assessment. The techniques examined included, amongst others, intraoperative US, optical spectroscopy, imprint cytology and frozen section. The results showed that the latter two were superior to all other approaches tested in the individual studies with sensitivity and specificity reaching as high as 91% and 95%, respectively [34]. Some, but not all, studies have shown that these good results from the frozen section assessment also translate to a reduction in the re-excision rates [35–37]. The frozen section of course requires an experienced pathologist, good margin sampling and assessment and can be time-consuming which translates to increased operative times, something that can prove to be challenging in time-restricted theatre setups.

One of the first, non-pathology approaches used to assess the margin status in the resected specimen was MarginProbe. The system uses radiofrequency spectroscopy to identify the presence of cancer cells on the resection margin. One of the earliest randomised controlled trials published in 2008 showed a 56% relative reduction in the re-excision rates [38]. A more recent, multi-centre RCT though revealed a false negative rate of 24.6% and a false-positive rate of 53.6% resulting in a relative reduction of the re-excision rates of 23% compared to the control arm [39]. Another approach that has gained some wider acceptance especially in certain countries is the cavity shaving, in which an extra rim of tissue is excised from the remaining cavity after the initial excision has taken place. In this case the actual resection margins are not assessed intraoperatively. Several studies have shown good results with this approach. A randomised controlled study involving 235 patients showed a reduction in the margin positivity from 34% in the control group to 19% in the cavity shaving group [40]. A more recent multi-centre RCT showed an even greater reduction in the margin positivity which translated to a reduction in the re-excision rated from 23.5% to 8.7% [41].

14.5 Flow Cytometry in Breast Lumpectomy

Each of the methods used and described previously have their merits but also their limitations. For example, frozen sections require an experienced pathologist and usually are time-consuming whereas margin probe comes at the additional cost of the equipment. A new approach that has been used in other cancers is intraoperative flow cytometry.

Flow cytometry as a method for the intraoperative assessment of the presence of tumour cells in central nervous system cancer surgery was first developed and tested independently by two research groups, one in Tokyo, Japan and one in Ioannina, Greece [42]. After the first very promising results of the method, its use was further tested in other areas of cancer surgery, amongst which in breast conserving surgery. With the importance of the resection margin in breast surgery already illustrated, it is more than clear why having an accurate but also quick tool is absolutely necessary. The Ioannina technique, described in detailed steps below, includes a thorough sampling of the margins of resection. The samples are then assessed with flow cytometry with a DNA index and cell cycle fraction analysis, the principles of which are detailed earlier in this book.

14.5.1 The Technique

After the tumour has been resected and the specimen is orientated for the pathology assessment, all the surfaces (5 or 6 depending on whether the skin is included in the specimen) are meticulously and thoroughly sampled with a cytology brush

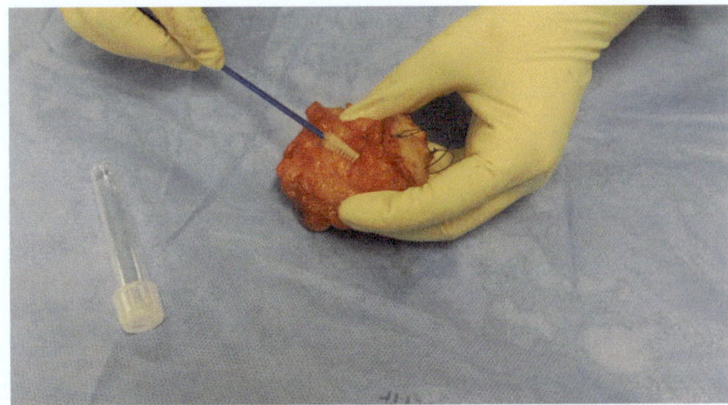

Fig. 14.1 Sampling the specimen margins with brushing

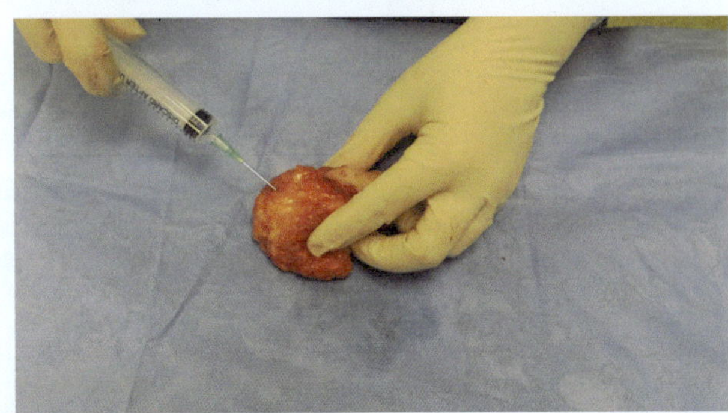

Fig. 14.2 FNA of the tumour

(Fig. 14.1). The tumour itself is sampled too with fine needle aspiration-FNA (Fig. 14.2). Depending on the DNA index the samples can be eu-, hypo- or hyperploid. As far as the cell cycle fraction is concerned, a cut-off of 5% of the malignancy index (S-phase fraction [SPF] + G2/M-phase fraction) was used to detect pathological samples. All the details of the sampling and cytometry analysis, the evolution of the technique and the process of defining the range of the accepted values can be found in Chaps. 4 and 5 of this book and also in the original article [33].

14.5.2   Results

The results from the use of intraoperative flow cytometry have been very promising. An initial assessment of 606 samples, retrieved from 99 patients who underwent breast conserving surgery, where intraoperative flow cytometry was compared to the final pathological assessment of the margins revealed that the technique had a sensitivity of 93.3% and a specificity of 92.4%. The sensitivity of the intraoperative cytology on the same samples was 82.3% [33]. The flow cytometry had a surprisingly low number of false negative findings (0.2% of the total number of samples) [33] and this is quite an important parameter, as the intraoperative false negative results will expose the patient to a second operation for re-excision. The role of the ploidy and the cell cycle fraction assessment in breast cancer has been widely

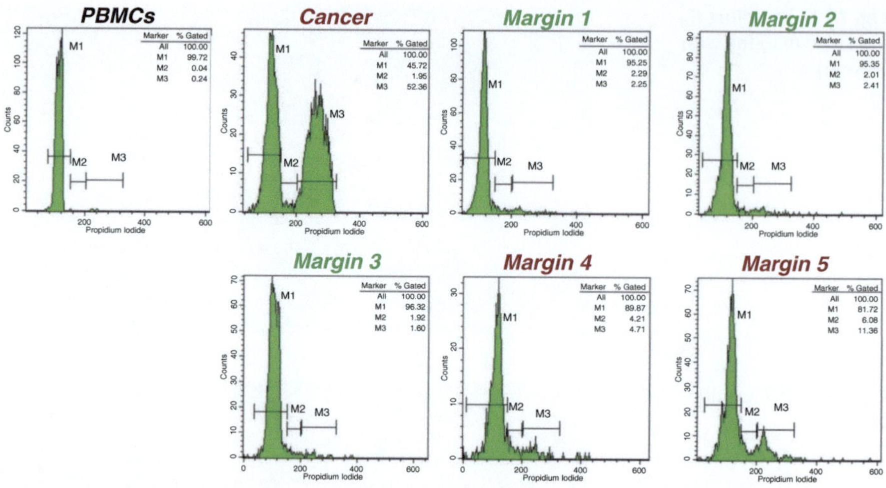

Fig. 14.3 A representative analysis of breast cancer using intraoperative flow cytometry. DNA content was quantified following propidium iodide staining. Markers M1, M2 and M3 denote cells in G0/G1, S and G2/M cell cycle phases, respectively. Percentage of cells in each phase is presented in the right corner of each individual histogram. Peripheral blood mononuclear cells ("PBMCs") were used as a control for normal diploid DNA peak. Tumour cells ("CANCER") are characterised by a high proliferative potential, quantified as a large fraction in S and G2/M cell cycle phases (denoted as tumour index). Among the five margins, number 4 and 5 appear as "tumour contaminated", since they exhibit a significantly higher fraction of proliferating cells. (Courtesy of Georgios Vartholomatos)

investigated and, albeit not unequivocally, it seems that both parameters can be used as prognostic factors in many cases [42].

The findings of intraoperative flow cytometry are explained in the example presented in Fig. 14.3 where the analysis of an excised tumour and its five margins have been evaluated.

One of the greatest merits of the technique, apart from its strength in detecting margin positivity and, even more importantly as mentioned above, minimising the number of false negative results, is the time it takes to give results. It has been consistently shown that a result for all-margin status can be available within 10 min, a time significantly shorter than most of the alternatives (e.g., intraoperative cytology or frozen section). Also, equally important, unlike the pathology-based methods, the cytometry assessment is operator independent.

14.5.3   End Note

The first results from the use of intraoperative flow cytometry in the assessment of the resection margins in breast conserving surgery show that it is a quick, accurate, easy to perform and adopt method. The comparison with the final pathology assessment in this initial series showed that only 0.2% of the positive margins were missed by the flow cytometry, which would essentially mean, although this still needs to be tested in a trial setting, that there would be only one re-excision in 99 patients, a number much lower than with other intraoperative assessment methods.

References

1. Cardoso F, Kyriakides S, Ohno S, Penault-Llorca F, Poortmans P, Rubio IT, et al. Early breast cancer: ESMO clinical practice guidelines for diagnosis, treatment and follow-up. Ann Oncol. 2019;30:1194–220.
2. Sarrazin D, Lê M, Rouëssé J, et al. Conservative treatment versus mastectomy in breast cancer tumors with macroscopic diameter of 20 millimeters or less. The experience of the Institut Gustave-Roussy. Cancer. 1984;53(5):1209–13.
3. Veronesi U, Saccozzi R, Del Vecchio M, et al. Comparing radical mastectomy with quadrantectomy, axillary dissection, and radiotherapy in patients with small cancers of the breast. N Engl J Med. 1981;305(1):6–11.
4. Veronesi U, Banfi A, Salvadori B, et al. Breast conservation is the treatment of choice in small breast cancer: long-term results of a randomized trial. Eur J Cancer. 1990;26(6):668–70.
5. Fisher B, Bauer M, Margolese R, et al. Five-year results of a randomized clinical trial comparing total mastectomy and segmental mastectomy with or without radiation in the treatment of breast cancer. N Engl J Med. 1985;312(11):665–73.
6. van Dongen JA, Voogd AC, Fentiman IS, et al. Long-term results of a randomized trial comparing breast-conserving therapy with mastectomy: European Organization for Research and Treatment of cancer 10801 trial. J Natl Cancer Inst. 2000;92(14):1143–50.
7. Fisher B, Anderson S, Redmond CK, Wolmark N, Wickerham DL, Cronin WM. Reanalysis and results after 12 years of follow-up in a randomized clinical trial comparing total mastectomy with lumpectomy with or without irradiation in the treatment of breast cancer. N Engl J Med. 1995;333(22):1456–61.
8. Poggi MM, Danforth DN, Sciuto LC, et al. Eighteen-year results in the treatment of early breast carcinoma with mastectomy versus breast conservation therapy: the National Cancer Institute randomized trial. Cancer. 2003;98(4):697–702.
9. Hartmann-Johnsen OJ, Kåresen R, Schlichting E, Nygård JF. Survival is better after breast conserving therapy than mastectomy for early stage breast cancer: a registry-based follow-up study of Norwegian women primary operated between 1998 and 2008. Ann Surg Oncol. 2015;22(12):3836–45.
10. Agarwal S, Pappas L, Neumayer L, Kokeny K, Agarwal J. Effect of breast conservation therapy vs mastectomy on disease-specific survival for early-stage breast cancer. JAMA Surg. 2014;149(3):267–74.
11. Hofvind S, Holen Å, Aas T, Roman M, Sebuødegård S, Akslen LA. Women treated with breast conserving surgery do better than those with mastectomy independent of detection mode, prognostic and predictive tumor characteristics. Eur J Surg Oncol. 2015;41(10):1417–22.
12. Chen K, Liu J, Zhu L, Su F, Song E, Jacobs LK. Comparative effectiveness study of breast-conserving surgery and mastectomy in the general population: a NCDB analysis. Oncotarget. 2015;6(37):40127–40.
13. Hwang ES, Lichtensztajn DY, Gomez SL, Fowble B, Clarke CA. Survival after lumpectomy and mastectomy for early stage invasive breast cancer: the effect of age and hormone receptor status. Cancer. 2013;119(7):1402–11.
14. Fredriksson I, Liljegren G, Palm-Sjövall M, et al. Risk factors for local recurrence after breast-conserving surgery. Br J Surg. 2003;90(9):1093–102.

15. Park CC, Mitsumori M, Nixon A, et al. Outcome at 8 years after breast-conserving surgery and radiation therapy for invasive breast cancer: influence of margin status and systemic therapy on local recurrence. J Clin Oncol. 2000;18(8):1668–75.

16. Bodilsen A, Bjerre K, Offersen BV, et al. Importance of margin width in breast-conserving treatment of early breast cancer. J Surg Oncol. 2016;113(6):609–15.

17. Fortin A, Larochelle M, Laverdière J, Lavertu S, Tremblay D. Local failure is responsible for the decrease in survival for patients with breast cancer treated with conservative surgery and postoperative radiotherapy. J Clin Oncol. 1999;17(1):101–9.

18. Fisher B, Anderson S, Fisher ER, et al. Significance of ipsilateral breast tumour recurrence after lumpectomy. Lancet. 1991;338(8763):327–31.

19. Cowen D, Houvenaeghel G, Bardou V, et al. Local and distant failures after limited surgery with positive margins and radiotherapy for node-negative breast cancer. Int J Radiat Oncol Biol Phys. 2000;47(2):305–12.

20. Vos EL, Gaal J, Verhoef C, Brouwer K, van Deurzen CHM, Koppert LB. Focally positive margins in breast conserving surgery: predictors, residual disease, and local recurrence. Eur J Surg Oncol. 2017;43(10):1846–54.

21. Sarrazin D, Lê MG, Arriagada R, et al. Ten-year results of a randomized trial comparing a conservative treatment to mastectomy in early breast cancer. Radiother Oncol. 1989;14(3):177–84.

22. Fisher ER, Anderson S, Tan-Chiu E, Fisher B, Eaton L, Wolmark N. Fifteen-year prognostic discriminants for invasive breast carcinoma: National Surgical Adjuvant Breast and bowel project Protocol-06. Cancer. 2001;91(8 Suppl):1679–87.

23. Schwartz GF, Veronesi U, Clough KB, et al. Consensus conference on breast conservation. J Am Coll Surg. 2006;203(2):198–207.

24. Taghian A, Mohiuddin M, Jagsi R, Goldberg S, Ceilley E, Powell S. Current perceptions regarding surgical margin status after breast-conserving therapy: results of a survey. Ann Surg. 2005;241(4):629–39.

25. Houssami N, Macaskill P, Marinovich ML, et al. Meta-analysis of the impact of surgical margins on local recurrence in women with early-stage invasive breast cancer treated with breast-conserving therapy. Eur J Cancer. 2010;46(18):3219–32.

26. Moran MS, Schnitt SJ, Giuliano AE, Harris JR, Khan SA, Horton J, Klimberg S, et al. SSO-ASTRO consensus guideline on margins for breast- conserving surgery with whole breast irradiation in stage I and II invasive breast cancer. Int J Radiat Oncol Biol Phys. 2014;88(3):553–64.

27. Houssami N, Macaskill P, Marinovich ML, Morrow M. The association of surgical margins and local recurrence in women with early-stage invasive breast cancer treated with breast-conserving therapy: a meta-analysis. Ann Surg Oncol. 2014;21(3):717–30.

28. Havel L, Naik H, Ramirez L, Morrow M, Landercasper J. Impact of the SSO-ASTRO margin guideline on rates of re-excision after lumpectomy for breast cancer: a meta-analysis. Ann Surg Oncol. 2019;26(5):1238–44.

29. Landercasper J, Whitacre E, Degnim AC, Al-Hamadani M. Reasons for re-excision after lumpectomy for breast cancer: insight from the American Society of Breast Surgeons Mastery(SM) database. Ann Surg Oncol. 2014;21(10):3185–91.

30. Morrow M, Van Zee KJ, Solin LJ, et al. Society of Surgical Oncology-American Society for Radiation Oncology-American Society of Clinical Oncology consensus guideline on margins for breast-conserving surgery with whole-breast irradiation in ductal carcinoma in situ. Ann Surg Oncol. 2016;23(12):3801–10.

31. National Comprehensive Cancer Network: NCCN Clinical Practice Guidelines. 2022. Breast Cancer version 3.2022. https://www.nccn.org. Accessed 22 May 2022.

32. Wapnir IL, Dignam JJ, Fisher B, et al. Long-term outcomes of invasive ipsilateral breast tumor recurrences after lumpectomy in NSABP B-17 and B-24 randomized clinical trials for DCIS. J Natl Cancer Inst. 2011;103(6):478–88.

33. Vartholomatos G, Harissis H, Andreou M, et al. Rapid assessment of resection margins during breast conserving surgery using intraoperative flow cytometry. Clin Breast Cancer. 2021;21(5):e602–10.

34. St John ER, Al-Khudairi R, Ashrafian H, et al. Diagnostic accuracy of intraoperative techniques for margin assessment in breast cancer surgery: a meta-analysis. Ann Surg. 2017;265(2):300–10.
35. Osako T, Nishimura R, Nishiyama Y, et al. Efficacy of intraoperative entire-circumferential frozen section analysis of lumpectomy margins during breast-conserving surgery for breast cancer. Int J Clin Oncol. 2015;20(6):1093–101.
36. Jorns JM, Visscher D, Sabel M, et al. Intraoperative frozen section analysis of margins in breast conserving surgery significantly decreases reoperative rates: one-year experience at an ambulatory surgical center. Am J Clin Pathol. 2012;138(5):657–69.
37. Esbona K, Li Z, Wilke LG. Intraoperative imprint cytology and frozen section pathology for margin assessment in breast conservation surgery: a systematic review. Ann Surg Oncol. 2012;19(10):3236–45.
38. Allweis TM, Kaufman Z, Lelcuk S, et al. A prospective, randomized, controlled, multicenter study of a real-time, intraoperative probe for positive margin detection in breast-conserving surgery. Am J Surg. 2008;196(4):483–9.
39. Schnabel F, Boolbol SK, Gittleman M, et al. A randomized prospective study of lumpectomy margin assessment with use of MarginProbe in patients with nonpalpable breast malignancies. Ann Surg Oncol. 2014;21(5):1589–95.
40. Chagpar AB, Killelea BK, Tsangaris TN, et al. A randomized, controlled trial of cavity shave margins in breast cancer. N Engl J Med. 2015;373(6):503–10.
41. Dupont E, Tsangaris T, Garcia-Cantu C, et al. Resection of cavity shave margins in stage 0-III breast cancer patients undergoing breast conserving surgery: a prospective multicenter randomized controlled trial. Ann Surg. 2021;273(5):876–81.
42. Andreou M, Vartholomatos E, Harissis H, Markopoulos GS, Alexiou GA. Past, present and future of flow cytometry in breast cancer - a systematic review. EJIFCC. 2019;30(4):423–37.

Part V
Intraoperative Flow Cytometry in Head and Neck Malignancies

Chapter 15
Head and Neck Malignancies

Evangeli Lampri and Alexandra Papoudou-Bai

15.1 Introduction

The different types of cancer associated with head and neck are cancer of nasal cavity and paranasal sinuses, nasopharynx, hypopharynx, larynx and trachea, oral cavity and oropharynx, salivary glands, odontogenic tumors, ear, and paraganglionic System [1]. In practice, pathologists have to discriminate specimens from head and neck in three categories. Most of them are benign, such as sinus contents, tonsils, and extracted teeth. The second in frequency category includes squamous cell carcinoma, its precursor and mimics. All the other entities fall into the third category of a diverse spectrum of malignancies whose origin ranges from epithelial to mesenchymal, neuroectodermal, melanocytic, neuroendocrine, and hematolymphoid [2].

The risk factors in most malignancies include tobacco, alcohol abuse, and oncogenic viruses, such as human papillomavirus (HPV) and Epstein–Barr virus (EBV). Head and neck malignancies need a multidisciplinary approach, with surgery, radiotherapy, and systemic therapy, especially in advanced disease. In the era of personalized medicine, treatment in head and neck cancer is site-specific and histology-specific.

E. Lampri (✉) · A. Papoudou-Bai
Faculty of Medicine, Department of Pathology, School of Health Sciences, University of Ioannina, Ioannina, Greece
e-mail: elampri@uoi.gr; apapoudou@uoi.gr

G. Alexiou, G. Vartholomatos (eds.), *Intraoperative Flow Cytometry*,
https://doi.org/10.1007/978-3-031-33517-4_15

15.2 Squamous Cell Carcinoma (SCC)

SCC and its variants remain the most common form of neoplasia as they constitute more than 90% of all head and neck cancers, with a smaller proportion within the sinonasal tract [3–5].

There are clinical and biologic differences among SCC arising in different head and neck subsites. Carcinomas in the oral cavity are better differentiated in comparison to those in the hypopharynx. Tumors of true vocal cord present at a lower stage, because of early given symptoms, such as changes in voice quality, while a carcinoma of tonsilar crypt or hypopharynx is often diagnosed because of metastatic disease in cervical lymph nodes. Patients with oropharyngeal squamous cell carcinoma tend to be younger (less than 45 years of age) and usually non-smokers than those whose tumors arise in other head and neck sites. The same high-risk human papillomavirus (HR-HPV) types responsible for cervical cancer were frequently identified in the oropharyngeal and tonsillar tumors, which are more frequently of basaloid or papillary subtypes [3]. Moreover, EBV plays role in non-keratinizing carcinomas of the nasopharynx. Although SCC have similar appearance in different sites of head and neck, there are site-specific differences, revealing that SCC is not a single disease [2].

As SCC in any other site, has morphologic features of atypical squamous epithelium which, by definition, penetrates through the basement membrane, into the underlying connective tissue stroma. The extent of invasion is a component of tumor staging. The tumor is graded as well- (grade 1), moderately- (grade 2), or poorly differentiated (grade 3), based on the degree of maturation, presence of whorls of keratin, abnormal mitotic figures, mitotic activity, nuclear pleomorphism, and pattern of invasion (Figs. 15.1 and 15.2). Most of squamous carcinomas invade, arranged in irregular nests and cords, or as individual cells. The infiltrated stroma may be fibroblastic or inflamed [2].

SCC is subdivided into **keratinizing** and **non-keratinizing types**, based on the presence or absence of extracellular keratin pearls [2].

Non-keratinizing SCC in the sinonasal tract is much more likely than keratinizing SCC to be secondary to HR-HPV infection (41 vs. <5%) [4–8]. There are other variants of SCC, such as basaloid SCC, papillary SCC, spindle cell carcinoma, etc.). HR-HPV is associated with 45% of basaloid SCCs and 80% of papillary [4, 5, 9].

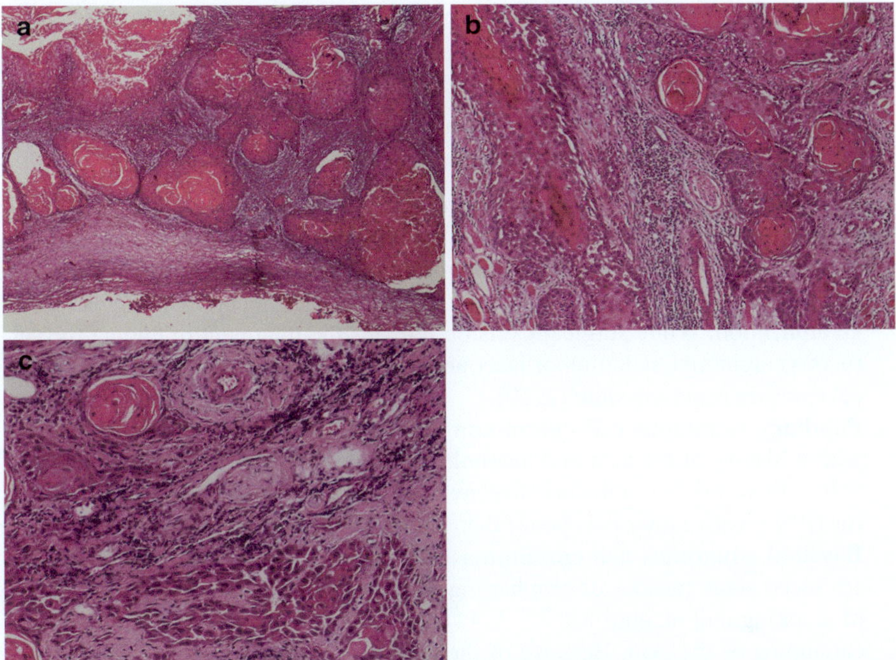

Fig. 15.1 Infiltrative keratinizing well-differentiated squamous cell carcinoma of the tongue. The presence of keratinization, intercellular bridges, and mild pleomorphism makes this lesion a well-differentiated SCC. ((**a**) H&E ×40, (**b**) H&E ×100, (**c**) H&E ×200)

Fig. 15.2 Lymph node metastasis from squamous cell carcinoma of the tongue (H&E ×40)

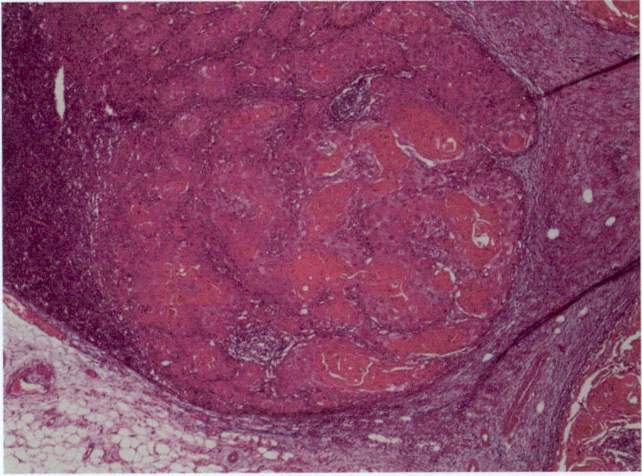

15.3   Other Variants of Squamous Cell Carcinoma

Other variants of squamous cell carcinoma include verrucous carcinoma, papillary squamous cell carcinoma, basaloid squamous cell carcinoma, spindle cell squamous cell carcinoma, and lymphoepithelial carcinoma.

- **Verrucous Carcinoma** most often involves the oral cavity and larynx of elderly male smokers, with limited metastatic potential. Its recognition may avoid overtreatment. Although its gross appearance may cause serious concern, its histology is bland, as it looks like a common wart with its "church-spire" pattern of keratinization. While surgical excision remains the treatment of choice for verrucous carcinoma, radiation or laser ablation are accepted therapies when surgical excision is not possible [2, 10].
- **Papillary squamous cell carcinoma** most often arises in the larynx of males with a history of tobacco and alcohol use. In one third of cases and more than half of those arising in the oropharynx, there is evidence of HPV. The prognosis for HPV-positive tumors is better than for HPV-negative cases [2, 9].
- **Basaloid squamous cell carcinoma** is an aggressive variant presenting as an advanced stage tonsilar or oropharyngeal tumor in elderly males with a history of smoking and alcohol use [2, 3, 11]. There is a resemblance with basal cell carcinoma of the skin. Because of the cell size, high mitotic rate and frequent presence of necrosis, the histologic differential includes small cell (neuroendocrine) carcinoma. The presence of co-existing conventional SCC, in situ or invasive and absence of neuroendocrine markers by immunohistochemistry helps in the diagnosis. HPV can be demonstrated in a proportion of tumors, generally in the oropharynx. HPV-positive tumors respond better to radiation therapy, improving prognosis [2].
- **Spindle cell (sarcomaroid) squamous cell carcinoma** (SCSCC) is an unusual variant of SCC characterized by predominant malignant spindle and/or pleomorphic cells intermingled with conventional SCC. It presents usually in elderly men. The tumor is presented as a polypoid mass arising in the oral cavity, oropharynx or larynx. There is not only conventional squamous carcinoma, but also fascicles of malignant spindle cells and in some cases, foci of malignant bone or cartilage [1, 2, 12].
- **Lymphoepithelial carcinoma** (LEC) describes an Epstein–Barr Virus (EBV)-related to non-keratinizing nasopharyngeal carcinoma, undifferentiated subtype, composed of nests or single cells, in a background rich of lymphocytes [1, 2].

15.4   Neuroendocrine Tumors of the Head and Neck

Neuroendocrine tumors, uncommon though, occurs in the head and neck region, such as in lung. It is about a high-grade carcinoma with morphological and immunohistochemical features of neuroendocrine differentiation and includes both small cell carcinoma and large cell neuroendocrine carcinoma. In rare cases, neuroendocrine carcinoma are combined with either squamous cell carcinoma or adenocarcinoma. There are tumors which are related to HR-HPV and previous irradiation, but no strong smoking association. However, squamous cell carcinoma or adenocarcinoma should not be regarded as neuroendocrine carcinoma based solely on the presence of focal neuroendocrine immunoreactivity in the absence of microscopic features of neuroendocrine differentiation [1, 2, 13–21]. The differential diagnosis includes olfactory neuroblastoma, sinonasal undifferentiated carcinoma, and NUT carcinoma [2, 13, 14].

Small Cell Neuroendocrine Carcinoma is identical to the lung, there is a male predominance with a significant smoking history and have metastatic disease at the time of diagnosis. Because of its rarity as a primary head and neck tumor, it is important to exclude metastatic disease. In addition to a lung primary, it should be taken into consideration **Merkel cell carcinoma**, a primary small cell neuroendocrine carcinoma of the skin. Like other small cell carcinomas, Merkel cell carcinoma is an aggressive tumor with frequent nodal and distant metastasis. This tumor has a predilection for the head and neck region and it seems that those arising from the lip are more aggressive than those arising in other head and neck skin sites [15]. Sun exposure, particularly ultraviolet radiation, and a recently described Merkel cell polyomavirus (MCPyV), appear to be important in the pathogenesis of this tumor. Merkel cell carcinoma, in contrast to other small cell carcinomas, commonly shows a perinuclear dot-like staining with cytokeratin 20. The MCPyV large T protein may be detected by immunohistochemistry in 7–97% of cases [2, 16].

15.5 Ewing's Sarcoma (ES)/Primitive Neuroectodermal Tumor (PNET)

ES/PNET is a family of small blue cell tumors with a characteristic t(11;22) translocation involving the EWS and FLI-1 genes. Ewing's sarcoma is predominantly limited to adolescents and young adults, with sheets of small uniform round cells with scant, glycogen-rich pale cytoplasm. PNET differs from Ewing's in that it may be seen in any age group, has a higher proliferative rate, and shows histologic or immunophenotypic evidence of neuroendocrine differentiation. These tumors show membranous staining for CD99, the product of the MIC2 gene. In the head and neck, it is often difficult to tell whether the tumor is arising in bone or from an extraosseous location. Those tumors arising from soft tissue of the sinonasal cavity appear to have a better prognosis than ES/PNET overall [2, 22].

15.6 Melanoma

Melanoma is called the great mimicker in pathology, as it enters the histologic differential of almost any tumor. Most of melanomas of the head and neck arise from sun-exposed skin and behave similar to those arising on skin elsewhere on the body.

Occasionally a melanoma is identified in periparotid lymph nodes. Up to 5% of head and neck melanomas arise from squamous mucosa, rather than skin. These are most commonly seen in the oral cavity but may arise anywhere from the paranasal sinuses to the larynx. Smoking, rather than UV radiation from sun exposure, may be a possible explanation for the occurrence of these tumors, however, their etiology remains uncertain [2, 23]. Mucosal melanoma (MM) arises from scattered melanocytes intrinsically present throughout the aerodigestive tracts, although most are confined to the sinonasal tract.

15.7 Tumors of the Nasal Cavity, Paranasal Sinuses and Skull Base

In addition to the SCC, the nasal cavity and paranasal sinuses are the sites of origin for a variety of tumors. The seromucinous glands lining the nasal passages can give rise to salivary gland carcinomas, and to a unique set of intestinal and non-intestinal type sinonasal adenocarcinomas.

There are a few new well-defined and emerging sinonasal neoplasms. Both NUT carcinomas and SMARCB1—deficient carcinomas were previously classified as poorly differentiated squamous cell carcinomas or sinonasal undifferentiated carcinoma. Although the tumors have almost similar, very poor, prognoses, the specific molecular abnormalities seen with them may make these tumors candidates to targeted therapies in the future. The recognition of biphenotypic sinonasal sarcoma as a distinct neoplasm helps to clean up the somewhat heterogeneous group of tumors previously classified as malignant peripheral nerve sheath tumors or fibrosarcomas at the site. Finally, the association of some carcinomas with HR-HPV can show differentiation reminiscent of salivary gland neoplasia expanding our understanding of the potential plasticity of sinonasal mucosa during oncogenesis [4].

The gender distribution varies between different tumor types, with a male-to-female ratio of up to 6:1 for intestinal-type adenocarcinomas (ITAC), 3:1 in sinonasal undifferentiated carcinoma (SNUC), 2:1 in squamous cell carcinoma (SCC), 1:1.5 in human papillomavirus (HPV)-related multiphenotypic carcinoma (HMSC), 1:2 in biphenotypic sinonasal sarcoma (BSNS), and 1:1 in melanoma and SMARCB1-deficient sinonasal carcinoma (SDSC) [24–31]. Similarly, the age distribution for sinonasal malignancies is wide with a median age of 67 years, although the more recently described SDSC and HMSC seem to present in the early 50's. The incidence of sinonasal malignancy varies in different studies between females and males, presumably due to differences in profession and the environmental risk factors for ITAC [31].

Patients present with nasal congestion, epistaxis, rhinorrhea, or midfacial pressure, causing for prolonged diagnostic latency as these symptoms largely overlap with those of benign disease. Involvement of the brain and orbit with diplopia and/

or exophthalmos can occur, especially in cases with involvement of the superior nasal cavity or ethmoid complex. Nodal involvement in salivary-type and ITAC is rare as compared to SCC of the nasal cavity (10%) and maxillary sinus (21%). The recently identified SDSC and HMSC rarely show nodal involvement, but the former show frequent metastatic spread and invasion into the skull base and orbital structures whereas the latter has a relatively indolent clinical course and is often confined to the sinonasal tract [24–31].

15.7.1 Adenocarcinoma

The most important distinction of adenocarcinomas is between intestinal-type adenocarcinomas (ITACs) which is morphologically similar to adenocarcinomas primary to the intestines and non-intestinal sinonasal adenocarcinomas (SNACs). This distinction is justified by the distinct histological and immunohistochemical features of ITAC as well as its very strong association with wood and other dust exposures [4, 23–28].

ITACs are sub-classified into papillary, tubular, solid or mucinous types. The last type is divided into colloid and signet ring cell [32–39].

SNACs remain a group of phenotypically diverse tumors, although there is much more homogeneity with the tumors classified as low-grade. Low-grade SNACs are typically papillary and/or tubular and composed of monomorphic cuboidal or columnar cells with rare mitosis and without necrosis [4]. As low-grade SNACs resemble normal seromucinous glands, their site of origin is obvious. However, sometimes distinguishing this tumor from normal seromucinous glands may need immunohistochemistry for revealing the absence of a second cell layer (myoepithelial cells). High grade SNACs have a variety of histologic appearances, which may be difficult to be distinguished from the other poorly differentiated or undifferentiated carcinomas. Many have abundant solid growth with only focal glandular differentiation with high mitotic index and frequently necrosis. This category may include some entities with unique morphology, such as sinonasal renal cell-like adenocarcinoma [1, 2, 4, 39–43]. As the name suggests, renal cell-like adenocarcinoma histologically resembles clear cell renal cell carcinoma, with nests and follicles of polyhedral cells with abundant optically clear cytoplasm [4]. Clearly, a diagnostic consideration for renal cell-like adenocarcinoma is metastatic renal cell carcinoma, which is not uncommon in the head and neck. Sinonasal renal cell-like adenocarcinoma is consistently negative for the immunohistochemical markers PAX8, RCC, and vimentin, unlike true renal cell carcinoma. Other diagnostic considerations include the minor salivary gland tumors hyalinizing clear cell carcinoma, mucoepidermoid carcinoma, and myoepithelial carcinoma. Sinonasal renal cell-like adenocarcinoma appears to be very indolent [4, 44, 45].

15.7.2   NUT Carcinoma

NUT carcinoma, also known as NUT midline carcinoma or t (15;19) carcinoma, is a rare, aggressive epithelial malignancy. Most cases (65%) in the head and neck are in the nasal cavity and paranasal sinuses, but rare cases involve the orbital region, nasopharynx, oropharynx, larynx, epiglottis, and major salivary glands, but can be encountered in numerous different sites outside this region [1, 46–48]. NUT carcinoma is a poorly differentiated carcinoma (often with evidence of squamous differentiation) defined by the presence of nuclear protein in testis (NUT) gene (NUTM1) rearrangement, on chromosome 15q14. It can affect patients of any age though is most common in children and young adults (median, 21.9 years), and has a slight female predominance [1, 49–56].

The etiology is unknown. There is no association with HPV, EBV, other viral infection; smoking; or other environmental factors.

Histologically, NUT carcinoma grows as undifferentiated cells in nests and sheets within the sinonasal submucosa. There is no carcinoma in situ component. The histology is that of an undifferentiated carcinoma or poorly differentiated squamous cell carcinoma. Two histologic hallmarks of NUT carcinoma are (1) monotonous tumor cells and (2) a peculiar pattern of keratinization often described as "abrupt." Rarely, foci of glandular or even mesenchymal differentiation may be encountered. The carcinoma is highly infiltrative and demonstrates necrosis and high mitotic rates. Intratumoural acute inflammation is common. Glandular and mesenchymal differentiation, although described, is infrequent. The diagnosis of NUT carcinoma is established by demonstration by rearrangement of nuclear protein in testis (NUT) gene (NUTM1), rather than by histology. The most common fusion partner is BRD4 (in about 70% of cases) [1, 49–56].

An unequivocal diagnosis can be made by demonstration of diffuse (>50%) nuclear staining with the NUT monoclonal antibody C52, which has a sensitivity of 87%. Other diagnostic tools include FISH, RT-PCR, conventional cytogenetics, and targeted next-generation sequencing approaches [1].

Due to the non-specific, poorly differentiated nature of NUT carcinoma, it is often confused with poorly differentiated squamous cell carcinoma, Ewing sarcoma, sinonasal undifferentiated carcinoma, leukemia, germ cell tumor, olfactory neuroblastoma), or SMARCB1-deficient carcinoma.

The prognosis of NUT carcinoma is poor, with a median overall survival of 9.8 months. There is some evidence that NUT carcinomas with variant rearrangements not involving BRD4 may have longer survival [54–59].

15.7.3   Sinonasal Undifferentiated Carcinoma (SNUC)

SNUC is an aggressive, rapidly growing tumor of uncertain etiology. It remains a diagnosis of exclusion, without squamous or glandular differentiation [4, 60]. No consistent etiology of SNUC has been identified. If EBV or HPV is detected, the diagnosis of SNUC should be questionesd [1].

15.7.4 SMARCB1 (INI-1) Deficient Sinonasal Sarcoma

SMARCB1 (INI-1) Deficient Sinonasal Sarcoma is a highly cellular lesion with high mitotic index and frequent necrosis, without focal keratinization. Tumor cells are uniform with monomorphic, hyperchromatic nuclei, and indistinctive borders. Two histologic variants are described; one variant composed of undifferentiated basaloid tumor cells ("blue cell tumor") and another with eosinophilic rhabdoid or plasmacytoid tumor cells ("pink cell tumor"). Because SMARCB1-deficient sinonasal carcinomas have biallelic inactivation of SMARCB1, immunohistochemical staining for SMARCB1 consistently demonstrates loss of nuclear expression, an important finding for distinguishing SMARCB1-deficient carcinoma from NUT carcinoma [2, 25].

SMARCB1 (INI-1) is a tumor suppressor gene located on chromosome 22q11.2; its inactivation has been implicated in the pathogenesis of a family of malignant neoplasms that includes pediatric atypical teratoid/rhabdoid tumor, rhabdoid tumors of the kidney and soft tissue, epithelioid sarcoma, renal medullary carcinoma, myoepithelial carcinoma of soft tissue, epithelioid malignant peripheral nerve sheath tumor, and extraskeletal myxoid chondrosarcoma [4].

It remains unclear, however, whether SMARCB1 (INI-1) deficient sinonasal carcinoma is a distinct entity, or rather a pattern that can be seen in a variety of tumor types.

15.7.5 Olfactory Neuroblastomas (ONBs)

ONBs are malignant neuroectodermal neoplasms with neuroblastic differentiation, most often localized in the superior nasal cavity. They must be distinguished from carcinomas, Ewing sarcoma/peripheral neuroectodermal tumor (PNET), and melanoma. ONBs show little or no expression of keratins by immunohistochemistry and do not have EWSR1 rearrangements as seen with Ewing sarcomas/PNETs [1, 61, 62].

15.7.6 Sinonasal Tract HPV-Related Carcinoma

The newly recognized sinonasal tract HPV-related carcinoma with adenoid cystic-like features is a distinctive HPV-related carcinoma of the sinonasal tract, with histological and immunophenotypic features of both surface-derived and salivary gland carcinoma, similar to a high-grade adenoid cystic carcinoma [1].

It may have an appearance like that of epithelial-myoepithelial carcinoma. Although there is not squamous differentiation in the invasive component, the surface epithelium may show features of dysplasia [1].

HPV-related carcinomas of the head and neck have a striking predilection for the oropharynx, where up to 80% of carcinomas are HPV-positive compared to 5% or fewer in sites like the oral cavity and larynx [4, 63–67]. In the oropharynx, HPV-related carcinomas are histologically and clinically distinct from their HPV-negative counterparts, and as a result, in the new edition of the WHO, squamous cell carcinomas of the oropharynx are classified by HPV status. In the new edition of the WHO classification, however, "HPV-related squamous cell carcinoma" is not regarded as a separate tumor entity as it is in the oropharynx, largely because it lacks clinical and pathologic distinctness. For example, while most HPV-related sinonasal carcinomas have a histologic appearance that conforms to the WHO entity of non-keratinizing squamous cell carcinoma, only about 41% of sinonasal non-keratinizing squamous cell carcinomas are HPV-positive [6–8].

The histologic variants of HPV-positive carcinoma that are encountered in the oropharynx (e.g., small cell carcinoma, adenosquamous carcinoma, papillary squamous cell carcinoma) have also been described in the sinonasal tract. There is one histologic variant, however, that has only been described in the sinonasal tract. This variant has features of both a surface-derived and salivary gland carcinoma and has been referred to as "sinonasal HPV-related carcinomas with adenoid cystic-like features."

At the histologic level, sinonasal HPV-related carcinoma with adenoid cystic like features consists of highly cellular proliferations of basaloid cells growing mostly as solid nests and trabeculae, with most cases also exhibiting focal cribriform structures with microcystic pseudoductal spaces, reminiscent of adenoid cystic carcinoma [4].

HPV-related carcinoma with adenoid cystic like features was considered as a possible new entity in the 4th edition of the WHO classification, but it was ultimately included as a provisional entity, listed in the differential diagnosis of non-keratinizing squamous cell carcinoma. The reservation for its inclusion focused on the low number of reported cases, its variable histology that often shows at least focal overlap with conventional non-keratinizing SCC, and its uncertain prognostic significance [4].

15.7.7 Teratocarcinoma

Teratocarcinoma is a malignant sinonasal neoplasm with combined histological features of teratoma and carcinosarcoma, lacking malignant germ cell components aside from those resembling teratoma. Thus, these tumors have carcinomatous components and sarcomatous elements. They seem to be clinically, histologically, and molecularly unique lesions mostly similar to carcinomas [67, 68].

15.7.8 Other Mesenchymal Neoplasms

There are also mesenchymal neoplasms involving the sinonasal tract which are classified as soft tissue tumors elsewhere. The exception here is the now well-recognized biphenotypic sinonasal sarcoma. Moreover, glomangiopericytomas are more often seen in the sinonasal tract than in soft tissue elsewhere. Recent research has shown recurrent CTNNB1 mutations in these lesions with beta-catenin nuclear accumulation seen by immunohistochemistry [69].

Biphenotypic sinonasal sarcoma (BSNS) is a rare "low-grade sinonasal sarcoma with neural and myogenic differentiation. It can arise anywhere in the sinonasal tract, with a predilection for the superior aspects of the nasal cavity and ethmoid sinuses. Affected patients present with non-specific symptoms like nasal obstruction and facial pressure. The histopathology of BSNS is that of an infiltrative proliferation of spindled cells arranged as fascicles or in a "herringbone" pattern. A characteristic feature of BSNS is its propensity to entrap benign downward invaginations of sinonasal epithelium. These glands can become proliferative and undergo squamous or oncocytic metaplasia, mimicking sinonasal papillomas. The nuclei of BSNS are pale, slender, and uniform. Mitotic figures are uncommon, and necrosis is absent. Before it was recognized, BSNS was likely to be misdiagnosed as cellular schwannoma, malignant peripheral nerve sheath tumor, solitary fibrous tumor, glomangiopericytoma, and synovial sarcoma. BSNS tends to demonstrate slow, progressive growth. [57, 70–73]

15.8 Nasopharyngeal Carcinoma

The World Health Organization separates squamous cell carcinomas arising in the nasopharynx into keratinizing nasopharyngeal carcinoma (NPC), non-keratinizing NPC, and non-keratinizing undifferentiated carcinoma (lymphoepithelioma). This classification has etiologic and prognostic basis. Keratinizing NPC is histologically identical to conventional squamous cell carcinoma and is not significantly related to EBV infection, while the other two NPC types are strongly associated with EBV. Any NPC found to be EBV-negative, or not limited to the nasopharynx should also be tested for HPV to exclude an oropharyngeal primary [74, 75].

15.9 Tumors of the Salivary Gland

Tumors of the salivary gland constitute a large number of different entities with the vast majority being of epithelial origin. Salivary gland malignancies are as varied in their appearance as the benign salivary gland tumors. Some are malignant counterparts of the benign tumor. For example, basal cell adenocarcinoma may be histologically identical to a basal cell adenoma, except for the presence of invasion into adjacent normal salivary tissue [2]. Sudden growth of a mass lesion that may have been present for more than 10 years is a common presentation of a carcinoma arising in a pleomorphic adenoma (carcinoma-ex-pleomorphic adenoma). For most salivary gland malignancies, relationships with normal cell types are seen.

Most of benign tumors in the parotid gland are pleomorphic adenoma (PA), whereas the sublingual gland and minor salivary glands mainly harbor carcinomas. The most frequent carcinoma type seems to be mucoepidermoid carcinoma (MEC).

For carcinomas there is an approximately even distribution between the genders, a median age of 62 years. The same age group is affected by parotid Warthin tumors with 2/3 occurring in males and cigarette smokers; in contrast, 2/3 of parotid PAs occur in women with a median age of 53 years [76–79]. Acinic cell carcinoma, MEC, and PA are the most frequent malignant and benign salivary gland tumors in children and adolescents, respectively [80, 81].

Patients present with a mass and accompanying symptoms depending on the site involved. For carcinomas, facial palsy may be a presenting symptom in case of parotid involvement, and ulceration of the overlaying mucosa can be seen in oral sites, including the sublingual gland [82, 83].

Salivary gland tumors are heterogeneous and the majority of these have histologically and genetically homologous tumors in the skin, breast, and lacrimal gland [84–87]. As normal salivary gland ducts and acini have two cell layers, an outer (or abluminal) layer composed of myoepithelial (with contractile muscle fibers) or basal (without muscle) cells, and an inner luminal cell layer. They are broadly divided into monophasic and biphasic tumors. Monophasic tumors can be composed of pure luminal (cells lining the luminal side of the salivary gland acini) (salivary duct carcinoma [SDC], secretory carcinoma, *acinic cell carcinoma*), myoepithelial (cells from the outer layer) (myoepithelioma and myoepithelial carcinoma), or basal (basal cell adenoma and basal cell adenocarcinoma) cell components. While biphasic tumors invariably contain a mixture of both luminal and abluminal (myoepithelial) cell components (e.g., ACC, epithelial-myoepithelial carcinoma), unlike those arising in the breast, prostate or other organ systems.

The number of carcinoma types have increased from 5 in the 1972 WHO classification to 22 in the 2017 edition, and, in the same period, the number of benign tumors have increased from 4 to 11 [88, 89].

15.9.1 *Adenoid Cystic Carcinoma*

Adenoid cystic carcinoma consists of relatively uniform neoplastic luminal and myoepithelial cells. The luminal component is the minor of the two, and the myoepithelial cells produce excess amounts of basal membrane-like extracellular material. Architecturally, ACC grows as tubules, cribriform structures or solid nests, all these patterns are often seen intermingled in varying proportions, with solid component being the determinant of the most common architectural grading system: >30% solid areas is considered poorly differentiated [2, 76, 90]. The propensity of ACC for intra- and perineural invasion enables ACC to invade beyond the clinically apparent lesion, with only intraneural invasion being associated with reduced overall and recurrence-free survival [76, 91]. In addition to the solid pattern, the presence of lymph node metastasis, particularly with extracapsular extension of the tumor, are risk factors for distant metastasis [2].

15.9.2 *Mucoepidermoid Carcinoma*

Mucoepidermoid carcinoma (MEC) is the most common malignant salivary gland tumor, comprising one third of all cases, and is seen in a wide age range. It is characterized by three principal cell populations: epidermoid, goblet (mucin-producing), and intermediate cells, whose frequency varies with the grade of the tumor. Grading of MEC relies on the extent of the cystic component, amount of goblet cells, nuclear atypia, lymphatic-vascular-perineural invasion, presence of necrosis, and extent of invasion, however, current WHO classification does not endorse the use of any specific grading system, possibly due to the lack of consensus criteria. PAS positive, PAS-D resistant intracytoplasmic mucous in goblet cells are mandatory for the diagnosis. The morphology of MEC show a wide spectrum with clear cell, oncocytic, sclerosing, and a recently described Warthin-like variant described [1, 2, 76, 92].

15.9.3 *Acinic Cell Carcinoma/Mammary Analog Secretory Carcinoma*

Acinic cell carcinoma generally arises as a circumscribed, slow-growing parotid mass, usually in adults, but may be seen in teenagers. A well-differentiated acinic cell carcinoma may closely mimic the normal parotid gland, with acini lined by polygonal cells with abundant basophilic granular cytoplasm and round dark nuclei. In such cases, recognizing an absence of ducts may be the only clue to the correct diagnosis. Tumors with solid, papillary, micro- or macrocystic architectures are less subtle. Most acinic cell carcinomas are low-grade tumors and may be cured with conservative excision with negative margins. These are not entirely benign tumors, as local recurrence has been reported in up to 15% and lymph node metastasis in 8% of cases. A proportion of tumors have foci with more significant nuclear pleomorphism and a higher mitotic rate, indicating transformation to a higher-grade tumor. Such tumors behave more aggressively, with a mean overall survival of 40 months vs. 125 months for cases without high-grade transformation [2, 93].

Recently a subset of adenoid cystic carcinomas with minimal cytoplasmic granules have been reclassified as **Mammary Analog Secretory Carcinoma (MASC)**, based on the presence of a t(12;15) translocation creating the same ETV6-NRTK2 fusion found in (juvenile) secretory carcinoma of the breast. In contrast to typical acinic cell carcinomas, these tumors lack zymogen granules and show strong immunoreactivity for S100 protein. They have a marked male predominance and may arise from major or minor salivary glands. While generally low-grade tumors, local recurrence is not uncommon and distant metastasis have been described [2, 94–96].

15.9.4   Basal Cell Adenocarcinoma

Basal cell adenocarcinoma (BAC) is a salivary gland malignancy with variable basal and myoepithelial neoplastic cells forming nests and glandular structures. A typical basal cell adenoma with even focal invasion into adjacent tissue is considered to be a basal cell adenocarcinoma. As with both pleomorphic and monomorphic adenomas, basal cell adenocarcinoma usually arises in the superficial lobe of the parotid, where it is composed of tubules, trabeculae or solid nests with palisading of the peripheral columnar cells. A prominent basement membrane is characteristic, as are scattered hyaline globules of basement membrane material scattered within the nests. With few exceptions, these are low-grade tumors that are adequately treated with complete surgical excision [2].

15.9.5   Epithelial-Myoepithelial Carcinoma

While many salivary gland carcinomas show luminal (epithelial) and abluminal (myoepithelial or basal cell) differentiation, epithelial-myoepithelial carcinoma (EMC) show the highest degree of this two-cell-type differentiation. EMC most often presents as a slow-growing, circumscribed parotid mass in an elderly patient. Rarely, a long-standing EMC begins rapidly enlarging, indicating transformation to a high-grade carcinoma. At low magnification, EMC appears as nodules invading into the surrounding tissue. Closer examination reveals at least focal areas containing bilayered ducts, with inner columnar epithelial cells and outer myoepithelial cells with prominent clear cytoplasm. Most EMCs are adequately treated with complete surgical excision, although late local recurrences have been reported [2, 97].

15.9.6   Salivary Duct Carcinoma

Salivary duct carcinoma is characterized by duct structures of different size, lined with eosinophilic tumor cells in usually cribriform architecture. Histologically, the tumor consists of infiltrating cords, papillae, and large circumscribed nests with central (comedo) necrosis, similar to a high-grade ductal carcinoma of the breast. Roman bridge formation is frequent, and apocrine differentiation with apical snouting is a hallmark. Salivary duct carcinoma is an intriguing tumor with morphologic similarities to breast carcinoma. Although a low-grade variant exists, most cases present as a rapidly growing parotid mass, frequently with metastatic disease involving regional lymph nodes and distant sites [2, 76].

15.9.7 Carcinoma Ex Pleomorphic Adenoma

Carcinoma ex pleomorphic adenoma (PA) is an epithelial and/or myoepithelial malignancy developing from primary or recurrent PA. The carcinoma component can be either purely epithelial or myoepithelial in presentation, with infiltration into the surrounding glandular and extraglandular tissue.

Up to 5% of untreated pleomorphic adenomas eventually enter a phase of rapid growth, denoting malignant transformation. Histologically the malignant component is usually an adenocarcinoma, thus termed Carcinoma ex Pleomorphic Adenoma. Rarely the malignant component is mesenchymal (sarcoma-ex-pleomorphic adenoma) or exceptionally has both malignant epithelial and mesenchymal components (a true malignant mixed tumor). While the diagnosis is usually straightforward, it can prove to be more difficult in cases where the malignant component overgrows and completely replaces the pre-existing pleomorphic adenoma. Extensive histologic sampling of the tumor is necessary to reveal some residual chondromyxoid matrix or a scar, suggesting the correct diagnosis. These were usually cured with complete surgical excision of the lesion. Postoperative radiation is useful in more advanced cases [1, 2, 98, 99].

15.9.8 Secretory Carcinoma (SC)

SC is a generally low-grade salivary gland carcinoma characterized by morphological resemblance to mammary secretory carcinoma and ETV6-NTRK3 gene fusion. SC was separated from mainly acinic cell carcinoma due to its homology to SC of the breast. Histologically, SC is characterized by eosinophilic tumor cells with granulated or vacuolated cytoplasm arranged in microcystic, solid, tubular, papillary, or follicular growth patterns. As implied by its name, SC is characterized by distinctive luminal secretions [76, 100].

15.9.9 Polymorphous Adenocarcinoma (PAC)

PAC is a malignant epithelial tumor characterized by cytological uniformity, morphological diversity, and an infiltrative growth pattern. It is a diagnosis encompassing what was previously known as polymorphous low-grade adenocarcinoma (PLGA) as well as cribriform adenocarcinoma of the tongue and minor salivary glands (CATSMG), originally termed cribriform adenocarcinoma of the tongue. These two entities are now collected under PAC as "classic variant" (i.e., PLGA) and "cribriform variant" (i.e., CATSMG). Due to an aggressive behavior of some classic PAC, the "low-grade" part is now abandoned. Classic PAC is most frequently encountered in the palate and intraoral minor salivary glands, and only very rarely in the major salivary glands [76, 101, 102]. Tumor cells are small and uniform with only rare mitoses. Various growth patterns can be encountered, including lobular, trabecular, microcystic, cribriform, solid, and papillary-cystic. Perineural invasion is common, and the neurotropism cause for a characteristic targetoid growth pattern.

Cribriform PAC is located intraorally and mainly affects the base of tongue and, in contrast to classic PAC, frequently present with neck metastases. Tumor cells are relatively uniformly sized with eosinophilic to clear cytoplasm and pale, or even clear, nuclei arranged in cribriform, microcribriform, or solid patterns [76].

15.10 Special Molecular Characteristics and Targeted Therapy

In PAC of classic type, the E710D hotspot mutation in exon 15 of the PRKD1 gene is unique to this tumor type, while rearrangement of the PRKD1-3 genes is described exclusively in PAC of cribriform type. The HTN3-MSANTD3 fusion in acinic cell carcinoma has not been described in any other tumor type [76, 103–105].

The most promising targeted therapy is in SC which consistently harbor fusions involving ETV6, with the most frequent fusion partner being NTRK3, and RET in a subset of cases. Use of the pan-Trk inhibitor entrectinib has given promising results, but while RET inhibition has not been employed in SC to date the RET inhibitor cabozantinib has given dramatic response in the rare SDC with NCOA4-RET fusion [106, 107]. A recent discovery in the management of ACC is the identification of targetable NOTCH1 mutations, which are especially prevalent in the solid type [108, 109]. However, only one case with partial response to treatment with the Notch1 inhibitor brontictuzumab has been reported.

Although limited, the most widespread use of targeted therapy in salivary gland carcinoma is in SDC. Here, the overexpression of androgen receptor (AR) and human epidermal growth factor receptor 2 (HER2) have been used in the treatments of mainly advanced disease, as both have well-documented effect in other cancers. Androgen deprivation therapy (ADT), otherwise mainly used in AR-positive prostate cancer, has shown clinical benefit in approximately 50% of AR+ SDC [110, 111]. The first randomized clinical trial (NCT01969578) investigating the effect of ADT in advanced salivary gland carcinoma is actively recruiting, but only small case series are currently available. In this context, it is noteworthy that the V7 isoform of the AR transcript, which confer resistance to ADT in prostate cancer, is known to be expressed in a subset of SDC [112].

HER2 inhibition is currently standard of care in HER2+ breast cancer, whereas this is not the case in SDC. The largest study on this to date reports on 48 HER2+ SDC patients, presenting results of a combination regimen of the HER2-inhibitor Trastuzumab in combination with Docetaxel, had an objective response rate of 76% [111, 113].

Although the advances in targeted therapies, the primary treatment of salivary gland carcinoma is T-site surgery and neck dissection in all patients with clinically involved lymph nodes and/or T3 or T4 tumors while taking into account the type of malignancy and location. Regardless of stage, elective neck dissection is recommended in case of high-grade histology [114, 115].

15.11 Tumors of the Oral Cavity

15.11.1 Malignant Surface Epithelial Tumors

Although human papillomavirus (HPV), particularly type 16, is mentioned as an etiologic factor in the development of oral cavity squamous cell carcinoma (OSCC), although HPV-driven OSCC accounts for a very small percentage (1–10%) of cancers [116–122]. The major risk factor remains smoking in connection with alcohol consumption [106, 107, 123].

15.11.2 Oral Potentially Malignant Disorders and Oral Epithelial Dysplasia

The name oral potentially malignant disorders (OPMD) recognizes that in some conditions the risk of malignant transformation is extremely low and even reversible [124]. The global malignant transformation rate of oral leukoplakia is estimated to be 1–2% [125].

The WHO dysplasia grade is three tiered: mild, moderate, and severe with severe dysplasia and carcinoma in situ considered to be synonymous. A binary system (high grade and low grade) is also proposed [1].

Using p16 as a surrogate marker of HPV status in oral cavity dysplasia and OSCC is discouraged. HPV-driven OSCC has a very low incidence. Studies have shown that up to a third of OSCC are p16 positive and viral DNA is detectable by polymerase chain reaction in up to 28% of cases [121, 122]. However, when studies use in situ hybridization, a more sensitive method of detecting HR-HPV, very few cases (1–10%) are positive [117–122]. Therefore, relying on p16 as a surrogate marker for HPV overestimates the number of HPV-related cancers in the oral cavity. In addition, studies have shown no survival benefit in p16 positive OSCC compared to p16 negative OSCC [121, 122].

In 2017, the College of American Pathologists (CAP) published evidence-based guidelines on HPV testing of histological and cytological specimens obtained from head and neck SCC. It is recommended that high-risk HPV testing should be performed either primary or metastatic lesions from all patients with newly diagnosed OPSCC regardless of histologic subtype. Importantly, HPV is preserved in

                                                E. Lampri and A. Papoudou-Bai

metastases and demonstration of HPV in cytologies from cervical lymph nodes in patients with SCC of unknown primary strongly raises the possibility for an oropharyngeal primary tumor [1].

15.11.3 Adenocarcinoma in Oral Cavity

Except for those originating in the salivary glands, adenocarcinomas involving the oral cavity are exceedingly rare. Through recently a peculiar type of adenocarcinoma resembling colonic adenocarcinoma has emerged, provisionally termed colonic-type adenocarcinoma of the tongue and oral cavity. The origin of these rare lesions is still unclear but is speculated to arise from embryonic endodermal remnants, explaining their frequent midline localization [126].

15.11.4 Mesechymal Neoplasm of Oral Cavity

Ectomesenchymal chondromyxoid tumor (ECMT) is a rare mesenchymal neoplasm of uncertain origin included in the current WHO classification, with a striking predilection for the anterior dorsal tongue and occasional local recurrence [1, 127, 128]. Histologically, these are lobulated lesions composed of pale to eosinophilic tumor cells with small nuclei and scant atypia in a chondromyxoid stroma. Immunohistochemically, tumor cells are characterized by dual expression of S100 and glial acidic fibrillary protein similar to myoepithelial carcinoma, which is likely to be the label most ECMTs have been given in the past. Recently, a RREB1-MKL2 gene fusion has been reported in 90% of cases, which further solidifies the distinctive nature of ECMT and facilitates its recognition among its mimics [129].

15.11.5 Tumors of the Ear

The 2017 fourth edition of the World Health Organization Classification of Tumors of the Head and Neck, lesions of the middle and inner ear were combined, as practical limitations of origin and imaging make a definitive separation artificial. Apart from SCC, another malignant tumor is ceruminous gland adenocarcinoma. This entity arises from glands lining the external auditory canal and has overlapping features with the salivary gland carcinomas. Typically presenting as a polypoid mass, the tumor grows as infiltrative cribriform nests or glands that may resemble mucoepidermoid carcinoma, adenoid cystic carcinoma, or have apocrine features and pink to brown cytoplasmic granules resembling normal ceruminous glands. The latter two patterns have a dual cell population, consisting of luminal epithelial cells and abluminal myoepithelial cells. These tumors are prone to local recurrence and are treated with surgical excision with or without postoperative radiation [2, 130].

15.11.6 *Malignant Odontogenic Tumors*

Odontogenic tumors are a heterogeneous group of lesions of diverse clinical behavior and histopathologic types, ranging from hamartomatous lesions to malignancy. They are epithelial or biphasic (epithelial and mesenchymal) tumors, arising from odontogenic epithelium and associated stroma. They are a complex group of lesions. Because odontogenic tumors arise from the tissues which make our teeth, they are unique to the jaws, and by extension almost unique to dentistry.

Malignant odontogenic tumors are quite rare and named similarly according to whether the epithelial or mesenchymal or both components are malignant.

This includes ameloblastic carcinoma, clear cell odontogenic carcinoma, primary intraosseous carcinoma, non-otherwise specified (NOS) sclerosing odontogenic carcinoma, ghost cell odontogenic carcinoma, odontogenic carcinosarcoma, and odontogenic sarcomas. All these tumors have the typical microscopic features of malignancy and can metastasize to regional lymph nodes or distant metastases.

The majority of ameloblastic carcinoma cases arise de novo and less commonly arise from pre-existing ameloblastoma. It is a rare tumor that represents less than 1% of all odontogenic tumors. Primary intraosseous carcinoma is another entity that can arise de novo or as a malignant transformation of an odontogenic cyst. Clear cell odontogenic carcinoma is another malignant intraosseous lesion of odontogenic origin previously thought to be distant metastasis from renal carcinoma.

Non otherwise specified (NOS) sclerosing odontogenic carcinoma has been recently added in the 4th edition of WHO classification for odontogenic tumors. It is a very rare, locally aggressive tumor with low potential for metastatic spread due to marked sclerosis in the surrounding stroma. Its origin is still unclear. Ghost cell odontogenic carcinoma is thought to originate from calcifying odontogenic cysts with some features of odontogenic ghost cells or calcifying odontogenic tumors. Odontogenic sarcoma and carcinosarcoma includes ameloblastic fibrosarcoma, fibro-odontosarcoma, and fibro-dentisarcoma [131–139].

15.12 Conclusions

Epithelial and related carcinomas of the head and neck show a wide range of appearances and behaviors. Refinements in the classification of these tumors continue to be made based on prognostic considerations. Carcinogens such as tobacco or virus

(HPV and EBV) have been considered responsible for these tumors. However, it would be helpful the discovery of new causative agents, or the discovery of specific molecular alterations, in order to provide more accurate prognosis and opportunity of new targeted therapies.

References

1. El-Naggar AK, Chan JKC, Grandis JR, Takata T, Slootweg PJ. WHO classification of head and neck tumours. WHO classification of tumours, vol. 9. 4th ed. Geneva: WHO; 2017.
2. Radosevich JA, editor. Head & neck cancer: current perspectives, 257 advances, and challenges. Dordrecht: Springer; 2013. https://doi.org/10.1007/978-94-007-5827-89.
3. Thariat J, Badoual C, Faure C, et al. Basaloid squamous cell carcinoma of the head and neck: role of HPV and implication in treatment and prognosis. J Clin Pathol. 2010;63:857–66.
4. Stelow EB, Bishop JA. Update from the 4th edition of the World Health Organization classification of head and neck tumours: tumors of the nasal cavity, paranasal sinuses and skull base. Head Neck Pathol. 2017;11:3–15.
5. Lewis JS Jr. Sinonasal squamous cell carcinoma: a review with emphasis on emerging histologic subtypes and the role of human papillomavirus. Head Neck Pathol. 2016;10:60–7.
6. Bishop JA, Guo TW, Smith DF, Wang H, Ogawa T, Pai SI, Westra WH. Human papillomavirus-related carcinomas of the sinonasal tract. Am J Surg Pathol. 2013;37:185–92.
7. El-Mofty SK, Lu DW. Prevalence of high-risk human papilloma-virus DNA in nonkeratinizing (cylindrical cell) carcinoma of the sinonasal tract: a distinct clinicopathologic and molecular disease entity. Am J Surg Pathol. 2005;29:1367–72.
8. Larque AB, Hakim S, Ordi J, Nadal A, Diaz A, del Pino M, Marimon L, Alobid I, Cardesa A, Alos L. High-risk human papillomavirus is transcriptionally active in a subset of sinonasal squamous cell carcinomas. Mod Pathol. 2014;27:343–51.
9. Jo VY, Mills SE, Stoler MH, Stelow EB. Papillary squamous cell carcinoma of the head and neck: frequent association with human papillomavirus infection and invasive carcinoma. Am J Surg Pathol. 2009;33:1720–4.
10. Devaney KO, Ferlito A, Rinaldo A, et al. Verrucous carcinoma (carcinoma cuniculatum) of the head and neck: what do we know now that we did not know a decade ago? Eur Arch Otorhinolaryngol. 2011;268:477–80.
11. Chernock RD, Sewis JS Jr, Zhang Q, et al. Human papillomavirus-positive basaloid squamous cell carcinomas of the upper aerodigestive tract: a distinct clinicopathologic and molecular subtype of basaloid squamous cell carcinoma. Hum Pathol. 2010;41(7):1016–23.
12. Spector ME, Wilson KF, Light E, et al. Clinical and pathologic predictors of recurrence and survival in spindle cell squamous cell carcinoma. Otolaryngol Head Neck Surg. 2011;145:242–7.
13. Lewis JS Jr, Ferlito A, Gnepp DR, et al. Terminology and classification of neuroendocrine neoplasms of the larynx. Laryngoscope. 2011;121:1187–93.
14. Lewis JS Jr, Spence DC, Chiosea S, et al. Large cell neuroendocrine carcinoma of the larynx: definition of an entity. Head Neck Pathol. 2010;4:198–207.
15. Smith VA, MaDan OP, Lentsch EJ. Tumor location is an independent prognostic factor in head and neck Merkel cell carcinoma. Head Neck Surg. 2012;146:403–8.
16. Erovic BM, Habeeb AA, Harris L, et al. Significant overexpression of the Merkel cell polyomavirus (MCPyV) large T antigen in Merkel cell carcinoma. Head Neck. 2012;35(2):184–9. https://doi.org/10.1002/hed.22942.
17. Perez-Ordonez B, Caruana SM, Huvos AG, Shah JP. Small cell neuroendocrine carcinoma of the nasal cavity and paranasal sinuses. Hum Pathol. 1998;29:826–32.

18. Weinreb I, Perez-Ordonez B. Non-small cell neuroendocrine carcinoma of the sinonasal tract and nasopharynx. Report of 2 cases and review of the literature. Head Neck Pathol. 2007;1:21–6.
19. Franchi A, Rocchetta D, Palomba A, Degli Innocenti DR, Castiglione F, Spinelli G. Primary combined neuroendocrine and squamous cell carcinoma of the maxillary sinus: report of a case with immunohistochemical and molecular characterization. Head Neck Pathol. 2015;9:107–13.
20. Thompson ED, Stelow EB, Mills SE, Westra WH, Bishop JA. Large cell neuroendocrine carcinoma of the head and neck: a clinicopathologic series of 10 cases with an emphasis on HPV status. Am J Surg Pathol. 2016;40:471–8.
21. Wang CP, Hsieh CY, Chang YL, Lou PJ, Yang TL, Ting LL, Ko JY. Postirradiated neuroendocrine carcinoma of the sinonasal tract. Laryngoscope. 2008;118:804–9.
22. Hafezi S, Seethala RR, Stelow EB, et al. Ewing's family of tumors of the sinonasal tract and maxillary bone. Head Neck Pathol. 2011;5:8–16.
23. Kerr HE, Hameed O, Lewis JS Jr, et al. Head and neck mucosal malignant melanoma: clinicopathologic correlation with contemporary review of prognostic indicators. Int J Surg Pathol. 2012;20:37–46.
24. Barnes L. Intestinal-type adenocarcinoma of the nasal cavity and paranasal sinuses. Am J Surg Pathol. 1986;10:192–202.
25. Agaimy A, Hartmann A, Antonescu CR, Chiosea SI, El-mofty SK, Geddert H, et al. SMARCB1 (INI-1)-deficient sinonasal carcinoma. A series of 39 cases expanding the morphologic and clinicopathologic spectrum of a recently described entity. Am J Surg Pathol. 2017;41:458–71.
26. Llorente JL, Lopez F, Suarez C, Hermsen MA. Sino-nasal carcinoma: clinical, pathological, genetic and therapeutic advances. Nat Rev Clin Oncol. 2014;11:460–72.
27. Cooper JS, Porter K, Mallin K, Hoffman HT, Weber RS, Ang KK, et al. National cancer database report on cancer of the head and neck: 10-year update. Head Neck. 2009;31:748–58.
28. Xu CC, Dziegielewski PT, McGaw WT, Seikaly H. Sinonasal undifferentiated carcinoma (SNUC): the Alberta experience and literature review. J Otolaryngol Head Neck Surg. 2013;42:2.
29. Bishop JA, Andreasen S, Hang JF, Bullock MJ, Chen TY, Franchi A, et al. HPV-related multipheno-typic sinonasal carcinoma. Am J Surg Pathol. 2017;41:1690–701.
30. Mikkelsen LH, Larsen AC, von Buchwald C, Drzewiecki KT, Prause JU, Heegaard S. Mucosal malignant melanoma – a clinical, oncological, pathological and genetic survey. APMIS. 2016;124:475–86.
31. Youlden DR, Cramb SM, Peters S, Porceddu SV, Møller H, Fritschi L, et al. International comparisons of the incidence and mortality of sinonasal cancer. Cancer Epidemiol. 2013;37:770–9.
32. Batsakis JG, Mackay B, Ordonez NG. Enteric-type adenocarcinoma of the nasal cavity. An electron microscopic and immunocytochemical study. Cancer. 1984;54:855–60.
33. Cathro HP, Mills SE. Immunophenotypic differences between intestinal-type and low-grade papillary sinonasal adenocarcinomas: an immunohistochemical study of 22 cases utilizing CDX2 and MUC2. Am J Surg Pathol. 2004;28:1026–32.
34. Acheson ED, Cowdell RH, Hadfield E, Macbeth RG. Nasal cancer in woodworkers in the furniture industry. Br Med J. 1968;2:587–96.
35. Hadfield EH. A study of adenocarcinoma of the paranasal sinuses in woodworkers in the furniture industry. Ann R Coll Surg Engl. 1970;46:301–19.
36. Hadfield EH, Macbeth RG. Adenocarcinoma of ethmoids in furniture workers. Ann Otol Rhinol Laryngol. 1971;80:699–703.
37. Franchi A, Palomba A, Fondi C, et al. Immunohistochemical investigation of tumorigenic pathways in sinonasal intestinal-type adenocarcinoma. A tissue microarray analysis of 62 cases. Histopathology. 2011;59:98–105.

38. Stelow EB, Mills SE, Jo VY, et al. Adenocarcinoma of the upper aerodigestive tract. Adv Anat Pathol. 2010;17:262–9.
39. Stelow EB, Jo VY, Mills SE, et al. A histologic and immunohistochemical study describing the diversity of tumors classified as sinonasal high-grade nonintestinal adenocarcinomas. Am J Surg Pathol. 2011;35:971–80.
40. Cordes B, Williams MD, Tirado Y, et al. Molecular and phenotypic analysis of poorly differentiated sinonasal neoplasms: an integrated approach for early deiagnosis and classification. Hum Pathol. 2009;40:283–92.
41. Heffner DK, Hyams VJ, Hauck KW, Lingeman C. Low-grade adenocarcinoma of the nasal cavity and paranasal sinuses. Cancer. 1982;50:312–22.
42. Jo VY, Mills SE, Cathro HP, Carlson DL, Stelow EB. Low-grade sinonasal adenocarcinomas: the association with and distinction from respiratory epithelial adenomatoid hamartomas and other glandular lesions. Am J Surg Pathol. 2009;33:401–8.
43. Kleinsasser O. Terminal tubulus adenocarcinoma of the nasal seromucous glands. A specific entity. Arch Otorhinolaryngol. 1985;241:183–93.
44. Zur KB, Brandwein M, Wang B, Som P, Gordon R, Urken ML. Primary description of a new entity, renal cell-like carcinoma of the nasal cavity: van Meegeren in the house of Vermeer. Arch Otolaryngol Head Neck Surg. 2002;128:441–7.
45. Storck K, Hadi UM, Simpson R, Ramer M, Brandwein-Gensler M. Sinonasal renal cell-like adenocarcinoma: a report on four patients. Head Neck Pathol. 2008;2:75–80.
46. Agaimy A, Fonseca I, Martins C, Thway K, Barrette R, Harrington KJ, et al. NUT carcinoma of the salivary glands: clinicopathologic and molecular analysis of 3 cases and a survery of NUT expression in salivary gland carcinomas. Am J Surg Pathol. 2018;42:877–84.
47. Andreasen S, French CA, Josiassen M, Hahn CH, Kiss K. NUT carcinoma of the sublingual gland. Head Neck Pathol. 2016;10:363–6.
48. Bishop JA, Westra WH. NUT midline carcinomas of the sinonasal tract. Am J Surg Pathol. 2012;36:1216–21.
49. French C. NUT midline carcinoma. Nat Rev Cancer. 2014;14:149–50.
50. French CA. The importance of diagnosing NUT midline carcinoma. Head Neck Pathol. 2013;7:11–6.
51. Stelow EB. A review of NUT midline carcinoma. Head Neck Pathol. 2011;5:31–5.
52. Bauer DE, Mitchell CM, Strait KM, Lathan CS, Stelow EB, Luer SC, Muhammed S, Evans AG, Sholl LM, Rosai J, Giraldi E, Oakley RP, Rodriguez-Galindo C, London WB, Sallan SE, Bradner JE, French CA. Clinicopathologic features and long-term outcomes of NUT midline carcinoma. Clin Cancer Res. 2012;18:5773–9.
53. Stelow EB, Bellizzi AM, Taneja K, Mills SE, Legallo RD, Kutok JL, Aster JC, French CA. NUT rearrangement in undifferentiated carcinomas of the upper aerodigestive tract. Am J Surg Pathol. 2008;32:828–34.
54. Solomon LW, Magliocca KR, Cohen C, Muller S. Retrospective analysis of nuclear protein in testis (NUT) midline carcinoma in the upper aerodigestive tract and mediastinum. Oral Surg Oral Med Oral Pathol Oral Radiol. 2014;119:213–20.
55. Fang W, French CA, Cameron MJ, Han Y, Liu H. Clinicopathological significance of NUT rearrangements in poorly differentiated malignant tumors of the upper respiratory tract. Int J Surg Pathol. 2013;21:102–10.
56. French CA, Ramirez CL, Kolmakova J, Hickman TT, Cameron MJ, Thyne ME, Kutok JL, Toretsky JA, Tadavarthy AK, Kees UR, Fletcher JA, Aster JC. BRD-NUT oncoproteins: a family of closely related nuclear proteins that block epithelial differentiation and maintain the growth of carcinoma cells. Oncogene. 2008;27:2237–42.
57. Huang SC, Ghossein RA, Bishop JA, Zhang L, Chen TC, Huang HY, Antonescu CR. Novel PAX3-NCOA1 fusions in biphenotypic sinonasal sarcoma with focal rhabdomyoblastic differentiation. Am J Surg Pathol. 2016;40:51–9.

58. Haack H, Johnson LA, Fry CJ, Crosby K, Polakiewicz RD, Stelow EB, Hong SM, Schwartz BE, Cameron MJ, Rubin MA, Chang MC, Aster JC, French CA. Diagnosis of NUT midline carcinoma using a NUT-specific monoclonal antibody. Am J Surg Pathol. 2009;33:984–91.
59. French CA. Pathogenesis of NUT midline carcinoma. Annu Rev Pathol. 2012;7:247–65.
60. Frierson HF Jr, Mills SE, Fechner RE, Taxy JB, Levine PA. Sinonasal undifferentiated carcinoma. An aggressive neoplasm derived from schneiderian epithelium and distinct from olfactory neuroblastoma. Am J Surg Pathol. 1986;10:771–9.
61. Kumar S, Perlman E, Pack S, Davis M, Zhang H, Meltzer P, Tsokos M. Absence of EWS/FLI1 fusion in olfactory neuroblastomas indicates these tumors do not belong to the Ewing's sarcoma family. Hum Pathol. 1999;30:1356–60.
62. Taxy JB, Bharani NK, Mills SE, Frierson HF Jr, Gould VE. The spectrum of olfactory neural tumors. A light-microscopic immunohistochemical and ultrastructural analysis. Am J Surg Pathol. 1986;10:687–95.
63. Singhi AD, Westra WH. Comparison of human papillomavirus in situ hybridization and p16 immunohistochemistry in the detection of human papillomavirus-associated head and neck cancer based on a prospective clinical experience. Cancer. 2010;116:2166–73.
64. Bishop JA, Ma XJ, Wang H, Luo Y, Illei PB, Begum S, Taube JM, Koch WM, Westra WH. Detection of transcriptionally active high-risk HPV in patients with head and neck squamous cell carcinoma as visualized by a novel E6/E7 mRNA in situ hybridization method. Am J Surg Pathol. 2012;36:1874–82.
65. Poling JS, Ma XJ, Bui S, Luo Y, Li R, Koch WM, Westra WH. Human papillomavirus (HPV) status of non-tobacco related squamous cell carcinomas of the lateral tongue. Oral Oncol. 2014;50:306–10.
66. Lewis JS Jr, Ukpo OC, Ma XJ, Flanagan JJ, Luo Y, Thorstad WL, Chernock RD. Transcriptionally-active high-risk human papillomavirus is rare in oral cavity and laryngeal/hypopharyngeal squamous cell carcinomas–a tissue microarray study utilizing E6/E7 mRNA in situ hybridization. Histopathology. 2012;60:982–91.
67. Heffner DK, Hyams VJ. Teratocarcinosarcoma (malignant teratoma?) of the nasal cavity and paranasal sinuses: a clinicopathologic study of 20 cases. Cancer. 1984;53:2140–54.
68. Salem F, Rosenblum MK, Jhanwar SC, Kancherla P, Ghossein RA, Carlson DL. Teratocarcinosarcoma of the nasal cavity and paranasal sinuses: report of 3 cases with assessment for chromosome 12p status. Hum Pathol. 2008;39:605–9.
69. Rooper LM, Huang SC, Antonescu CR, Westra WH, Bishop JA. Biphenotypic sinonasal sarcoma: an expanded immunoprofile including consistent nuclear beta-catenin positivity and absence of SOX10 expression. Hum Pathol. 2016;55:44–50.
70. Lewis JT, Oliveira AM, Nascimento AG, Schembri-Wismayer D, Moore EA, Olsen KD, Garcia JG, Lonzo ML, Lewis JE. Low-grade sinonasal sarcoma with neural and myogenic features: a clinicopathologic analysis of 28 cases. Am J Surg Pathol. 2012;36:517–25.
71. Wang X, Bledsoe KL, Graham RP, Asmann YW, Viswanatha DS, Lewis JE, Lewis JT, Chou MM, Yaszemski MJ, Jen J, Westendorf JJ, Oliveira AM. Recurrent PAX3-MAML3 fusion in biphenotypic sinonasal sarcoma. Nat Genet. 2014;46:666–8.
72. Powers KA, Han LM, Chiu AG, Aly FZ. Low-grade sinonasal sarcoma with neural and myogenic features-diagnostic challenge and pathogenic insight. Oral Surg Oral Med Oral Pathol Oral Radiol. 2015;119:e265–e9.
73. Wong WJ, Lauria A, Hornick JL, Xiao S, Fletcher JA, Marino-Enriquez A. Alternate PAX3-FOXO1 oncogenic fusion in biphenotypic sinonasal sarcoma. Genes Chromosomes Cancer. 2016;55:25–9.
74. Cheung F, Chan O, Ng WT, et al. The prognostic value of histological typing in nasopharyngeal carcinoma. Oral Oncol. 2012;48:429–33.
75. Singhi AD, Califano J, Westra WH. High-risk human papillomavirus in nasopharyngeal carcinoma. Head Neck. 2011;34:213–8.

76. Andreasen S, Kiss K, Mikkelsen LH, Channir HI, Plaschke CC, Melchior LC, Eriksen JG, Wessel I. An update on head and neck cancer: new entities and their histopathology, molecular background, treatment, and outcome. APMIS. 2019;127:240–64.
77. Bjørndal K, Krogdahl A, Therkildsen MH, Overgaard J, Johansen J, Kristensen CA, et al. Salivary gland carcinoma in Denmark 1990–2005: a national study of incidence, site and histology. Results of the Danish Head and Neck Cancer Group (DAHANCA). Oral Oncol. 2011;47:677–82.
78. Eveson JW, Cawson RA. Warthin's tumor (cystadenolymphoma) of salivary glands. A clinicopathological investigation of 278 cases. Oral Surg Oral Med Oral Pathol. 1986;61:256–62.
79. Andreasen S, Therkildsen MH, Bjørndal K, Homøe P. Pleomorphic adenoma of the parotid gland 1985–2010: a Danish nationwide study of incidence, recurrence rate, and malignant transformation. Head Neck. 2016;38(1):E1364–9.
80. Stevens E, Andreasen S, Bjørndal K, Homøe P. Tumors in the parotid are not relatively more often malignant in children than in adults. Int J Pediatr Otorhinolaryngol. 2015;79:1192–5.
81. Andreasen S, Stevens E, Bjørndal K, Homøe P. Salivary gland epithelial neoplasms in pediatric population: a single-institute experience with a focus on the histologic spectrum and clinical outcome. Hum Pathol. 2018;73:193–4.
82. Andreasen S, Bjørndal K, Agander TK, Wessel I, Homøe P. Tumors of the sublingual gland: a national clinicopathologic study of 29 cases. Eur Arch Otorhinolaryngol. 2016;273:3847–56.
83. Dhanuthai K, Boonadulyarat M, Jaengjongdee T, Jiruedee K. A clinico-pathologic study of 311 intra-oral salivary gland tumors in Thais. J Oral Pathol Med. 2009;38:495–500.
84. Geyer FC, Pareja F, Weigelt B, Rakha E, Ellis IO, Schnitt SJ, et al. The spectrum of triple-negative breast disease. High- and low-grade lesions. Am J Pathol. 2017;187:2139–51.
85. Andreasen S, Esmaeli B, Von Holstein SL, Mikkelsen LH, Rasmussen PK, Heegaard S. An update on tumors of the lacrimal gland. Asia Pac J Ophthalmol. 2017;6:159–72.
86. Hyrcza MD, Andreasen S, Melchior LC, Tucker T, Heegaard S, White VA. Primary secretory carcinoma of the lacrimal gland: report of a new entity. Am J Ophthalmol. 2018;193:178–83.
87. Ihrler S, Weiler C, Eckert F, Mollenhauer M. Cutaneous adnexal and salivary gland tumours. Similarities and differences. Pathologe. 2014;35:476–86.
88. Thackray AC, Sobin LH. Histological typing of salivary gland tumours. Geneva: WHO; 1972.
89. Slootweg P. Tumours of the salivary glands. In: El-Naggar A, Chan J, Grandis J, Takata T, Slootweg P, editors. World Health Organization classification of tumours. 4th ed. Lyon: IARC Press; 2017. p. 159–201.
90. Szanto PA, Luna MA, Tortoledo ME, White RA. Histologic grading of adenoid cystic carcinoma of the salivary glands. Cancer. 1984;54:1062–9.
91. Amit M, Binenbaum Y, Trejo-Leider L, Sharma K, Ramer N, Ramer I, et al. International collaborative validation of intraneural invasion as a prognostic marker in adenoid cystic carcinoma of the head and neck. Head Neck. 2015;37:1038–45.
92. Ishibashi K, Ito Y, Masaki A, Fujii K, Beppu S, Sakakibara T, et al. Warthin-like mucoepidermoid carcinoma: a combined study of fluorescence in situ hybridization and whole-slide imaging. Am J Surg Pathol. 2015;39:1479–87.
93. Chiosea SI, Griffith C, Assaad A, et al. The profile of acinic cell carcinoma after recognition of mammary analog secretory carcinoma. Am J Surg Pathol. 2012;36:343–50.
94. Skálová A, Vanecek T, Sima R, et al. Mammary analogue secretory carcinoma of salivary glands, containing the ETV6-NTRK3 fusion gene: a hitherto undescribed salivary gland tumor entity. Am J Surg Pathol. 2010;34:599–608.
95. Connor A, Perez-Ordoñez B, Shago M, et al. Mammary analog secretory carcinoma of salivary gland origin with the ETV6 gene rearrangement by FISH: expanded morphologic and immunohistochemical spectrum of a recently described entity. Am J Surg Pathol. 2012;36:27–34.
96. Chiosea SI, Griffith C, Assaad A, et al. Clinicopathologic characterization of mammary analogue secretory carcinoma of salivary glands. Histopathology. 2012;61:387–94.

97. Roy P, Bullock MJ, Perez-Ordoñez B, et al. Epithelial-myoepithelial carcinoma with high grade transformation. Am J Surg Pathol. 2010;34:1258–65.
98. El-Naggar AK, Callender D, Coombes MM, et al. Molecular genetic alterations in carcinoma ex-pleomorphic adenoma: a putative progression model? Genes Chromosomes Cancer. 2000;27:162–8.
99. Weiler C, Zengel P, van der Wal JE, et al. Carcinoma ex pleomorphic adenoma with special reference to the prognostic significance of histologic progression: a clinicopathologic investigation of 41 cases. Histopathology. 2011;59:741–50.
100. Skalova A, Vanecek T, Sima R, Laco J, Weinreb I, Perez-Ordonez B, et al. Mammary analogue secretory carcinoma of salivary glands, containing the ETV6-NTRK3 fusion gene: a hitherto undescribed salivary gland tumor entity. Am J Surg Pathol. 2010;34:599–608.
101. Patel TD, Vazquez A, Marchiano E, Park RC, Baredes S, Eloy JA. Polymorphous low-grade adenocarcinoma of the head and neck: a population-based study of 460 cases. Laryngoscope. 2015;125:1644–9.
102. Nagao T, Gaffey TA, Kay PA, Minato H, Serizawa H, Lewis JE. Polymorphous low-grade adenocarcinoma of the major salivary glands: report of three cases in an unusual location. Histopathology. 2004;44:164–71.
103. Weinreb I, Piscuoglio S, Martelotto LG, Waggott D, Ng CK, Perez-Ordonez B, et al. Hotspot activating PRKD1 somatic mutations in polymorphous low-grade adenocarcinomas of the salivary glands. Nat Genet. 2014;46:1166–9.
104. Barasch N, Gong X, Kwei KA, Varma S, Biscocho J, Qu K, et al. Recurrent rearrangements of the Myb/SANT-like DNA-binding domain containing 3 gene (MSANTD3) in salivary gland acinic cell carcinoma. PLoS ONE. 2017;12:e0171265.
105. Andreasen S, Varma S, Barasch N, Thompson LDR, Miettinen M, Rooper L, et al. The HTN3MSANTD3 fusion gene defines a subset of acinic cel carcinoma of the salivary gland. Am J Surg Pathol. 2018;43(4):489–96. https://doi.org/10.1097/pas.0000000000001200.
106. Bagnardi V, Rota M, Botteri E, et al. Alcohol consumption and site-specific cancer risk: a comprehensive dose-response meta-analysis. Br J Cancer. 2015;112:580–93.
107. Goldstein BY, Chang SC, Hashibe M, et al. Alcohol consumption and cancers of the oral cavity and pharynx from 1988 to 2009: an update. Eur J Cancer Prev. 2010;19:431–65.
108. Ferrarotto R, Mitani Y, Diao L, Guijarro I, Wang J, Zweidler-McKay P, et al. Activating NOTCH1 mutations define a distinct subgroup of patients with adenoid cystic carcinoma who have poor prognosis, propensity to bone and liver metastasis, and potential responsiveness to notch1 inhibitors. J Clin Oncol. 2016;35:352–60.
109. Andreasen S, Agander TK, Bjørndal K, Erentaite D, Heegaard S, Larsen SR, et al. Genetic rearrangements, hotspot mutations, and microRNA expression in the progression of metastatic adenoid cystic carcinoma of the salivary gland. Oncotarget. 2018;9:19675–87.
110. Boon E, van Boxtel W, Buter J, Baatenburg de Jong RJ, van Es RJJ, Bel M, et al. Androgen deprivation therapy for androgen receptor-positive advanced salivary duct carcinoma: a nationwide case series of 35 patients in The Netherlands. Head Neck. 2018;40:605–13.
111. Schmitt NC, Kang H, Sharma A. Salivary duct carcinoma: an aggressive salivary gland malignancy with opportunities for targeted therapy. Oral Oncol. 2017;74:40–8.
112. Dalin MG, Desrichard A, Katabi N, Makarov V, Walsh LA, Lee KW, et al. Comprehensive molecular characterization of salivary duct carcinoma reveals actionable targets and similarity to apocrine breast cancer. Clin Cancer Res. 2016;22:4623–33.
113. Takahashi H, Masubuchi T, Fushimi C, Matsuki T, Inomata T, Okada T, et al. Trastuzumab and docetaxel for Her2-positive unresectable salivary gland carcinoma: updated results of a phase II trial. In: AHNS Annual Meeting, 2016, p. S207.
114. Seethala RR. An update on grading of salivary gland carcinomas. Head Neck Pathol. 2009;57:69–77.
115. Bentzen J, Toustrup K, Eriksen JG, Primdahl H, Andersen LJ, Overgaard J. Locally advanced head and neck cancer treated with accelerated radiotherapy, the hypoxic modifier nimora-

zole and weekly cisplatin. Results from the DAHANCA 18 phase II study. Acta Oncol. 2015;54:1001–7.

116. Müller S. Update from the 4th edition of the World Health Organization of head and neck tumours: tumours of the oral cavity and mobile tongue. Head Neck Pathol. 2017;11:33–40.

117. Dahlgren L, Dahlstrand HM, Lindquist D, et al. Human papillomavirus is more common in base of tongue than in mobile tongue cancer and is a favorable prognostic factor in base of tongue cancer patients. Int J Cancer. 2004;112:1015–9.

118. Gillison ML, Chaturvedi AK, Anderson WF, Fakhry C. Epidemiology of human papillomavirus-positive head and neck squamous cell carcinoma. J Clin Oncol. 2015;33:3235–42.

119. Lingen MW, Xiao W, Schmitt A, et al. Low etiologic fraction for high-risk human papillomavirus in oral cavity squamous cell carcinomas. Oral Oncol. 2013;49:1–8.

120. Sgaramella N, Coates PJ, Strindlund K, et al. Expression of p16 in squamous cell carcinoma of the mobile tongue is independent of HPV infection despite presence of the HPV-receptor syndecan-1. Br J Cancer. 2015;113:321–6.

121. Zafereo ME, Xu L, Dahlstrom KR, Viamonte CA, et al. Squamous cell carcinoma of the oral cavity often overexpresses p16 but is rarely driven by human papillomavirus. Oral Oncol. 2016;56:47–53.

122. Reuschenbach M, Kansy K, Garbe K, et al. Lack of evidence of human papillomavirus-induced squamous cell carcinomas of the oral cavity in southern Germany. Oral Oncol. 2013;49(9):937–42.

123. IARC. Alcohol consumption and ethyl carbamate. IARC Monogr Eval Carcinog Risks Hum. 2010;96:1–1428.

124. Kuribayashi Y, Tsushima F, Morita K, et al. Long-term outcome of non-surgical treatment in patients with oral leukoplakia. Oral Oncol. 2015;51:1020–5.

125. Petti S. Pooled estimate of world leukoplakia prevalence: a systematic review. Oral Oncol. 2003;39:770–80.

126. Agaimy A. Colonic-type adenocarcinoma of the tongue and oral cavity (CATOC). Head Neck Pathol. 2017;12:291–3.

127. Smith BC, Ellis GL, Meis-Kindblom JM, Williams SB. Ectomesenchymal chondromyxoid tumor of the anterior tongue. Nineteen cases of a new clinicopathologic entity. Am J Surg Pathol. 1995;19:519–30.

128. Bishop J, Gnepp D, Ro J. Ectomesenchymal chondromyxoid tumour. In: El-Naggar A, Chan J, Grandis J, Takata T, Slootweg P, editors. WHO classification of head and neck tumours. Lyon: IARC Press; 2017. p. 119–20.

129. Dickson BC, Antonescu CR, Argyris PP, Bilodeau EA, Bullock MJ, Freedman PD, et al. Ectomesenchymal chondromyxoid tumor a neoplasm characterized by recurrent RREB1-MKL2 fusions. Am J Surg Pathol. 2018;42:1297–305.

130. Crain N, Nelson BL, Barnes EL, et al. Ceruminous gland carcinomas: a clinicopathologic and immunophenotypic study of 17 cases. Head Neck Pathol. 2009;3:1–17.

131. Hertog D, Bloemena E, Aartman IHA, et al. Histopathology of ameloblastoma of the jaws; some critical observations based on a 40 years single institution experience. Med Oral Pathol Oral Cir Bucal. 2012;1:e76–82.

132. Labib A, Adlard RE. Odontogenic tumors of the jaws. In: StatPearls. Treasure Island: StatPearls Publishing; 2022. https://www.ncbi.nlm.nih.gov/books/NBK572116/.

133. Rizzitelli A, Smoll NR, Chae MP, Rozen WM, Hunter-Smith DJ. Incidence and overall survival of malignant ameloblastoma. PLoS One. 2015;10(2):e0117789.

134. Dissanayake RK, Jayasooriya PR, Siriwardena DJ, Tilakaratne WM. Review of metastasizing (malignant) ameloblastoma (METAM): pattern of metastasis and treatment. Oral Surg Oral Med Oral Pathol Oral Radiol Endod. 2011;111(6):734–41.

135. Iezzi G, Rubini C, Fioroni M, Piattelli A. Clear cell odontogenic carcinoma. Oral Oncol. 2002;38(2):209–13. https://doi.org/10.1016/s1368-8375(01)00038-0. PMID: 11854070.

136. Irié T, Ogawa I, Takata T, Toyosawa S, Saito N, Akiba M, Isobe T, Hokazono C, Tachikawa T, Suzuki Y. Sclerosing odontogenic carcinoma with benign fibro-osseous lesion of the mandible: an extremely rare case report. Pathol Int. 2010;60(10):694–700.
137. Wood A, Young F, Morrison J, Conn BI. Sclerosing odontogenic carcinoma presenting on the hard palate of a 43-year-old female: a case report. Oral Surg Oral Med Oral Pathol Oral Radiol. 2016;122(6):e204–8.
138. Mosqueda Taylor A, Meneses García A, Ruíz Godoy Rivera LM, de Suárez Roa ML, Luna OK. Malignant odontogenic tumors. A retrospective and collaborative study of seven cases. Med Oral. 2003;8(2):110–21.
139. Goldenberg D, Sciubba J, Koch W, Tufano RP. Malignant odontogenic tumors: a 22-year experience. Laryngoscope. 2004;114(10):1770–4.

Chapter 16
Current Techniques for Intraoperative Application

Ioannis Kastanioudakis and Lentiona Basiari

Radical excision with tumor free margins is the main goal of surgical treatment in oncologic surgery. The head and neck region has a unique anatomy when compared to the rest of the body. Many vital structures, such as large vessels, cranial nerves, and important organs, are located in the head and neck area. Close or involved margins affect patient prognosis, survival and postoperative decision about adjuvant chemoradiotherapy, whereas wider margins may impact normal function and increase morbidity. Due to the great impact of surgical margins, scientists worldwide are developing different methods for the intraoperative evaluation of resection margins. Although frozen section analysis remains the most applicable method, many other in vivo optical technologies are being applied in the operating room.

16.1   Frozen Section Analysis in Head and Neck Margins

The complete surgical excision of cancers with negative margins impacts significantly local tumor recurrence and overall survival for patients with head and neck squamous cell carcinomas [1]. Intraoperative frozen section analysis of surgical margins is a widely used practice in head and neck surgery and remains the most common and standard technique for assessment of surgical margins, even though its applicability is seriously influenced by the surgeon's and pathologist's experience, tumor site and size, and specific hospital facilities [2]. Frozen section techniques have significantly improved in quality and accuracy through the years. Standard frozen section evaluation begins with fresh tissue specimens embedded in optimal cutting temperature compound which are frozen using a cryostat machine, thinly

I. Kastanioudakis · L. Basiari (✉)
Department of Otorhinolaryngology, Head and Neck Surgery, University Hospital of Ioannina, Ioannina, Greece

G. Alexiou, G. Vartholomatos (eds.), *Intraoperative Flow Cytometry*, https://doi.org/10.1007/978-3-031-33517-4_16

sectioned to an average thickness of 7 µm, and fixed to glass slides. Next step is staining with hematoxylin and eosin, and finally evaluation by a pathologist [3]. When frozen section reveals infiltrated margin than the surgeon performs additional resection. Many differences exist between surgeons, institutions, and pathologists regarding how tissue is sampled and how specimens are processed [2, 3]. In the hands of experienced pathologists frozen section diagnoses tend to have high accuracy. DiNardo et al. found an overall accuracy rate of 98.3% [4]. Cooley et al. found that 2% to 10% of margins that are negative intraoperatively are later diagnosed as positive on permanent histopathology [5]. There are two types of frozen section errors. The first type can be interpretive error and the second type is sampling error. Interpretive errors occur when the pathologist makes an incorrect diagnosis due to poor staining, distortion of tissue during freezing and uneven sectioning. On the other hand, sampling errors can occur at multiple points. A positive margin can be missed if it is never sampled. According to Gandour-Edwards et al. sampling errors are more common than interpretive ones and most errors occur due to superficial sectioning and missing deeper lesions [6]. Also discrepancies between frozen section analysis and permanent histopathology are related to whether the sample is specimen driven or tumor bed driven. Black and colleagues found that most surgeons send fragments of tissue from the surgical bed to be read as frozen sections because this approach is faster. But with this approach is not possible to measure the distance of the margin from the tumor [3]. In the specimen-driven approach, tissue is sampled from the resected specimen, and the margin distance from the tumor is measured. Intraoperative sampling via a specimen-driven approach has many advantages such as an improved accuracy of final margin status, a reduced rate of local recurrence, and patient survival. Yahalom and colleagues proved that frozen section sampling from the resected specimen correlated best with final margin status, local recurrence, and overall patient survival [7]. Meier et al. [8] and Maxwell et al. [9] described three methods for evaluating margin status: (1) sampling of main specimen edges without tumor bed sampling, (2) intraoperative evaluation of main specimen margins by a pathologist with extra tissue taken if these samples are positive for carcinoma, and (3) tumor bed sampling only without intraoperative sampling of the main specimen. They found that the 3-year recurrence-free survival was poorest for the third method [8].

Disadvantages of frozen section analysis include the fact that are costly in terms of time and personnel. In case of tumor bone involvement, frozen section evaluation of decalcified cortical bone is not practical and does not add any improvement to margins assessment accuracy [10]. Also oversampling can increase cost, the size of the surgical defect, and operative time. Undersampling, on the other hand, can lead to missed positive margins. Positive margins have significant impact on patient prognosis and often necessitate adjuvant chemotherapy or radiation treatment [11].

Frozen section analysis is the gold standard and an important tool for head and neck surgeons. Its value is quite clear in cases where patients are spared repeat operations or additional therapy.

16.2   In Vivo Optical Imaging in Head and Neck Margins

Complete surgical resection with clear margins remains the basis of therapy for patients with head and neck squamous cell carcinoma. In head and neck area very radical approaches are considered undesirable because of related morbidity, loss of function, and esthetics. Achieving clear resection margins is the main goal of surgical oncology, as inadequate resection margins are associated with increased recurrence rates and poorer survival [12, 13]. Despite the burden on patients and the healthcare system, inadequate margins continue to occur frequently in head and neck cancers [12].

Surgeons depend on their own skills and judgment to decide which tissues to resect because common imaging techniques only reveal anatomical structures and do not offer real-time intraoperative guidance. After resection, the specimen and wound bed are inspected macroscopically, often followed by a (time-consuming) frozen section. It is practically and technically impossible to evaluate the whole resection margin with frozen thus having the risk of sampling errors. The result of this approach is positive margins in 12–30% of cases [14–16]. Due to the negative effect of positive margins in prognosis, there is a need for improved intraoperative detection and visualization of HNSCC [17]. In order to reduce the number of inadequate margins and associated consequences, there has been wide interest in imaging techniques for intraoperative margin analysis.

Anatomic or metabolic changes in the tissue are the bases of current imaging strategies commonly used for cancer detection and pretreatment planning. The evolution in optical hardware and reagents has made possible real-time cancer imaging in the clinic or operating room. New techniques with real-time applicability have been used in order to better delineate primary HNSCC for the purpose of either mucosal or deep margin assessment intraoperatively. Also advances in the understanding of the biology and tumorigenesis of head and neck cancer such as identification of specific biomarker expression in tumor cells lead to the development of new diagnostic methods and instruments. Optical imaging and light-based imaging techniques use specific properties of light to image anatomical or chemical characteristics of tissue and permit real-time diagnosis and margin discrimination [18]. Optical imaging techniques in the head and neck include: autofluorescence imaging (AFI) [19], targeted fluorescence imaging (TFI) [19], high-resolution microendoscopy (HRME) [20], narrow band imaging (NBI) [21], and the Raman spectroscopy (RS) [22]. Optical coherence tomography, elastic scattering spectroscopy, confocal laser endomicroscopy, and confocal reflectance microscopy, have also been used in the head and neck region [23, 24].

The various optical imaging techniques function optimally within a certain range of the light spectrum. The optimal window for fluorescent dyes is in the near infrared (NIR) spectrum (700–900 nm), in which light may travel up to millimeters rather than micrometers [25].

16.2.1   Non-fluorescent Visualization

Several mucosal non-fluorescent tissue dyes such as Lugol's iodine solution that stains normal mucosa brown but leaves dysplastic epithelium white or pink have been applied for tumor delineation and visualization [26] (Fig. 16.1). Lugol can only be used in non-keratinized epithelium and poses the risk of aspiration into the airway, that is why this method has not been applied widely in the oral cavity [26]. Another dye that has been used is Toluidine blue which has an affinity for nucleic acids. Dysplastic and abnormal tissues have higher RNA and DNA content and as a result they show more intense staining than healthy tissues [28]. Toluidine blue, like Lugol, has limited clinical benefits with a 75% sensitivity and 60% specificity for the detection of oral lesion.

16.2.2   Fluorescence Imaging

Different fluorescent agents can be used in the real-time identification of primary HNSCC. In optical image-guided surgery, the tumor-to-background ratio (TBR) is an important parameter to distinguish tumor from normal tissues [29]. Fluorescence imaging has become a booming research area during the last decades. Fluorescent agents such as methylene blue, indocyanine green (ICG), and 5-aminolevulinic acid

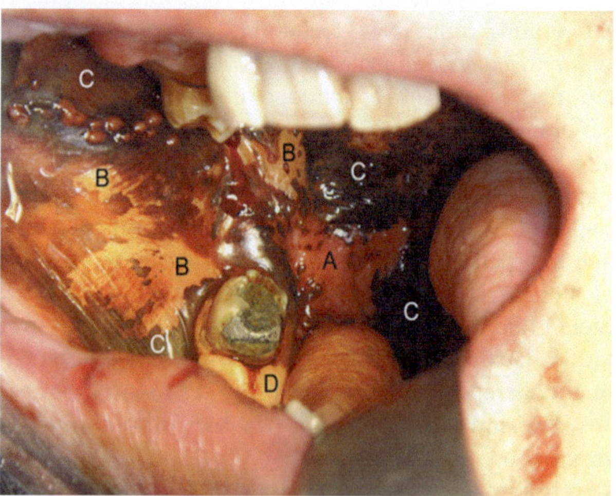

Fig. 16.1 (**a**) Invasive squamous cell carcinoma of oral cavity and oropharynx not stained after the application of lugol iodine in the field; (**b**) areas with dysplasia not stained by iodine; (**c**) normal parakeratinized mucosa stained brown or black by iodine; and (**d**) normal orthokeratinized mucosa not stained by iodine. (Reprinted from Use of Lugol's iodine in the resection of oral and oropharyngeal squamous cell carcinoma. Br J Oral Maxillofac Surg. 2009;48:84–7. McMahon J, Devine JC, McCaul JA, McLellan DR, Farrow A., with permission from Elsevier) [27]

(ALA) have been used as untargeted agents leading to non-specific fluorescence, higher background signals, and faster clearance, reducing the time window for surgery [30]. Therefore, efforts have been made to conjugate fluorescent molecules to specific tumor-targeting agents for increased accuracy and efficacy. Cancer cells are characterized by higher expression of growth factor receptors such as EGFR and VEGFR that can serve as potential targets for molecular imaging [31]. The use of targeted molecules can result in higher specificity lowering the required dose of the fluorescent agent and leading to better TBRs. Another benefit is the increased binding time of these agents that could result in a prolonged time window to perform surgery, compared to ICG where peak fluorescence decreased after 1 hour. Fluorophores such as Cy5.5 and IRDye800CW have frequently been described in HNSCC and can be conjugated to targeting molecules [32–34]. Cetuximab is a monoclonal antibody that binds with high affinity to EGFR. Several studies have used cetuximab-IRDye800CW for fluorescence imaging of HNSCC [35, 36]. On the other hand autofluorescence which emits between 450 and 650 nm and disappears beyond 1500 nm can be detected due to endogenous fluorophores, such as structural proteins. The endogenous fluorophores appear in green when excited by ultraviolet light in contrast to precancerous and malignant lesions which appear as red-violet caused by an altered metabolism in tumor cells [29, 30]. Autofluorescence is characterized by low specificity caused by interpretation errors of images due to variety in autofluorescence caused by scar formation, minimal amounts of blood, bacterial overgrowth, and inflammation [29]. Also autofluorescence is best suited to evaluate superficial margins because the penetrating depth of autofluorescence illumination is relatively shallow (Fig. 16.2).

Narrow Band imaging (NBI) is an endoscopic optical imaging technique that has gained attention over the past two decades. During carcinogenesis the structure and organization of vasculature may change due to angiogenesis, forming intraepithelial papillary capillary loops (IPCL) [38]. Enhanced visualization of these new abnormal blood vessels using two narrow band filters of blue and green leads to increased and earlier detection of precancerous and cancerous lesions [39]. These filters have a bandwidth of 30 nm with central wavelengths of 415 nm and 540 nm, respectively, which are maximally absorbed by hemoglobin [40]. The superficial

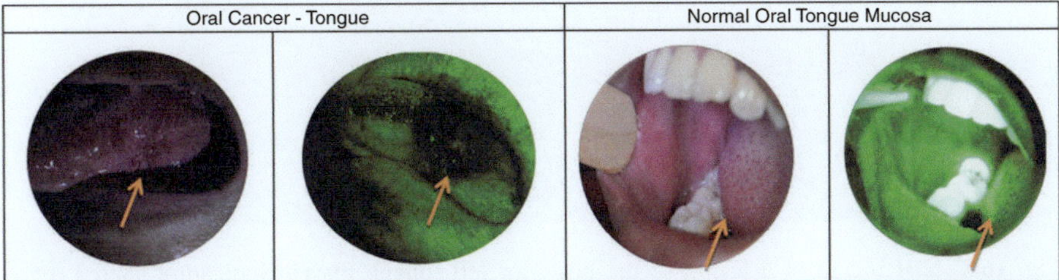

Fig. 16.2 Images of oral cancer of the tongue and normal oral tongue mucosa with wight light and fluorescence visualization. (Reprinted from Novel quantitative analysis of autofluorescence images for oral cancer screening. Oral Oncol 2017;68: 20–6. Huang T, Huang J, Wang Y, Chen K, Wong T, Chen Y, et al. with permission from Elsevier) [37]

vessels are displayed in brown and submucosal vessels in cyan, increasing the contrast between vasculature and surrounding mucosa. As a result, neoplastic areas with rich vascularity are characterized by a hypointense signal. NBI seems to be a promising technique in the detection of laryngeal, pharyngeal, and oral malignancies with an overall sensitivity of 89% and specificity of 96% [41, 42]. Tirelli et al. compared white light (WL) examination and NBI guided resection of oral and oropharyngeal tumors demonstrating that resection margins status improves when NBI is used [43] (Figs. 16.3 and 16.4). A follow-up study conducted by Farah et al. showed that the use of NBI in resections of oral and oropharyngeal squamous cell carcinoma is associated with improved 5-year local recurrence rates and disease-free survival [44]. On the other hand difficulties related to the intraoperative application of NBI have been reported. An experienced team should be created because a learning curve has been reported for this technique [45]. Preoperative evaluation of tumor extent is necessary in order to limit an increase in operating time but in certain areas this proves to be difficult sometimes because of location and poor patient compliance. In addition, it is recommended to perform NBI application before surgical actions because the presence of blood in the surgical field alters NBI evaluation. Moreover, superficial mucosal margins can only be evaluated with NBI [43]. Large prospective studies or randomized controlled trials are necessary to provide evidence on the influence of NBI on clinical outcome or health care costs.

Intraoral ultrasound is a method that is increasingly used recently for determining the mucosal and deep resection margins of oral tongue squamous cell carcinoma with promising results. A systematic review showed a significant correlation between ultrasonographically measured and histologic tumor thickness [46].

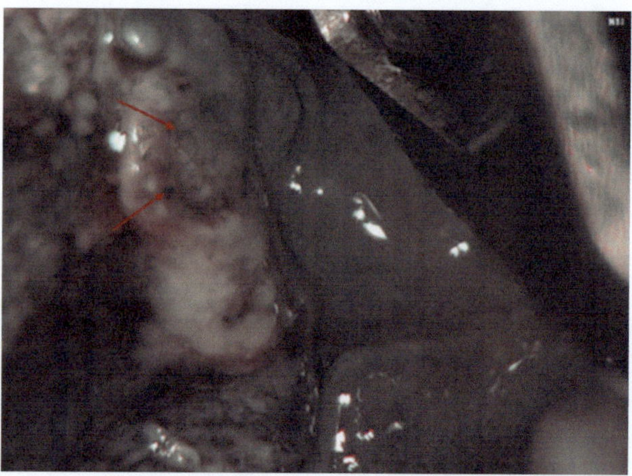

Fig. 16.3 NBI image of a lesion of the posterior left tongue margin indicating altered intrapapillary capillary loops (IPCL) defined as positive for malignancy. Histopathology confirmed the presence of squamous cell carcinoma. (Reproduced from Tirelli G, Piovesana M, Gatto A, Tofanelli M, Biasotto M, Boscolo Nata F. Narrow band imaging in the intraoperative definition of resection margins in oral cavity and oropharyngeal cancer. Oral Oncol 2015;51: 908–913 with permission from Elsevier) [43]

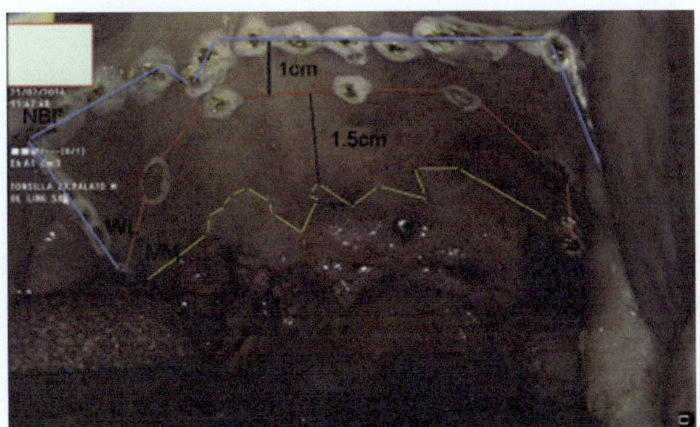

Fig. 16.4 Squamous cell carcinoma of the oropharynx. Delineation of gross tumor edge (green line), delineation of resection margin obtained after evaluation with white light and palpation (red line) and resection margin drawn after NBI evaluation (blue line). (Reproduced from Tirelli G, Piovesana M, Gatto A, Tofanelli M, Biasotto M, Boscolo Nata F. Narrow band imaging in the intraoperative definition of resection margins in oral cavity and oropharyngeal cancer. Oral Oncol 2015;51: 908–913 with permission of Elsevier) [43]

Optical coherence tomography (OCT) is an emerging non-invasive technology that uses reflecting coherent light to provide cross-sectional images of the underlying tissue structure on the micron scale and in real time with a penetration depth of 0.5–2 mm [47]. This technology widely used in the field of ophthalmology, provides a map of the mucosal epithelium. Due to accessibility reasons, it is mostly used in the oral cavity where epithelial thickening may indicate malignancy [48]. Sensitivity and specificity rates of 100% have been reported for the detection of oral SCC, compared to 93% and 69% for dysplastic lesions, respectively [49] (Fig. 16.5). Huang et al. described the basic principle of OCT [50]. In head and neck, OCT has been applied most often to detect early epithelial changes of the oropharyngeal mucosa. Prestin et al. [51] used OCT to measure oral tissue epithelium thickness and concluded that it was possible to recognize oral malignancy and determine the grade of dysplasia. However, this method has limited accuracy in the differentiation between malignancy and inflammation [48].

High-Resolution Microendoscopy (HRME) is a non-invasive optical imaging technology which is performed by placing a flexible fiber-optic probe in direct contact with the suspicious mucosal surface that has been previously stained with a fluorescent contrast agent. Microscopic images of the cellular architecture of selected tissue are provided to evaluate cellular pleomorphism, nuclear size, nuclear to cytoplasm ratio, and crowding. Based on these criteria specialists can distinguish benign epithelium from neoplastic tissue [20]. Miles et al. found a sensitivity and specificity of 96% and 95%, respectively, of HRME in distinguishing benign from malignant mucosa in patients with squamous cell carcinoma of the upper aerodigestive track [52]. An important limitation of this method is the narrow field of view.

Raman spectroscopy is a vibrational spectroscopic technique that was first applied in the head and neck by Stone et al. [53] in 2000 to analyze laryngeal mucosa ex vivo

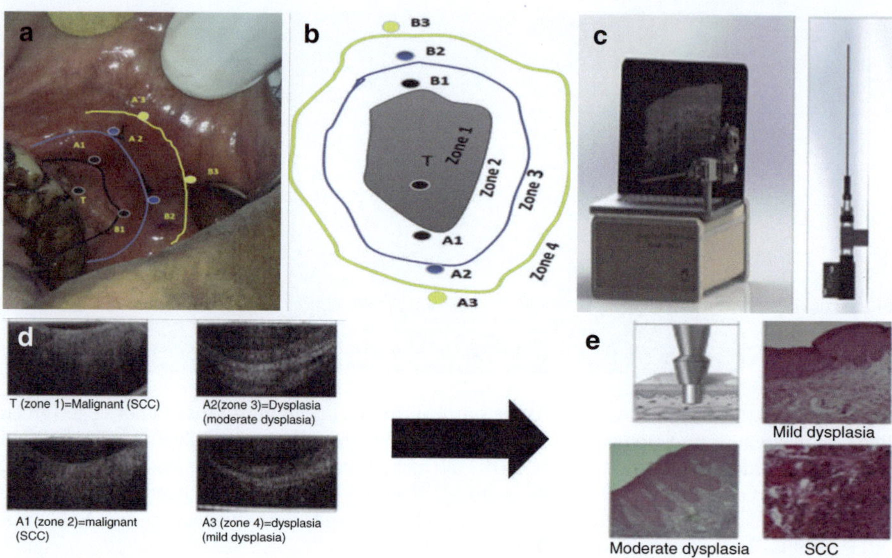

Fig. 16.5 Application of optical coherence tomography for optimal intraoperative surgical margin delineation. (**a**) Clinical photograph with tumor and resection margin mapping. (**b**) Schematic representation of tumor and resection margin mapping. [tumor: T & Zone 1, black outline: tumor margin (Zone 2), blue outline: surgical-excision margin , which is 1 cm away from clinical tumor margin (Zone 3) and yellow outline: the region 1 cm away from the surgical margin (Zone 4: 2 cm from the clinical tumor margin)]. (**c**) Portable OCT device. (**d**) OCT images from different zones with OCT diagnosis. (**e**) Histopathology images and diagnosis. (Reproduced from Sunny SP, Agarwal S, James BL, Heidari E, Muralidharan A, Yadav V, et al. Intraoperative point-of-procedure delineation of oral cancer margins using optical coherence tomography. Oral Oncol. 2019;92:12–9 with permission from Elsevier) [49]

using biopsy specimens from 15 patients with 90% sensitivity and 92% specificity reported for the detection of laryngeal squamous cell carcinoma. This technology is based on the fact that photons are scattered at a different wavelength due to energy loss while interacting with the vibrational modes of certain molecules and it can provide quantitative and qualitative information about the molecular structure of tissue. The Raman spectrum provides information about the content of lipids, nucleic acids, proteins, and water of biological tissue. Specific molecules, such as keratin, an epithelial cellular structural protein, are abnormally expressed in tumors, and can be used as cancer molecular indicators [54]. With Raman spectroscopy it is possible to assess not only superficial mucosa, but also deep soft tissue layers [55–60]. Barroso et al. applied Raman spectroscopy to analyze changes in water concentration between tumor border and healthy surrounding tissue on freshly excised specimens from the oral cavity [61].

Guze et al. [62] reported a 100% sensitivity and 77% specificity of Raman spectroscopy in distinguishing (pre)malignant oral lesions from normal tissue. Krishna et al. [63] accomplished to classify the Raman spectra of oral tissue sites into four categories including normal tissue, oral submucous fibrosis, oral leukoplakia, and oral squamous cell carcinoma using a specified diagnostic algorithm. However, analyzing an entire specimen may take up to several hours. Also in vivo accessibility is

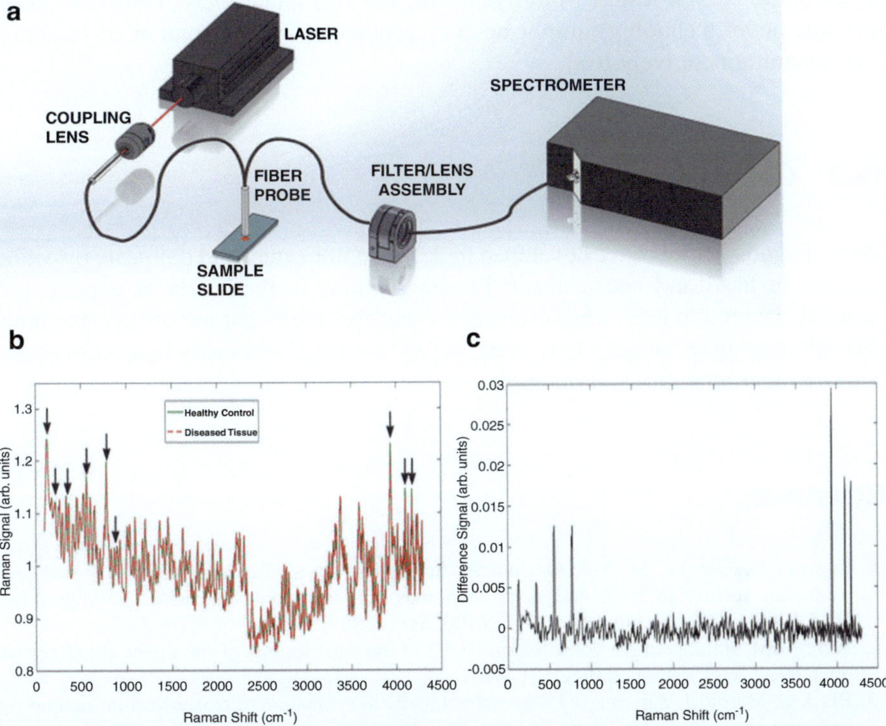

Fig. 16.6 (**a**) A 785 nm laser directed into the Raman probe via the objective lens which illuminates the tissue sample and collects the scattered light. A long pass filter removes the elastically scattered signal and the light is transmitted into spectrometer for dispersion and storage. (**b**) Raman spectra from one healthy and one cancerous sample over the entire ~4000 cm⁻¹ Raman shift signal. The arrows indicate the peaks that show differences between the healthy tissue and the cancerous tissue. (**c**) The difference spectrum obtained by withdrawing the cancerous spectrum from the healthy spectrum in panel (**b**). (Reproduced from Holler et al. Raman Spectroscopy of Head and Neck Cancer: Separation of Malignant and Healthy Tissue Using Signatures Outside the "Fingerprint" Region. Biosensors (Basel). CC BY 4.0) [64]

difficult because only rigid scopes can be used, and interpretation of results is more mathematical than visual (Fig. 16.6).

Concofocal laser microendoscopy is a new, non-invasive technique that allows high-resolution, microanatomical analysis of lining mucosa in real time. It is also referred as optical biopsies [65, 66]. It has been widely used in gastroenterology and its application in other specialties is recently being investigated. This technology can differentiate tissue types based on mucosal histologic characteristics and submucosal vasculature [67]. In this way it might be possible to identify lesions that need further treatment and to delineate the extent of neoplastic lesions in order to guide a more precise resection. Pogorzelski et al. applied intraoperative confocal laser microendoscopy in combination with fluorescence imaging intraoperatively for diagnostic and therapeutic purposes in fifteen patients with squamous cell carcinoma of head and neck. Scoring systems were used in order to differentiate benign lesion from dysplastic and malignant ones. They concluded that this novel technology might be very promising for delineation of resection margins intraoperatively [68].

16.3 Conclusion

Many diagnostic tools have developed to detect tumor extent and delineate resection margins in head and neck cancer. Frozen sections in the hands of experienced pathologists tend to have a high sensitivity and specificity but are time-consuming. Optical imaging techniques have been widely used but are mostly limited to evaluation of superficial mucosal margins.

References

1. Eugenie D, Ow TJ, Lo Y-T, Gersten A, Schiff BA, et al. Refining the utility and role of frozen section in head and neck squamous cell carcinoma resection. Laryngoscope. 2015;126(8):1768–75. https://doi.org/10.1002/lary.25899.
2. Wenig BM. Intraoperative consultation (IOC) in mucosal lesions of the upper aerodigestive tract. Head Neck Pathol. 2008;2:131–44.
3. Black C, Marotti J, Zarovnaya J, Paydarfar J. Critical evaluation of frozen section margins in head and neck cancer resections. Cancer. 2006;107:2792–800.
4. DiNardo LJ, Lin J, Karageorge LS, Powers CN. Accuracy, utility, and cost of frozen section margins in head and neck cancer surgery. Laryngoscope. 2000;110:1773–6.
5. Cooley ML, Hoffman HT, Robinson RA. Discrepancies in frozen section mucosal margin tissue in laryngeal squamous cell carcinoma. Head Neck. 2002;24:262–7.
6. Gandour-Edwards RF, Donald P, Wiese DA. Accuracy of intraoperative frozen section diagnosis in head and neck surgery: experience at a University Medical Center. Head Neck. 1993;1:373–6.
7. Yahalom R, Dobriyan A, Vered M, et al. A prospective study of surgical margin status in oral squamous cell carcinoma: a preliminary report. J Surg Oncol. 2008;98:572–8.
8. Meier JD, Oliver DA, Varvares MA. Surgical margin determination in head and neck oncology: current clinical practice. The results of an International American Head and Neck Society Member Survey. Head Neck. 2005;27(11):952–8.
9. Maxwell JH, Thompson LD, Brandwein-Gensler MS, Weiss BG, Canis M, Purgina B, Prabhu AV, Lai C, Shuai Y, Carroll WR, Morlandt A, Duvvuri U, Kim S, Johnson JT, Ferris RL, Seethala R, Chiosea SI. Early oral tongue squamous cell carcinoma: sampling of margins from tumor bed and worse local control. JAMA Otolaryngol Head Neck Surg. 2015;141(12):1104–10.
10. Robbins KT, Triantafyllou A, Suarez C, et al. Surgical margins in head and neck cancer: intra- and postoperative considerations. Auris Nasus Larynx. 2019;46:10–7.
11. Shapiro M, Salama A. Margin analysis squamous cell carcinoma of the oral cavity. Oral Maxillofacial Surg Clin N Am. 2017;29:259–67.
12. Smits RWH, Koljenovic S, Hardillo JA, et al. Resection margins in oral cancer surgery: room for improvement. Head Neck. 2016;38(1):E2197–203.
13. Stojadinovic A, Leung DHY, Hoos A, Jaques DP, Lewis JJ, Brennan MF. Analysis of the prognostic significance of microscopic margins in 2,084 localized primary adult soft tissue sarcomas. Ann Surg. 2002;235:424–34.

14. Woolgar JA, Triantafyllou A. A histopathological appraisal of surgical margins in oral and oropharyngeal cancer resection specimens. Oral Oncol. 2005;41:1034–43.
15. Van Keulen S, Van den Berg NS, Nishio N, Birkeland A, Zhou Q, Lu G, et al. Rapid, non-invasive fluorescence margin assessment: optical specimen mapping in oral squamous cell carcinoma. Oral Oncol. 2019;88:58–65.
16. Wong LS, McMahon J, Devine J, McLellan D, Thompson E, Farrow A, et al. Influence of close resection margins on local recurrence and disease-specific survival in oral and oropharyngeal carcinoma. Br J Oral Maxillofac Surg. 2011;50:102–8.
17. Hinni ML, Ferlito A, Brandwein-Gensler MS, Takes RP, Silver CE, Westra WH, et al. Surgical margins in head and neck cancer: a contemporary review. Head Neck. 2013;35:1362–70.
18. Warram JM, et al. Fluorescence imaging to localize head and neck squamous cell carcinoma for enhanced pathological assessment. J Pathol Clin Res. 2016;2:104–12.
19. Zhang RR, et al. Beyond the margins: real-time detection of cancer using targeted fluorophores. Nat Rev Clin Oncol. 2017;14:347–64.
20. Vila PM, et al. Discrimination of benign and neoplastic mucosa with a high resolution micro-endoscope (HRME) in head and neck cancer. Ann Surg Oncol. 2012;19:3534–9.
21. Vu A, Farah CS. Narrow band imaging: clinical applications in oral and oropharyngeal cancer. Oral Dis. 2016;22:383–90.
22. Harris AT, et al. Raman spectroscopy in head and neck cancer. Head Neck Oncol. 2010;2:26.
23. Green B, Cobb AR, Brennan PA, Hopper C. Optical diagnostic techniques for use in lesions of the head and neck: review of the latest developments. Br J Oral Maxillofac Surg. 2014;52:675–80.
24. Green B, Tsiroyannis C, Brennan PA. Optical diagnostic systems for assessing head and neck lesions. Oral Dis. 2016;22:180–4.
25. Vahrmeijer AL, Hutteman M, van der Vorst JR, van de Velde CJH, Frangioni JV. Image-guided cancer surgery using near-infrared fluorescence. Nat Rev Clin Oncol. 2013;10:507–18.
26. Muto M, Hironaka S, Nakane M, Boku N, Ohtsu A, Yoshida S. Association of multiple Lugol-voiding lesions with synchronous and metachronous esophageal squamous cell carcinoma in patients with head and neck cancer. Gastrointest Endosc. 2002;56:517–21.
27. McMahon J, Devine JC, McCaul JA, McLellan DR, Farrow A. Use of Lugol's iodine in the resection of oral and oropharyngeal squamous cell carcinoma. Br J Oral Maxillofac Surg. 2009;48:84–7.
28. Sridharan G, Shankar AA. Toluidine blue: a review of its chemistry and clinical utility. J Oral Maxillofac Pathol. 2012;16:251–5.
29. Keereweer S, Kerrebijn JDF, Mol IM, Mieog JSD, Van Driel PBAA, Baatenburg de Jong RJ, et al. Optical imaging of oral squamous cell carcinoma and cervical lymph node metastasis. Head Neck. 2012;34:1002–8.
30. Wang C, Wang Z, Zhao T, Li Y, Huang G, Sumer BD, et al. Optical molecular imaging for tumor detection and image-guided surgery. Biomaterials. 2018;157:62–75.
31. Yokoyama J, Fujimaki M, Ohba S, Anzai T, Yoshii R, Ito S, et al. A feasibility study of NIR fluorescent image-guided surgery in head and neck cancer based on the assessment of optimum surgical time as revealed through dynamic imaging. Onco Targets Ther. 2013;6:325–30.
32. Rosenthal EL, Kulbersh BD, Duncan RD, Zhang W, Magnuson JS, Carroll WR, et al. In vivo detection of head and neck cancer orthotopic xenografts by immunofluorescence. Laryngoscope. 2006;116:1636–41.
33. Withrow KP, Newman JR, Skipper JB, Gleysteen JP, Magnuson JS, Zinn K, et al. Assessment of bevacizumab conjugated to Cy5.5 for detection of head and neck cancer xenografts. Technol Cancer Res Treat. 2008;7:61–6.
34. Heath CH, Deep NL, Sweeny L, Zinn KR, Rosenthal EL. Use of panitumumab-IRDye800 to image microscopic head and neck cancer in an orthotopic surgical model. Ann Surg Oncol. 2012;19:3879–87.

35. Rosenthal EL, Moore LS, Tipirneni K, de Boer E, Stevens TM, Hartman YE, et al. Sensitivity and specificity of cetuximab-IRDye800CW to identify regional metastatic disease in head and neck cancer. Clin Cancer Res. 2017;23:4744–52.
36. Moore LS, Rosenthal EL, de Boer E, Prince AC, Patel N, Richman JM, et al. Effects of an unlabeled loading dose on tumor-specific uptake of a fluorescently labeled antibody for optical surgical navigation. Mol Imaging Biol. 2017;19:610–6.
37. Huang T, Huang J, Wang Y, Chen K, Wong T, Chen Y, et al. Novel quantitative analysis of autofluorescence images for oral cancer screening. Oral Oncol. 2017;68:20–6.
38. Kumagai Y, Toi M, Inoue H. Dynamism of tumour vasculature in the early phase of cancer progression: outcomes from oesophageal cancer research. Lancet Oncol. 2002;3:604–10.
39. Ni X, He S, Xu Z, Gao L, Lu N, Yuan Z, et al. Endoscopic diagnosis of laryngeal cancer and precancerous lesions by narrow band imaging. J Laryngol Otol. 2011;125:288–96.
40. Nonaka S, Saito Y. Endoscopic diagnosis of pharyngeal carcinoma by NBI. Endoscopy. 2008;40:347–51.
41. Cosway B, Drinnan M, Paleri V. Narrow band imaging for the diagnosis of head and neck squamous cell carcinoma: a systematic review. Head Neck. 2016;38:E2358–67.
42. Zhou H, Zhang J, Guo L, Nie J, Zhu C, Ma X. The value of narrow band imaging in diagnosis of head and neck cancer: a meta-analysis. Sci Rep. 2018;8:515. https://doi.org/10.1038/s41598-017-19069-0.
43. Tirelli G, Piovesana M, Gatto A, Tofanelli M, Biasotto M, Boscolo NF. Narrow band imaging in the intra-operative definition of resection margins in oral cavity and oropharyngeal cancer. Oral Oncol. 2015;51:908–13.
44. Farah CS. Narrow band imaging-guided resection of oral cavity cancer decreases local recurrence and increases survival. Oral Dis. 2018;24:89–97.
45. Piazza C, Cocco D, De Benedetto L, Del Bon F, Piero P, Peretti G. Narrow band imaging and high definition television in the assessment of laryngeal cancer: a prospective study on 279 patients. Eur Arch Otorhinolaryngol. 2010;267(3):409–14.
46. Tarabichi O, Bulbul MG, Kanumuri VV, Faquin WC, Juliano AF, Cunnane ME, et al. Utility of intraoral ultrasound in managing oral tongue squamous cell carcinoma: systematic review. Laryngoscope. 2019;129:662–70.
47. De Leeuw F, Abbaci M, Casiraghi O, Ben Lakhdar A, Alfaro A, Breuskin I, et al. Value of full-field optical coherence tomography imaging for the histological assessment of head and neck cancer. Lasers Surg Med. 2020;52(8):768–78.
48. Hamdoon Z, Jerjes W, McKenzie G, Jay A, Hopper C. Optical coherence tomography in the assessment of oral squamous cell carcinoma resection margins. Photodiagn Photodyn Ther. 2015;13:211–7.
49. Sunny SP, Agarwal S, James BL, Heidari E, Muralidharan A, Yadav V, et al. Intraoperative point-of-procedure delineation of oral cancer margins using optical coherence tomography. Oral Oncol. 2019;92:12–9.
50. Huang D, Swanson EA, Lin CP, Schuman JS, Stinson WG, Chang W, et al. Optical coherence tomography. Science. 1991;254:178–81.
51. Prestin S, Rothschild SI, Betz CS, Kraft M. Measurement of epithelial thickness within the oral cavity using optical coherence tomography. Head Neck. 2012;34(12):1777–81.
52. Miles BA, Patsias A, Quang T, Polydorides AD, Richards-Kortum R, Sikora AG. Operative margin control with high-resolution optical microendoscopy for head and neck squamous cell carcinoma. Laryngoscope. 2015;125(10):2308–16.
53. Stone N, Stavroulaki P, Kendall C, Birchall M, Barr H. Raman spectroscopy for early detection of laryngeal malignancy: preliminary results. Laryngoscope. 2000;110(10):1756–63.
54. Singh S, Alam H, Dmello C, Vaidya MM, Krishna CM. Raman spectroscopic study of keratin 8 knockdown oral squamous cell carcinoma derived cells. In: Imaging, manipulation, and analysis of biomolecules, cells, and tissues. Bellingham: International Society for Optics and Photonics; 2012.

55. Malini R, et al. Discrimination of normal, inflammatory, premalignant, and malignant oral tissue: a Raman spectroscopy study. Biopolymers. 2006;81:179–93.
56. Oliveira AP, et al. Near-infrared Raman spectroscopy for oral carcinoma diagnosis. Photomed Laser Surg. 2006;24:348–53.
57. Su L, et al. Raman spectral properties of squamous cell carcinoma of oral tissues and cells. Laser Phys. 2012;22:311–6.
58. Nijsen A, Koljenović S, Schut TCB, Caspers PJ, Puppels GJ. Towards oncological application of Raman spectroscopy. J Biophotonics. 2009;2:29–36.
59. Cals FLJ, Schut TCB, Hardillo JA, Baatenburg de Jong RJ, Koljenović S, Puppels GJ. Investigation of the potential of Raman spectroscopy for oral cancer detection in surgical margins. Lab Investig. 2015;95(10):1186–96.
60. Harris AT, Rennie A, Waqar-Uddin H, Wheatley SR, Ghosh SK, Martin-Hirsch DP, et al. Raman spectroscopy in head and neck cancer. Head Neck Oncol. 2010;2:26.
61. Barroso EM, Smits RW, van Lanschot CG, Caspers PJ, Ten Hove I, Mast H, Sewnaik A, Hardillo JA, Meeuwis CA, Verdijk R, Noordhoek Hegt V, Baatenburg de Jong RJ, Wolvius EB, Bakker Schut TC, Koljenović S, Puppels GJ. Water concentration analysis by Raman spectroscopy to determine the location of the tumor border in oral cancer surgery. Cancer Res. 2016;76(20):5945–53.
62. Guze K, Pawluk HC, Short M, Zeng H, Lorch J, Norris C, et al. Pilot study: Raman spectroscopy in differentiating premalignant and malignant oral lesions from normal mucosa and benign lesions in humans. Head Neck. 2015;37:511–7.
63. Krishna H, Majumder SK, Chaturvedi P, Sidramesh M, Gupta PK. In vivo Raman spectroscopy for detection of oral neoplasia: a pilot clinical study. J Biophotonics. 2014;7(9):690–702.
64. Holler S, Mansley E, Mazzeo C, Donovan MJ, Sobrero M, Miles BA. Raman spectroscopy of head and neck cancer: separation of malignant and healthy tissue using signatures outside the "fingerprint" region. Biosensors. 2017;7(2):20.
65. Paull PE, Hyatt BJ, Wassef W, Fischer AH. Confocal laser endomicroscopy: a primer for pathologists. Arch Pathol Lab Med. 2011;135:1343–8.
66. Goetz M, Watson A, Kiesslich R. Confocal laser endomicroscopy in gastrointestinal diseases. J Biophotonics. 2011;4:498–508.
67. Humphris J, Swartz D, Egan BJ, Leong RWL. Status of confocal laser endomicroscopy in gastrointestinal disease. Trop Gastroenterol. 2012;33:9–20.
68. Pogorzelski B, Hanenkamp U, Goetz M, Kiesslich R, Gosepath J. Systematic intraoperative application of confocal endomicroscopy for early detection and resection of squamous cell carcinoma of the head and neck: a preliminary report. Arch Otolaryngol Head Neck Surg. 2012;138(4):404–11.

Chapter 17
Intraoperative Flow Cytometry in Head and Neck Malignancies

Ioannis Kastanioudakis and Lentiona Basiari

17.1 Head and Neck Cancer

Head and neck malignancy is a heterogeneous disease and includes cancers originating from the oral cavity, nasopharynx, oropharynx, larynx, and hypopharynx. Each subtype within the disease group is associated with different epidemiology, etiology, and therapy [1]. The most common histological type is squamous cell carcinoma of head and neck (SCCHN) which represents the sixth most common cancer worldwide [2, 3]. The incidence rates in men are higher comparing with those in women and the median age at diagnosis is approximately 60 years [4].

The risk factors for developing head and neck cancer include tobacco exposure, alcohol use, infectious agents such as HPV especially in oropharyngeal carcinoma and EBV in nasopharyngeal carcinoma, gastroesophageal reflux, diet, radiation, and occupational exposure especially for malignancies of sinonasal region [5].

At the time of diagnosis, 29% of cases are categorized as localized cases, 47% as regional cases, and 20% as distant cases [5].

Treatment of SCCHN depends on the site and stage of disease. Over the past decades great advances have been made in the treatment of head and neck cancer. Surgery, radiotherapy, chemotherapy, targeted therapy, and immunotherapy are the available treatment modalities [6]. In general, early stage tumors can be treated with single modality therapy, either surgery or radiotherapy. For more advanced stages of disease a multimodality therapy is applied which consists of definitive chemoradiotherapy or combination of surgery and chemoradiotherapy [7]. For metastatic disease standard treatment consists of combinatory use of chemotherapy with a monoclonal antibody targeting epidermal growth factor receptor or immune

I. Kastanioudakis · L. Basiari (✉)
Department of Otorhinolaryngology, Head and Neck Surgery, University Hospital of Ioannina, Ioannina, Greece

© The Author(s), under exclusive license to Springer Nature Switzerland AG 2023
G. Alexiou, G. Vartholomatos (eds.), *Intraoperative Flow Cytometry*,
https://doi.org/10.1007/978-3-031-33517-4_17

checkpoint inhibitor [8]. Immunotherapy by anti-PD-1 or anti-PD-L1 antibodies significantly prolongs disease-free survival and overall survival in advanced stages [9]. However, treatment response is characterized by great disparities [10].

Even though many treatment protocols are applied, locoregional recurrences still occur in 30–40% of advanced stage patients [11]. Despite radical surgery aiming the complete tumor removal, the development of local and regional recurrences remains a persistent problem. After resection the surgical specimen is transferred to a pathology laboratory and screened by microscopy to confirm that the tumor has been removed completely. Strangely, even when the surgical margins are histologically tumor-free, local recurrences may still occur in 10–30% of patients [11]. Researchers trying to explain the cause of these unexpected local recurrences have concluded in two mechanisms. The first mechanism known as minimal residual disease refers to the fact that even after microscopic examination of the resected specimen, tumor cells that appear to be too small to be detected by routine histopathology may stay behind unnoticed and develop into a recurrence [12]. The second mechanism is related to the presence of premalignant mucosal changes characterized by genetic and morphological changes, mostly not visible to the naked eye. These precancerous lesions often surround the primary tumor and can stay behind unnoticed after excision of the tumor causing local relapse [12].

17.2 The Concept of Surgical Margins in Head and Neck Cancer

The concept of "surgical margins" was born in the second century from the observation that a tumor can early return in areas adjacent to where it was completely excised. Galen was the first to assume that cancer can infiltrate surrounding tissue even beyond the sensitivity of the naked eye [13]. Virchow and Lebert in the nineteenth century observed that in the early phase cancer cells can invade neighboring tissues without yet producing macroscopic morphologic changes [13]. It was Halsted one of the most distinguished oncologic surgeons to concretely apply this concept to surgical practice at the end of the nineteenth century [14].

Even though biological comprehension of cancer has evolved a lot since then, the basic concept of surgical margins has remained unchanged with the goal of removing enough tissue to ensure that all cancer cells are included in the surgical specimen.

Achieving adequately and homogeneously wide margins in the head and neck area is quite challenging. The need to preserve several vital functions most commonly compete with the demarcation of a wide margin all along the tumor surface. The presence of vital organs such as the eyes, the tongue, the pharynx, the larynx, the brain, and the dense neurovascular system place the surgeon in front of dilemmas on preservation versus ablation. Another element of complexity characterizing tumors of the head and neck is biological heterogeneity. Tumors pertaining to the same histological category can present with several degrees of biological aggressiveness [15, 16]. The 3-dimensional shape of the tumor also effects adequate and regular delineation of margins. Advanced tumors of the head and neck acquire a 3-dimensional morphology that mirrors the complexity of subsite anatomy. Cancers with no superficial components are not rare in head and neck which can increase the chance of resection to be misled [17]. Finally, the presence of recurrence within an irradiated area follows a multifocal pattern and increases remarkably the chance of leaving microscopic residual disease in surgical margins. Considering all the above-mentioned elements together, surgical margins have been obviously a hot topic in head and neck oncology over the last decades [18].

17.3 Defining an Adequate Margin in Head and Neck Cancer

Complete surgical excision with adequate resection margins is essential for local tumor control. Microscopically positive margins, R1 resections, have a high rate of local recurrence. Close margins also carry an increased risk of recurrence over the widely free surgical resection margin [19, 20]. Even though the concept of margin adequacy may seem simple, significant confusion surrounds the definition of adequate margins. Many discrepancies also exist regarding the extent of surgery, and the method of determining margin status. Thus, achieving resection margin adequacy is highly dependent on surgeons and pathologists.

Many critical factors such as the way margins are sampled: from the en bloc specimen versus only from the surgical defect, the subsite in the head and neck, the methods used to determine distance to margins, and the communication between the pathologist and surgeon involving the specimen, orientation, and areas of concern can impact the adequacy of surgical margins [21].

In general, according to the National Comprehensive Cancer Network (NCCN) a clear margin is >5 mm from the invasive tumor, a close margin is 1–5 mm from the invasive tumor, and a positive margin combines invasive carcinoma and carcinoma in situ at a margin and distance <1 mm from the invasive tumor [22].

In terms of margin sampling there are two methods for tissue submission termed en face and perpendicular that differ in the information that can be obtained. In en face tissue sections the entire microscopic slide represents the true margin, which is flat peripheral tissue, parallel to the margin of interest. However, in these sections, the distance of the margin from the invasive tumor cannot be accessed microscopically, and the results are either positive or negative for tumor. On the other hand, in perpendicular margins the tissue section represents a cross section through the tumor toward the margin and allows for the distance from the tumor cells to the resection margin in millimeters to be measured.

Tissue shrinkage can also affect the adequacy of surgical margins. Studies conducted in patients with oral squamous cell carcinoma demonstrated margin shrinkage rates ranging from 21% to 75%. Also, tumors located in areas like the buccal mucosa, retro-molar trigone, and mandibular alveolar ridge underwent a significantly greater degree of shrinkage than did tumors of the maxilla and tongue, suggesting that a wider resection in these areas is necessary to obtain a clear surgical margin [23, 24].

The anatomical subsite is an important factor that can affect what we consider an adequate surgical margin. For example, in the glottis region the need for balancing preservation of function with oncologic resection requires reconsideration of widely negative margins for early stage disease. Thus, margins of 1–2 mm in glottic tumors have been proposed [25]. Similarly, the evolution of transoral robotic surgery in oropharyngeal tumors and the better prognosis of HPV-associated squamous cell carcinomas has led to focused studies for margin assessment in this subgroup [26].

The definition of a clear margin paradoxically can be altered according to the technique used for the excision of the primary tumor. According to this a cancer of the upper aerodigestive tract would be defined as completely resected with a threshold of 5 mm of pathologically uninvolved tissue if open surgery was performed, 2–5 mm in case of transoral robotic surgery, 0.5–2 mm if resection was performed via transoral laser surgery, and regardless of metric measurements if adjacent structures are not infiltrated in case endoscopic transnasal resection has been performed [27–30].

It is more difficult for surgeons to achieve adequate margins for deep connective tissue planes as compared with mucosal margins. In a review of 301 patients with oral and oropharyngeal cancers that underwent surgical resection with curative intent, the percentage of inadequate deep margins was a lot higher than superficial mucosal inadequate margins [31]. A possible explanation might be that anatomic boundaries may limit the surgeon's ability to achieve adequate deep resection margins. Also, on the mucosal surface the tumor is visible whereas during excision of the tumor in the soft tissues the tumor is not visible but only palpable when one attempts an "en bloc" resection [31].

A more accurate and standardized approach to resection margins would be of great importance for the surgical management of HNSCC. An ideal approach should account for various anatomic and tumor factors such as the 3-dimensional aspects of tumor extension and pathologic factors such as the pattern of tumor invasion. Different surgical practices impact the optimal method of margin surveillance. Open or transoral en bloc resections are open to complete "specimen driven" tumor mapping and margin surveillance but the same approach may not be possible for endoscopic or multibloc laser microscopic resections. More sophisticated imaging and in vivo optical techniques are now being developed to allow surgeons, before and during surgery, to delineate tumor borders more precisely. The problem with these optical techniques is that they are limited to the surface mucosa and cannot assess deep resection margins. Recently has been proved that phenotypically normal mucosal cells can be genetically damaged. This has been proposed as the basis for novel molecular assays as a form of margin assessment, which has been termed "molecular margins analysis."

17.4   The Concept of Molecular Margin Analysis

The concept of field cancerization, first described by Slaughter et al. [32] in 1953, is important in any discussion of surgical margins and mucosal margins in particular. According to this theory HNSCCs arise from a "field" of genetically damaged or "condemned" mucosa. When considering surgical margins, the concept of field cancerization can be useful in explaining tumor recurrence after apparently a "complete" surgical excision with negative margins [33]. Even though the tissue may appear morphologically intact, it may have undergone genetic alteration beyond the excised margin that is not visible to the pathologist histologically. Considering the disturbing trend of local recurrence despite "adequate" histologic surgical excision and due to the growing lack of confidence in the pathologist's ability to recognize the presence and extent of the neoplastic process in patients at risk for HNSCC, researchers have turned to biochemical analysis of the surgical margin to help characterize the true status of the margin using novel biomarkers. The presence of genetically damaged cells can be detected in histologically normal mucosal margins with a variety of strategies for detecting genetic alterations including TP53 mutations [34], loss of heterozygosity [35], promoter hypermethylation [36, 37], eIF4E proto-oncogene overexpression [37], and mitochondrial DNA mutations [38].

Brennan et al. investigated the presence of an altered p53 gene at histologically normal surgical margins in oral squamous cell carcinoma. According to this study in more than half of the patient's molecular analysis was positive for a p53 mutation in at least one margin. 38% of those with an altered p53 gene developed local recurrence, in contrast to none of the patients who did not have the alteration [39]. In another study by Nathan and colleagues the presence of eIF4E, a well-known proto-oncogene that is activated in nearly all head and neck squamous cell carcinoma, at histologically negative surgical margins was investigated. They found that 55% of patients had elevated levels of eIF4E in histologically negative margins and 56% of those patients developed local recurrence. Only 7% of patients with eIF4E-negative margins developed local recurrence [40]. Many other mutated tumor suppressor genes correlated with local recurrence despite negative margins have been identified including p15, p16, and 9p21 [41, 42]. Alterations in gene promoter methylation patterns also have been investigated. Despite the variety of biomarkers available for characterization of apparently negative margins, there are very few real-time assays at this point that allow for intraoperative detection of biomarkers. Goldenberg and colleagues developed a novel method using the quantitative methylation-specific polymerase chain reaction protocol that allows for the detection of methylation-positive margins in less than 5 h, which could be useful in oral squamous cell resection cases that require combined primary tumor resection, cervical lymphadenectomy, and complex reconstruction [36]. Molecular margin analysis has been studied widely with promising results, but it remains investigational and not widely used in clinical practice due to practical, financial, and even ethical conflicts. A significant limitation of these molecular analyses of surgical margins is the considerable time required to perform them, which limits their intraoperative efficacy. Unlike in vivo optical imaging techniques using vital dyes or autofluorescence, molecular genetic analysis does not provide rapid results.

17.5 Intraoperative Flow Cytometry in Head and Neck Margins: Fast Cell Cycle Analysis

Flow cytometry is a laser-based technique that permits rapid analysis of large populations of cells with a high reproducibility. Flow cytometry represents an indispensable tool in basic research and can be performed using a flow cytometer, specific reagents, and data analysis system [43]. Multiparametric measurements of each cell such as size, protein content, DNA content, lipid content, antigenic properties, and enzyme activity are assessed using flow cytometry. It is widely used for the diagnosis and classification of hematologic malignancies. Its value in the analysis of solid tumors has gained a lot of interest because flow cytometry permits the assessment of a tumor's ploidy, which is associated with poor prognosis in several cancers [44]. Vijayavel and Aswath [45] reported that DNA ploidy assessment may play role as a prognostic factor in evaluation of oral premalignant diseases to carcinomatous progression and staging of neoplastic lesions. Other studies showed that DNA index shows a good correlation with the histological features of oral squamous cell carcinoma and that high S-phase fraction of primary oral squamous cell carcinoma assessed by flow cytometry was significantly associated with decrease disease-free survival rates [46].

Over the last few years Alexiou et al. also developed an intraoperative protocol for rapid cell cycle analysis, named Ioannina Protocol that could measure the tumor DNA content within 6 min and calculate the malignant index (MI) of the analyzed cells. Based on this protocol, cell cycle fractions, namely G0/G1, S, and G2/M, were used as an index of malignancy. DNA index was also calculated in order to distinguish diploid from aneuploid lesions [47].

This protocol was performed on 78 patients with head and neck lesions intraoperatively and we found that a cut-off value of 88% for G_0/G_1 phase had a 97.4% sensitivity and 90% specificity for the diagnosis of malignancy, for S-phase fraction the cut-off value was higher or equal to 6% (97.4% sensitivity and 73.3% specificity) and for G_2/M phase fraction a value higher or equal to 5% (80% sensitivity and 86.7% specificity). A tumor index ($S + G_2/M$) higher of 10% had a 97.4% sensitivity and 90% specificity for the detection of malignancy. Also, all aneuploid lesions were malignant and malignant lesions had lower G_0/G_1 and higher S-phase and G_2/M phase fractions than benign lesions (78.5% ± 11.5 vs 92.4% ± 2.1, $p <$ 0.0001, 9.7 ± 5 vs 4 ± 1.4, $p < 0.0001$ and 11.8 ± 9.9 vs 3.75 ± 1.8, $p < 0.0001$ respectively).

17.6 Presentation of Cases Using Intraoperative Flow Cytometry in Head and Neck Surgery

17.6.1 Case Presentation 1

A 50-year-old woman presented to our clinic with a vocal cord polyp. Microlaryngoscopy under general anesthesia was performed and the lesion was resected. A small tissue specimen from the lesion underwent analysis with intraoperative flow cytometry (iFC) according to Ioannina protocol and the rest was sent for histological evaluation. iFC analysis showed a benign lesion which was confirmed histologically (Fig. 17.1).

17.6.2 Case Presentation 2

A 38-year-old woman presented to our department with neck lymphadenopathy and a lesion of nasopharynx. Biopsy of nasopharynx was performed endoscopically and followed by iFC analysis. According to iFC the lesion was characterized as malignant due to pathologic cell cycle $G_0/G_1 = 72\%$, S-phase = 8%, $G_2/M = 20\%$ and high tumor index = 28%. Histopathology confirmed showing a low-grade neuroendocrine tumor (Fig. 17.2).

17.6.3 Case Presentation 3

A 79-year-old man with voice hoarseness presented to the emergency department. Endoscopy of the larynx showed an extended lesion of the left vocal cord. During microlaryngoscopy biopsy was taken and the same procedure described in the two

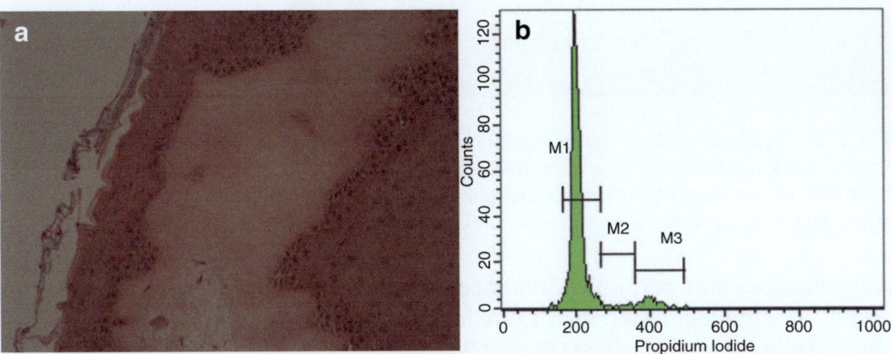

Fig. 17.1 (**a**) Histopathology microscopical image of a vocal cord polyp (H&E ×400). (**b**) DNA histogram acquired after iFC analysis showing a G_0/G_1 phase (*M*1) = 91%, *S*-phase(*M*2) = 4%, G_2/M phase(*M*3) = 5%. Tumor Index (TI = 9%) DNA Index = 1 (L. Basiari thesis)

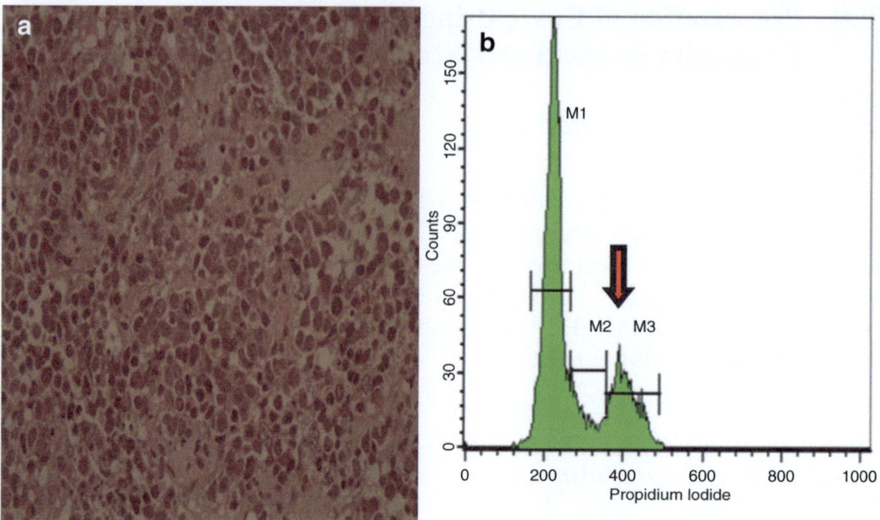

Fig. 17.2 (**a**) Histopathology microscopical image of a low-grade neuroendocrine tumor of nasopharynx (H&E ×400). (**b**) DNA histogram after iFC indicating a diploid lesion with an abnormal cell cycle: G_0/G_1 phase (*M1*) = 72%, S-phase fraction (*M2*) = 8%, G_2/M phase (*M3*) = 20%, TI = 28% and DNA Index =1. The red arrow shows the cancer cells in the analyzed specimen (L. Basiari thesis)

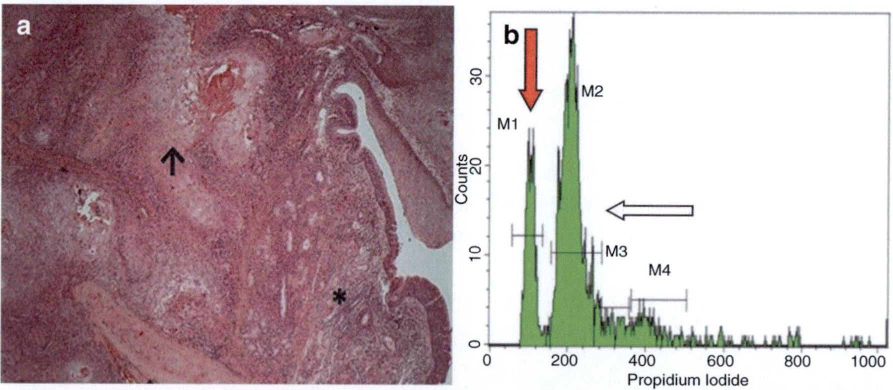

Fig. 17.3 (**a**) Histopathology microscopical image of an invasive squamous cell carcinoma of the larynx (black arrow tumor, asterisk normal mucosa) (H&E ×40) (**b**) DNA histogram after iFC indicating the presence of an aneuploid/tetraploid lesion (white arrow) with DNA Index = 2. Red arrow indicates cell from the normal mucosa (L. Basiari thesis)

previous cases was performed. Intraoperative flow cytometry analysis showed an aneuploid/tetraploid lesion with DNA index = 2. Histopathology showed an invasive squamous cell carcinoma (Fig. 17.3).

17.6.4 Case Presentation 4

A 75-year-old man with an ulcerative lesion of the nostril and nasolabial fold who underwent a wide resection under general anesthesia. Tissue specimen from the center of the lesion was analyzed with iFC which showed the presence of malignancy due to high tumor index. Tissue specimen from resection margin was also sent for iFC analysis which indicated the presence of cancer cells in the resection margin. Histopathology showed a squamous cell carcinoma with R1 resection. The patient was scheduled for reoperation (Fig. 17.4).

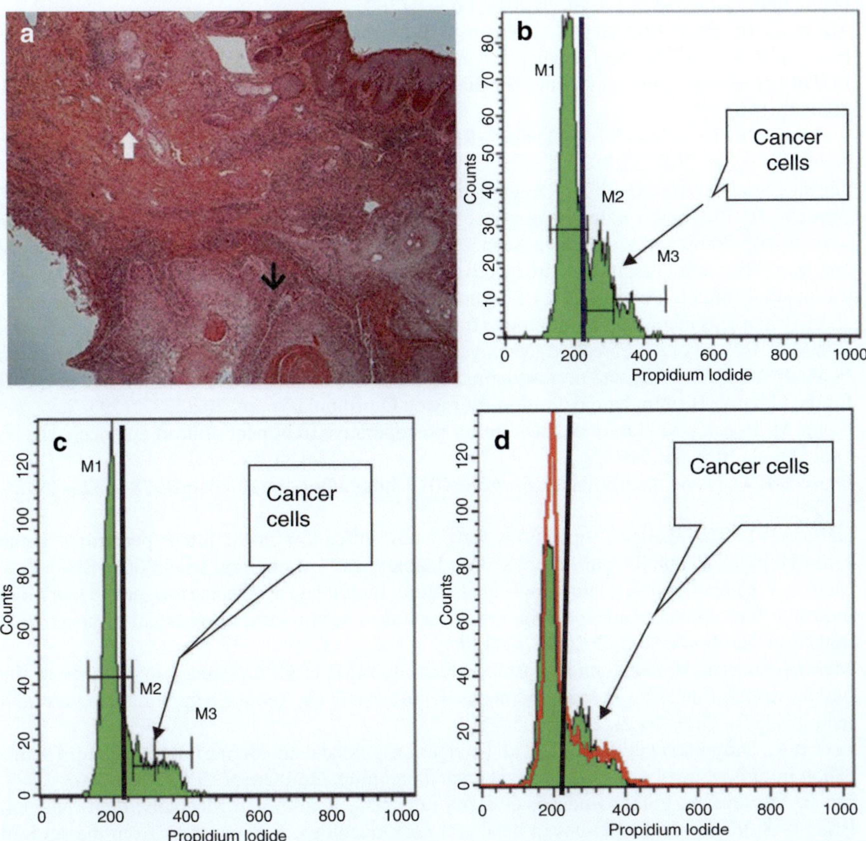

Fig. 17.4 (**a**) Histopathology microscopical image of an involved resection margin (black arrow indicating tumor cells and white arrow normal mucosa) (H&E ×40). (**b**) DNA histogram from iFC analysis of the specimen from tumor core showing the pathological cancer cells with abnormal cell cycle and increased tumor index (TI). G_0/G_1 ($M1$) = 66%, S-phase fraction ($M2$) = 23%, G_2/M = 11%, TI = 34%. (**c**) DNA histogram acquired after iFC analysis of specimen from resection margin also indicating the presence of tumor cells. G_0/G_1 ($M1$) = 82%, S-phase fraction ($M2$) = 10%, G_2/M = 8%, TI = 18%. As we can observe the amount of cancer cells at the resection margin is lower than at the tumor core. (**d**) Overlay of DNA histograms from the tumor (green) and from the margin (red) (L. Basiari thesis)

References

1. Zandberg DP, Bhargava R, Badin S, Cullen KJ. The role of human papillomavirus in nongenital cancers. CA Cancer J Clin. 2013;63(1):57–81.
2. Lo Nigro C, Denaro N, Merlotti A, Merlano M. Head and neck cancer: improving outcomes with a multidisciplinary approach. Cancer Manag Res. 2017;9:363–71.
3. Ciardiello F, Tortora G. A novel approach in the treatment of cancer: targeting the epidermal growth factor receptor. Clin Cancer Res. 2001;7(10):2958–70.
4. SEER cancer statistics review 1973-1999. 2003. http://seer.cancer.gov/.
5. Sturgis EM, Wei Q, Spitz MR. Descriptive epidemiology and risk factors for head and neck cancer. Semin Oncol. 2004;31:726–33.
6. Wang S, Liu Y, Feng Y, et al. A review on curability of cancers: more efforts for novel therapeutic options are needed. Cancer. 2019;11(11):1782.
7. Machiels JP, René Leemans C, Golusinski W, Grau C, Licitra L, Gregoire V. Squamous cell carcinoma of the oral cavity, larynx, oropharynx and hypopharynx: EHNS-ESMO-ESTRO clinical practice guidelines for diagnosis, treatment and follow-up 2020. Ann Oncol. 2020;31:1462–75.
8. Leemans CR, Braakhuis BJ, Brakenhoff RH. The molecular biology of head and neck cancer. Nat Rev Cancer. 2011;11:9–22.
9. Ghosh-Laskar S, Mummudi N, Rangarajan V, Purandare N, Gupta T, Budrukkar A, Murthy V, Agarwal JP. Prognostic value of response assessment fluorodeoxyglucose positron emission tomography-computed tomography scan in radically treated squamous cell carcinoma of head and neck: long-term results of a prospective study. J Cancer Res Ther. 2019;15:596–603.
10. Cadoni G, Giraldi L, Petrelli L, et al. Prognostic factors in head and neck cancer: a 10-year retrospective analysis in a single-institution in Italy. Acta Otorhinolaryngol Ital. 2017;37(6):458–66.
11. Rohde M, Rosenberg T, Pareek M, Nankivell P, Sharma N, Mehanna H, Godballe C. Definition of locally recurrent head and neck squamous cell carcinoma: a systematic review and proposal for the Odense–Birmingham definition. Eur Arch Otorhinolaryngol. 2020;277:1593–9.
12. Evans M, Beasley M. Target delineation for postoperative treatment of head and neck cancer. Oral Oncol. 2018;86:288–95.
13. Fonseca R. Oral and maxillofacial. Surgery. 2017. https://doi.org/10.1016/B978-0-323-26278-1.00011-8.
14. Halsted WS. The results of operations for the cure of cancer of the breast performed at the Johns Hopkins Hospital from June, 1889, to January, 1894. Ann Surg. 1894;20(5):497–555.
15. Maffeis V, Cappellesso R, Galuppini F, et al. Tumor budding is an adverse prognostic marker in intestinal-type sinonasal adenocarcinoma and seems to be unrelated to epithelial-mesenchymal transition. Virchows Arch. 2020;477:241–8.
16. Martins-Andrade B, Dos Santos Costa SF, Santana MSP, et al. Prognostic importance of the lymphovascular invasion in head and neck adenoid cystic carcinoma: a systematic review and meta-analysis. Oral Oncol. 2019;93:52–8.
17. Ferrari M, Daly MJ, Douglas CM, et al. Navigation-guided osteotomies improve margin delineation in tumors involving the sinonasal area: a preclinic. Oral Oncol. 2019;99:104463.
18. Jan B. Vermorken, Volker Budach, C. René Leemans, Jean-Pascal Machiels, Piero Nicolai, Brian O'Sullivan. Critical issues in head and neck oncology. Key concepts from the seventh THNO meeting. https://doi.org/10.1007/978-3-030-63234-2.
19. Batsakis JG. Surgical excision margins: a pathologist's perspective. Adv Anat Pathol. 1999;6(3):140–8.
20. Sutton DN, Brown JS, Rogers SN, Vaughan ED, Woolgar JA. The prognostic implications of the surgical margin in oral squamous cell carcinoma. Int J Oral Maxillofac Surg. 2003;32(1):30–4.
21. Williams MD. Determining adequate margins in head and neck cancers: practice and continued challenges. Curr Oncol Rep. 2016;18:54. https://doi.org/10.1007/s11912-016-0540-y.
22. NCCN-principles of surgery-margins SURG-A page 3 of 9 v1.2015, National Comprehensive Cancer Network Inc. Head and Neck Cancers.

23. Mistry RC, Qureshi SS, Kumaran C. Post-resection mucosal margin shrinkage in oral cancer: quantification and significance. J Surg Oncol. 2005;91(2):131–3.
24. Cheng A, Cox D, Schmidt BL. Oral squamous cell carcinoma margin discrepancy after resection and pathologic processing. J Oral Maxillofac Surg. 2008;66(3):523–9.
25. Ansarin M, Santoro L, Cattaneo A, Massaro MA, Calabrese L, Giugliano G, et al. Laser surgery for early glottic cancer: impact of margin status on local control and organ preservation. Arch Otolaryngol Head Neck Surg. 2009;135(4):385–90.
26. Weinstein GS, Quon H, Newman HJ, Chalian JA, Malloy K, Lin A, et al. Transoral robotic surgery alone for oropharyngeal cancer: an analysis of local control. Arch Otolaryngol Head Neck Surg. 2012;138(7):628–34.
27. Nichols AC, Theurer J, Prisman E, et al. Radiotherapy versus transoral robotic surgery and neck dissection for oropharyngeal squamous cell carcinoma (ORATOR): an open-label, phase 2, randomised trial. Lancet Oncol. 2019;20(10):1349–59.
28. Benazzo M, Canzi P, Mauramati S, et al. Transoral robot-assisted surgery in supraglottic and oropharyngeal squamous cell carcinoma: laser versus monopolar electrocautery. J Clin Med. 2019;8(12):2166.
29. Persky MJ, Albergotti WG, Rath TJ, et al. Positive margins by oropharyngeal subsite in transoral robotic surgery for T1/T2 squamous cell carcinoma. Otolaryngol Head Neck Surg. 2018;158(4):660–6.
30. Cracchiolo JR, Roman BR, Kutler DI, Kuhel WI, Cohen MA. Adoption of transoral robotic surgery compared with other surgical modalities for treatment of oropharyngeal squamous cell carcinoma. J Surg Oncol. 2016;114(4):405–11.
31. Woolgar JA, Triantafyllou A. A histopathological appraisal of surgical margins in oral and oropharyngeal cancer resection specimens. Oral Oncol. 2005;41:1034–43.
32. Slaughter DP, Southwick HW, Smejkal W. "Field cancerization" in oral stratified squamous epithelium. Clinical implications of multicentric origin. Cancer. 1953;6(5):963–8.
33. Westra WH, Sidransky D. Phenotypic and genotypic disparity in premalignant lesions: of calm water and crocodiles. J Natl Cancer Inst. 1998;90(20):1500–1.
34. van Houten VM, Leemans CR, Kummer JA, et al. Molecular diagnosis of surgical margins and local recurrence in head and neck cancer patients: a prospective study. Clin Cancer Res. 2004;10:3614–20.
35. Sardi I, Franchi A, Ferriero G, et al. Prediction of recurrence by microsatellite analysis in head and neck cancer. Genes Chromosomes Cancer. 2000;29:201–6.
36. Goldenberg D, Harden S, Masayesva BG, et al. Intraoperative molecular margin analysis in head and neck cancer. Arch Otolaryngol Head Neck Surg. 2004;130:39–44.
37. Nathan CO, Liu L, Li BD, Abreo FW, Nandy I, De Benedetti A. Detection of the proto-oncogene eIF4E in surgical margins may predict recurrence in head and neck cancer. Oncogene. 1997;15:579–84.
38. Dasgupta S, Koch R, Westra WH, et al. Mitochondrial DNA mutation in normal margins and tumors of recurrent head and neck squamous cell carcinoma patients. Cancer Prev Res. 2010;3:1205–11.
39. Brennan JA, Mao L, Hruban RH, et al. Molecular assessment of histopathological staging in squamous-cell carcinoma of the head and neck. N Engl J Med. 1995;332(7):429–35.
40. Nathan CO, Franklin S, Abreo FW, et al. Analysis of surgical margins with the molecular marker eIF4E: a prognostic factor in patients with head and neck cancer. J Clin Oncol. 1999;17(9):2909–14.
41. Hayashi M, Wu G, Roh JL, et al. Correlation of gene methylation in surgical margin imprints with locoregional recurrence in head and neck squamous cell carcinoma. Cancer. 2015;121:1957–65.
42. Wang X, Chen S, Chen X, et al. Tumor-related markers in histologically normal margins correlate with locally recurrent oral squamous cell carcinoma: a retrospective study. J Oral Pathol Med. 2016;45(2):83–8.

43. Woo J, Baumann A, Arguello V. Recent advancements of flow cytometry: new applications in hematology and oncology. Expert Rev Mol Diagn. 2014;14:67–81.
44. Kawamoto K, Nishiyama T, Ikeda Y, Yamanouchi Y, Kawamura Y, Matsumura H, et al. Flow cytometric studies of human brain tumors. Part I: human malignant brain tumors. No Shinkei Geka. 1980;8:723–8.
45. Vijayavel T, Aswath N. Correlation between histological grading and ploidy status in potentially malignant disorders of the oral mucosa: a flow cytometric analysis. J Oral Maxillofac Pathol. 2013;17:169–75.
46. El-Deftar MF, El Gerzawi SM, Abdel-Azim AA, Tohamy SM. Prognostic significance of ploidy and S-phase fraction in primary intraoral squamous cell carcinoma and their corresponding metastatic lymph nodes. J Egypt Natl Canc Inst. 2012;24:7–14.
47. Alexiou GA, Vartholomatos G, Goussia A, Batistatou A, Tsamis K, Voulgaris S, Kyritsis AP. Fast cell cycle analysis for intraoperative characterization of brain tumor margins and malignancy. J Clin Neurosci. 2015;22:129–32.

Part VI
Intraoperative Flow Cytometry in Gastrointestinal Malignancies

Chapter 18
Pathology of Digestive System Malignancies

Ioannis Parthymos, Redi Bumci, and Anna C. Goussia

18.1 Colorectal Cancer

Colorectal cancer (CRC) is the most common gastrointestinal cancer type. According to the GLOBOCAN data base of the World and Health organization (WHO), CRC is the second and third most common malignancy diagnosed in females and males, respectively, worldwide. Globally, there is extensive variation in its incidence. Higher rates are recorded in Europe, North America, Australia, and New Zealand, while lower rates are found in Africa and South-Central Asia [1, 2]. In the USA, 151,030 cases of CRC are diagnosed and 52,580 individuals die annually [1]. Incidence is increasing with age and most cases are detected between the ages of 40 and 50. Of note, mortality rates have declined in the USA and several European countries [1]. This fact can be attributed to several factors including prevention strategies, early recognition, and resection of colonic polyps, earlier diagnosis and surgical removal of CRC lesions.

18.1.1 Etiology-Risk Factors

Several risk factors associated with increased risk for tumor developing have been described. Some genetic disorders, most of which are autosomal-dominant inherited, are associated with increased risk for CRC. The main disorders are familial adenomatous polyposis (FAP) and Lynch syndrome [3, 4]. Inflammatory bowel

I. Parthymos · R. Bumci · A. C. Goussia (✉)
Department of Pathology, University Hospital of Ioannina, Ioannina, Greece
e-mail: agoussia@uoi.gr

G. Alexiou, G. Vartholomatos (eds.), *Intraoperative Flow Cytometry*,
https://doi.org/10.1007/978-3-031-33517-4_18

diseases including ulcerative colitis and Crohn disease are also established risk factors for developing CRC. Pancolitis due to both disorders seem to confer a 5- to 15-fold increase in risk for malignant transformation [5, 6]. Obesity, insulin resistance and diabetes mellitus are also associated with elevated risk for CRC [7]. Long-term consumption of red meat seems to enhance the risk for CRC, specifically for left colon tumors [8]. Finally, cigarette smoking and elevated alcohol intake are both associated with elevated incidence and mortality.

18.1.2 Pathology

The gross appearance of colorectal carcinoma is variable. Some tumors may be polypoid and eventually form large obstructive masses, while others present as ulcerative lesions with raised, irregular borders.

Histologically, more than 90% of CRCs are adenocarcinomas, well to moderately differentiated (Fig. 18.1). Most lesions consist of variably sized glands lined by tall columnar cells. Glandular spaces may be filled with mucus or nuclear and cellular debris. The neoplastic glands may be surrounded by a variable amount of desmoplastic stroma. Based on the WHO classification of digestive system tumours, several histopathological subtypes have been described including mucinous, signet ring, medullary, serrated, micropapillary, adenoma-like, adenosquamous, carcinoma with sarcomatoid components, and undifferentiated carcinoma (Figs. 18.2 and 18.3) (Table 18.1).

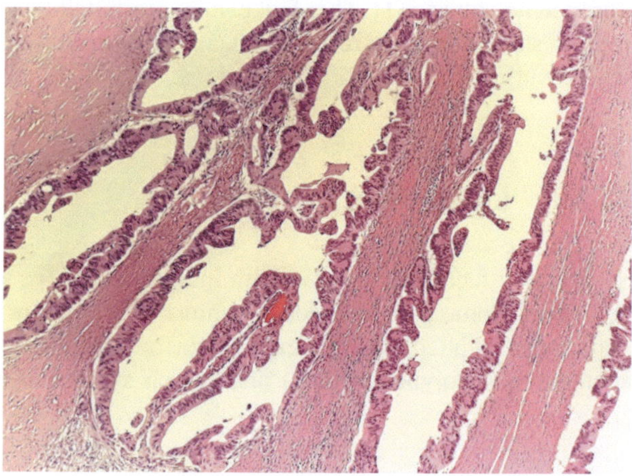

Fig. 18.1 Colorectal adenocarcinoma, moderately differentiated (low grade) (Hematoxylin-Eosin stain, original magnification ×200)

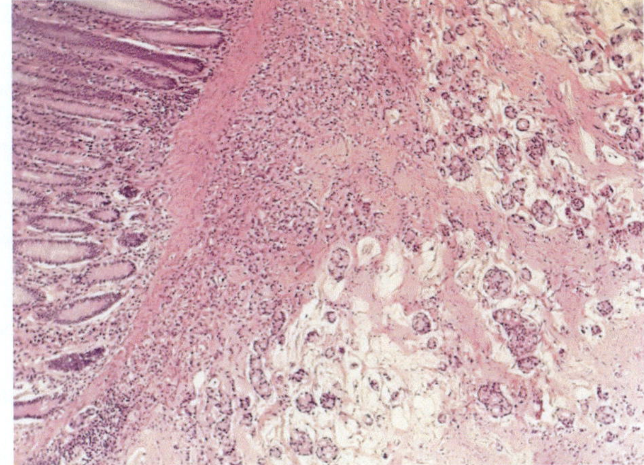

Fig. 18.2 Colorectal mucinous adenocarcinoma. Tumor cells are embedded in pools of extracellular mucin (Hematoxylin-Eosin stain, original magnification ×200)

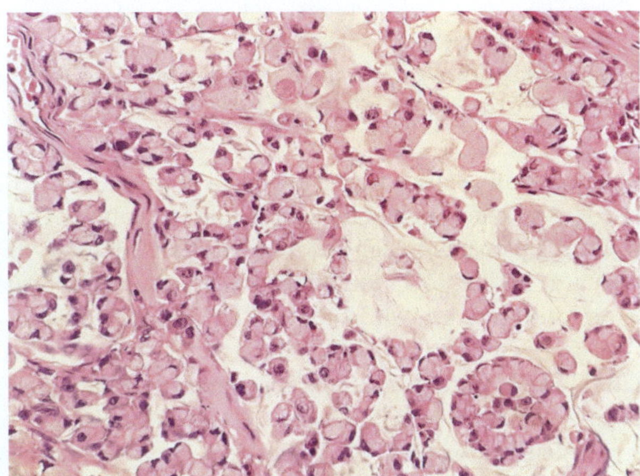

Fig. 18.3 Colorectal adenocarcinoma with signet-ring morphology (Hematoxylin-Eosin stain, original magnification ×200)

18.1.3 Molecular Pathology

The majority of CRCs derive from adenomatoid lesions either conventional or sessile. One well characterized molecular pathway is the adenoma-carcinoma sequence. Adenomas arise as a result of impaired major cellular function including DNA and cell proliferation. The evolution of normal epithelium of the crypts to hyperplastic and eventually dysplastic is stepwise and includes several genetic alterations [10]. Among them mutations of the Adenomatous Polyposis Coli (*APC*) gene, which acts as tumor suppressor gene, are the most common earlier molecular aberrations [11]. Subsequently, other mutations should be accumulated for the evolution to high-grade dysplastic lesions and finally to invasive carcinoma.

The serrated neoplasia pathway is another described route of colorectal carcinogenesis. The key molecular event in this pathway is the V600E mutation in *BRAF* gene [12]. This mutation results in the activation of intracellular kinase pathways

Table 18.1 Histological subtypes of colorectal adenocarcinoma [9]

Histological subtype	Major histological findings
Mucinous	>50% of the tumor is composed of extracellular mucin with individual tumor cells or strips of cells to be found into the mucin
Signet ring	>50% of tumor cells have signet-ring appearance; intracytoplasmic mucin with nucleus displacement at the periphery of the cell
Medullary	Sheets of polygonal cells with vesicular nuclei, prominent nucleoli, abundant cytoplasm and increased number of infiltrating lymphocytes
Serrated	Neoplastic glands resembling serrated adenomas
Micropapillary	>5% of tumor consists of clusters of tumor cells into stromal spaces mimicking vessels
Adenoma-like	>50% of tumor contains invasive areas with villous-like architecture resembling adenomas
Adenosquamous	Tumors with coexisting features of adenocarcinoma and squamous cell carcinoma
Carcinoma with sarcomatoid component	Tumors with spindle cell component or cells with rhabdoid morphology
Undifferentiated carcinoma	Tumors lacking morphological and immunohistochemical features related to epithelial cell origin

that eventually cause uncontrolled cell proliferation [13]. After *BRAF* mutation, sessile lesions can follow the microsatellite instability (*MSI*) pathway due to disorders in DNA mismatch repair (*MMR*) [14]. In other cases *BRAF*-mutant serrated adenomas also harbor TP53 mutations that eventually activate oncogenic pathways such as transforming growth factor B (*TGFB*) and Wnt [14].

The recent WHO classification has described two distinct molecular subtypes of CRC. The hypermutated type represents approximately 15% of CRCs and is characterized mainly by MSI. A major molecular disorder of this subtype is the diffuse hypermethylation of CpG nucleotides located in the promoters of several genes [15]. This hypermethylation, which is an epigenetic alteration, results in inactivation of tumor suppressor genes and mainly the MutL Homolog 1(*MLH1*) gene. On the other hand, the most common subtype is the non-hypermutated that is characterized by amplifications or deletions of chromosomal material. Genes that are typically involved include *APC, TP53,* and *KRAS* [16].

18.2　Liver Cancer

Primary liver cancer is the seventh most common malignancy worldwide and the second cause of neoplasia-related death in 2018 according to the GLOBOCAN database [17]. In most cases there is a linear association between incidence of liver cancer and age. Prognosis is generally poor and only surgical resection of small tumors may achieve long survival. Recent advances in genomics and epigenomics can provide new insights in diagnostic approach, histological, and molecular classification. Integrating new molecular findings with histopathological features may lead to novel therapeutic approaches for personalized treatment. Herein, we review and provide updates about the most common histologic type, hepatocellular carcinoma (HCC).

18.2.1 Epidemiology

HCC is the most common primary liver cancer [18]. It is estimated that it accounts approximately for 75–85% of primary liver neoplasms. The incidence of HCC differs across several geographic areas, with a lower incidence in Europe and North America and higher in Asia, China, and Africa [18]. Globally, the reported incidence rate is 9.3 per 10,000, while the mortality rate reaches up to 8.5 [18]. The median age of diagnosis is between 60 and 64 years for men while the estimated ages for women fluctuate from 65 to 69 years [18]. The incidence is greater in males than in females. In the USA, at 2016 the age-adjusted incidence was 10.4 per 100,000 for men 2.9 per 100,000 for women [18].

18.2.2 Clinical Features

The presenting clinical features are variable. Many patients may be asymptomatic for a long period. Frequent symptoms include abdominal pain, weight loss, malaise, and fever. In more advanced cases, patients are presented with large masses that exhibit rupture and hemorrhage. Moreover, many individuals can present complications due to an underlying liver disease, including jaundice and ascites [19].

18.2.3 Etiology-Risk Factors

Over 90% of patients diagnosed with HCC suffer from an underlying chronic disease [20]. The most common causes of chronic liver disease include hepatitis B, hepatitis C, autoimmune disorders, alcoholic hepatitis, non-alcoholic fatty liver disease in the context of diabetes and obesity as well as several genetic diseases (haemochromatosis, Wilson disease, glycogen storage diseases). In addition, aflatoxin B1 is an important cause of HCC mainly in tropical regions [21]. In most cases HCC develops in a chronically diseased liver and it often coexists with cirrhosis.

18.2.4 Pathology

During gross examination, HCC is white, yellow or green in color. According to the recent World and Health Organization Classification of the Digestive System Tumors [9], there are four major patterns of HCC. HCC can present as a single nodule or it may take the form of a large major nodule accompanied by smaller lesions. Another macroscopic feature is the diffuse growth where the lesion is consisted of multiple small nodules that resemble cirrhotic nodules. Moreover, HCC can be presented as multiple distinct nodules.

Based on the WHO classification of tumors, four major growth patterns of HCC have been reported: trabecular, pseudoglandular (acinar), solid (compact), and macrotrabecular [9].

The trabecular pattern, which is the most common, consists of cell plates that resemble those of normal liver. However, cell plates in the case of trabecular variant are thicker (three or more cells thick) and the reticulin framework is completely absent or severely reduced. Cell plates are typically lined by endothelial cells, although in some cases, trabeculae may be separated by bands of connective tissue. The pseudoglandular pattern is comprised of relatively round spaces resembling glands (acini) lined by tumor cells. The differential diagnosis of acinar variant of HCC with an adenocarcinoma may be challenging. In the solid variant tumor cells are arranged in sheets with no visible cell plates and loss of reticulin framework. The macrotrabecular pattern is defined by large and thick (more than ten cells thick) trabeculae. It should be noted that the above-mentioned patterns may coexist within a tumor.

Several histologic subtypes of HCC have been described including steatohepatic, clear cell, scirrhous, chromophobe, fibrolamellar, neutrophil-rich, and lymphocyte-rich (Table 18.2) (Fig. 18.4). Distinct morphological changes of neoplastic cells include bile production, lipofuscin and glycogen deposits, hyaline bodies, and Mallory-Denk bodies (Fig. 18.5).

Table 18.2 Morphological subtypes of Hepatocellular carcinoma [9]

Hepatocellular carcinoma subtypes	Histological description
Steatohepatic	Tumor cells with features of steatohepatitis including steatosis, fibrosis, cell ballooning, Mallory-Denk bodies, inflammation
Clear cell	Tumor cells (>80% of total tumor) with abundant, vacuolated and foamy cytoplasm due to glycogen and fat accumulation
Scirrhous	>50% of tumor contains areas of fibrosis
Chromophobe	Cells with clear cytoplasm and outlined cell borders. Nuclei are generally bland, however areas of increased nuclear pleomorphism may be observed
Macrotrabecular massive	>50% of tumor cells exhibit macrotrabecullar morphology (trabeculae >10 cells thick)
Fibrolamellar carcinoma	Tumor cells are large, polygonal with eosinophilic cytoplasm, and large prominent nucleoli. A characteristic feature is the presence of thick fibrous collagen bands
Neutrophil-rich	Numerous tumors infiltrating neutrophils. Tumors are often poorly differentiated, with occasional sarcomatoid areas
Lymphocyte-rich	Generally poorly differentiated tumors and prominent lymphocytic infiltrates

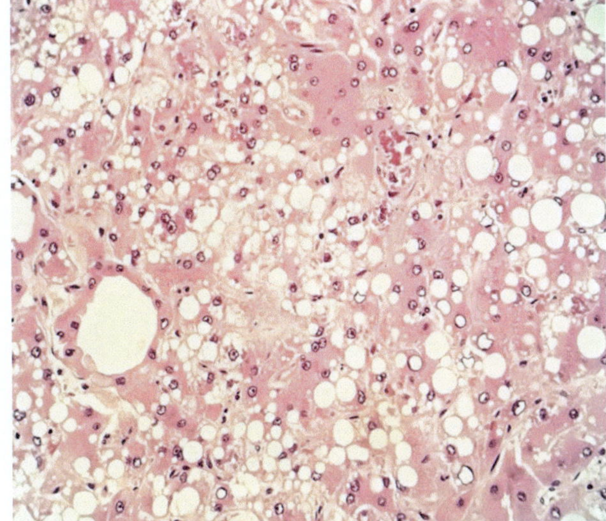

Fig. 18.4 Hepatocellular carcinoma of steatohepatic subtype. The tumor cells contain fat and are arranged in pseudoacinar and in trabecular structures. (Hematoxylin-Eosin stain, original magnification ×400)

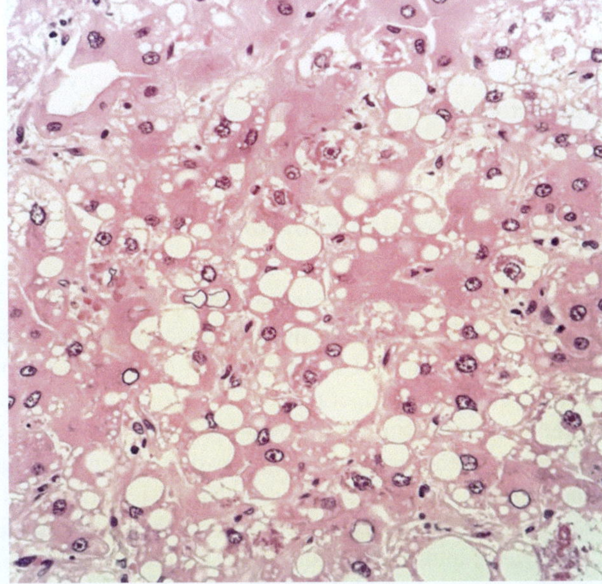

Fig. 18.5 Hepatocellular carcinoma. There are Mallory-Denk bodies in the cytoplasm of neoplastic cells (arrowheads) (Hematoxylin-Eosin stain, original magnification ×400)

Grading of HCC refers to the degree of differentiation of the tumor compared to the normal hepatocytes. Therefore, tumors can be classified into well, moderately, and poorly differentiated. In well differentiated carcinomas, neoplastic cells resemble normal hepatocytes and there is minimal to mild nuclear atypia. In moderately differentiated tumors neoplastic cells are clearly malignant but hepatocytic differentiation is preserved, while in poorly differentiated neoplasms hepatocytic features are not retained [22, 23].

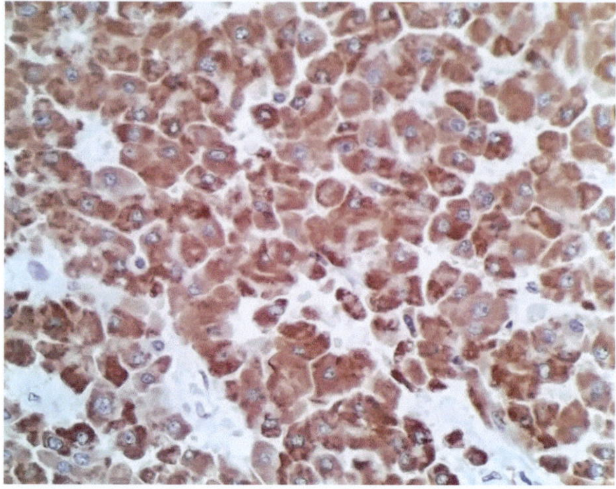

Fig. 18.6 Hepatocellular carcinoma. Immunohistochemically, the tumor cells are positive for Hep par-1 (Avidin-Biotin-Complex, ABC, original magnification ×400)

In cases of well and moderately differentiated tumors confirmation of hepatocellular origin through immunohistochemical analysis is not required. However, tissue biomarkers for hepatocytic differentiation are warranted in cases of poorly differentiated carcinomas. The most common markers include arginase-1, hepatocyte-paraffin-1 (Hep par-1), polyclonal carcinoembryonic antigen (CEA), CD10, and alpha fetoprotein (AFP) [24] (Fig. 18.6).

18.2.5 Molecular Pathology

Several somatic mutations and epigenetic modifications are implicated in the pathogenesis of HCC. Mutations in telomerase reverse transcriptase (*TERT*) promoter are frequently encountered in HCC (up to 60%) [25]. Hepatitis B infection also possesses a mutogenic effect upon *TERT* [26, 27]. Other common molecular disorders include the activation of the Wnt-β-catenin pathway activation and inactivation of p53 gene. Furthermore, receptor tyrosine kinase (*TRK*) and phosphatidylinositol-3-kinase (*PI3K*) are commonly activated [28]. Another pathway carrying mutations is that of the oxidative stress. Activation of the nuclear factor erythroid 2-related factor 2 (*NFE2L2*) and inactivation of the Kelchlike ECH-associated protein 1 (*KEAP1*) have been described [29]. Finally, disorders in chromatin structure and epigenetic alterations have been reported.

In recent years, based on the findings from molecular analyses, a molecular classification of HCC has been proposed, although it has not been established in clinical practice. According to the literature, two molecular subtypes have been proposed: the proliferation and the nonproliferation subtype. In the proliferation subtype activation of tyrosine kinase pathways, *p53* inactivation and chromosome instability have been described, while the nonproliferation type is characterized by *TERT* promoter mutations [29].

18.3 Pancreatic Cancer

Pancreatic ductal adenocarcinoma (PDA) is the most common type of pancreatic malignancy. It is an extremely lethal disease with a survival time following surgical tumor resection 10–20 months. At the time of diagnosis only a minority of patients possesses resectable tumors. As a result there is an increasing need for improving our understanding of tumor underlying biology in order to achieve stratification of patients with different prognosis. Up to now, histopathological grading, staging, and the status of resection margins (R0 vs R1) are factors with prognostic relevance.

18.3.1 Epidemiology

PDA accounts for 80–90% of all primary pancreatic tumors. According to GLOBOCAN, in 2020, 495,773 new cases were described making PDA the fourteenth most common cancer worldwide [30]. Of note, 466,003 deaths per year were recorded [31]. As a result, PDA is the seventh leading cause of cancer associated deaths. The incidence of this cancer is variable among countries; higher rates have been recorded in Europe and North America in contrast to Africa and Central Asia [31]. Specifically the incidence in North America is 9.9 per 100,000 and 6.7 per 100,000 for men and women, respectively [31], while in West Africa the incidence rates approximate 2.2 per 100,000 for men and 1.8 per 100,000 for women. The overall incidence of PDA is higher among men (5.7 per 100,000) compared to women (4.1 per 100,000) [31]. Mortality rates also differ across countries. Higher rates are recorded in Europe with 7.2 deaths per 100,000 people, while the lowest rate is recorded in East Africa (1.2 deaths per 100,000) [31].

18.3.2 Etiology-Risk factors

Several risk factors have been associated with the development of PDA. Hereditary pancreatitis due to mutations in cationic tryspinogen (*PRSS1*) and serine protease inhibitor Kazal-type 1 (*SPINK1*) genes, increases risk of PDA by 60 to 87-fold [32]. Patients with mutations in the breast cancer gene (*BRCA1/2*) that are likely to develop breast or ovarian cancer, also carry an increased risk for developing PDA by 3.5–10 times [33, 34]. Chronic pancreatitis may also contribute to the pathogenesis of PDA. In a meta-analysis of *Raimondi* et al. patients with chronic pancreatitis were found having a 13.3-fold greater risk for PDA compared to the general population [35]. Obesity and diabetes mellitus are also considered risk factors of PDA [30]. Moreover, a correlation with alcohol consumption has been emphasized in some studies [36].

18.3.3 Clinical Findings

Patients may be asymptomatic for a long period, mainly in tumors arising in the body and tail. In head located lesions, a frequent clinical sign is jaundice due to the obstruction of the common bile duct. General symptoms may also include fever, malaise, and weight loss.

18.3.4 Pathology

In over two-thirds of the cases, PDA is located in the head of the pancreas. Grossly, most tumors are firm, whitish in color and have ill-defined borders. Carcinomas of the pancreatic head directly invade the common bile and pancreatic duct, the ampulla of Vater, and the duodenal wall. In cases of pancreatic body and tail carcinomas, invasion of the common bile duct is not frequently seen but these tumors may extend to the stomach, spleen or to the left colon.

Histologically, most PDAs consist of small to medium sized tubular structures lined by a single layer of cyboidal to columnar epithelial cells that haphazardly infiltrate the pancreatic parenchyma and the peripancreatic tissues. The cell cytoplasm is eosinophilic, foamy or clear, and the nuclei are round to oval. The epithelial cells often produce mucin that is visible with hemotoxylin and eosin stain or with histochemical stains [periodic acid stain (PAS), Alcian blue] (Fig. 18.7).

Well differentiated tumors consist of structures that resemble both architecturally and cytologically the normal pancreatic ducts. In these cases, differential diagnosis can be challenging. In moderately differentiated tumors the glandular architecture is clearly malignant with cribriform or papillary structures, lined by pleomorphic cells. Finally, poorly differentiated carcinomas are characterized by

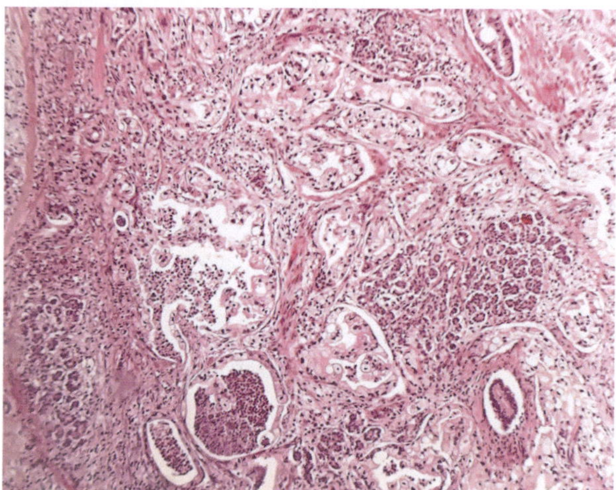

Fig. 18.7 Pancreatic ductal adenocarcinoma, moderately differentiated (Hematoxylin-Eosin stain, original magnification ×200)

solid nests or sheets of highly pleomorphic cells with little or no mucin production. A common feature in many tumors is the abundant desmoplastic stroma, consisting of collagen fibers, fibroblasts and scattered inflammatory cells.

At the time of diagnosis most tumors are extended beyond the pancreas. As a result neoplastic glands infiltrate the peripancreatic fat tissue, the duodenal wall, and the ampulla of Vater. Perineural invasion is a common finding of PDA (Fig. 18.8). Lymphatic and blood vessel infiltrations are also observed.

According to the World and Health Organization (WHO) classification of digestive system tumors several histological subtypes of PDA have been described, including adenosquamous, colloid, hepatoid, medullary, invasive micropapillary, signet ring, and undifferentiated carcinoma (Table 18.3).

18.3.5 Molecular Pathology

Extensive research in order to improve our understandings in the molecular biology of pancreatic cancer is undergoing. As a result, driver mutations in four major genes have been described; these include Kirsten rat sarcoma viral oncogene homolog (*KRAS*), *TP53*, Mothers against decapentaplegic homolog 4 (*SMAD4*), and Cyclin-dependent kinase inhibitor (*CDKN2A*) and they have been identified in over 50% of pancreatic cancer cases [37–39]. Epigenetic alterations may also contribute to pancreatic tumorigenesis. For instance, *CDKN2* is often mutated in pancreatic cancer due to methylation of its promoter [40, 41].

Trancriptomic analyses have described two distinct subtypes; the classical subtype that expresses several transcription factors including GATA6 (member of the GATA family of transcription factors), Pancreas/Duodenum Homeobox (*PDX1*),

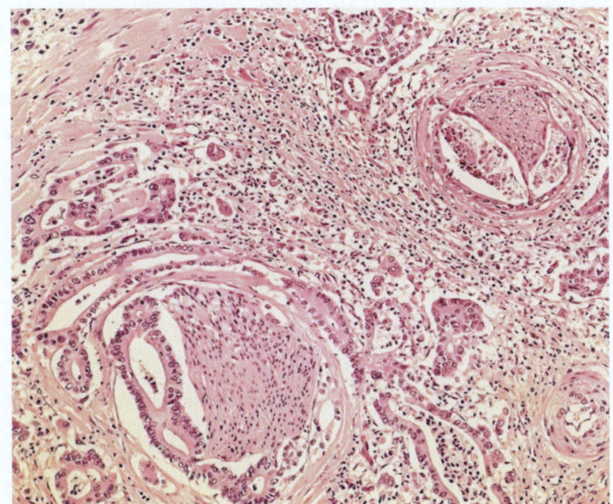

Fig. 18.8 Pancreatic ductal adenocarcinoma with perineural invasion (Hematoxylin-Eosin stain, original magnification ×200)

Table 18.3 Pancreatic ductal adenocarcinoma histological subtypes [9]

Histological type	Key histological features
Adenosquamous	>30% of tumor should possess squamous cell morphology (cells with distinct cellular borders, intracellular junctions, and areas of keratinization)
Colloid	>80% of tumor cells are embedded in mucin substrate
Hepatoid	>50% of the tumor presents morphological and immunohistochemical characteristics of hepatocellular origin. The cells are typically large, polygonal with eosinophilic cytoplasm
Medullary	Sheets of poorly differentiated cells, absence of glandular structures, prominent lymphocytic infiltration
Micropapillary	>50% of cells with micropapillary morphology. Intraepithelial neutrophils are frequently observable
Signet-ring cell	>80% of tumor consists of discohesive cells with intracellular mucin and peripherally located nuclei
Undifferentiated carcinoma	**Anaplastic**: >80% of the tumor is characterized by solid sheets of cells without glandular formation. Common neutrophilic infiltration **Sarcomatoid**: >80% of the tumor cells exhibit spindle morphology with or without the presence of a heterologous component **Carcinosarcoma**: Biphasic neoplasm with both epithelial and sarcomatoid component

and Hepatocyte Nuclear Factor-1 alpha (*HNF1A*) and the Basal-like one, where the expression of the above-mentioned factors is attenuated or lost [42–45]. Of note, Basal-like tumors are characterized by increased macrophage infiltrates, meaning that macrophages could constitute a potential therapeutic target [46].

Recently, several studies have attempted to identify molecular alterations in premalignant lesions including pancreatic intraepithelial neoplasia (PanIN), intraductal papillary mucinous neoplasm (IPMN), and mucinous cystic neoplasms (MCN). The major molecular defect in PanIN lesions includes *KRAS* mutations that are accompanied by inactivation of tumor suppressor genes. At later stages, other mutated genes such *CDKN2A* accumulate resulting in higher grades of dysplasia [47]. IPMN also harbors *KRAS* mutations as well as activating mutations in the guanine nucleotide binding protein (*GNAS*) that acts as an oncogene and induces protein kinase A activation [48]. MCN are also characterized by frequent *KRAS* mutations [49].

References

1. Siegel RL, Miller KD, Fuchs HE, Jemal A. Cancer statistics, 2022. CA Cancer J Clin. 2022;72(1):7–33.
2. Fitzmaurice C, Allen C, Barber RM, Barregard L, Bhutta ZA, Brenner H, et al. Global, regional, and national cancer incidence, mortality, years of life lost, years lived with disability, and disability-adjusted life-years for 32 cancer groups, 1990 to 2015: a systematic analysis for the global burden of disease study. JAMA Oncol. 2017;3(4):524–48.

3. Yurgelun MB, Kulke MH, Fuchs CS, Allen BA, Uno H, Hornick JL, et al. Cancer susceptibility gene mutations in individuals with colorectal cancer. J Clin Oncol. 2017;35(10):1086–95.
4. Pearlman R, Frankel WL, Swanson B, Zhao W, Yilmaz A, Miller K, et al. Prevalence and spectrum of germline cancer susceptibility gene mutations among patients with early-onset colorectal cancer. JAMA Oncol. 2017;3(4):464–71.
5. Olen O, Erichsen R, Sachs MC, Pedersen L, Halfvarson J, Askling J, et al. Colorectal cancer in ulcerative colitis: a Scandinavian population-based cohort study. Lancet. 2020;395(10218):123–31.
6. Olen O, Erichsen R, Sachs MC, Pedersen L, Halfvarson J, Askling J, et al. Colorectal cancer in Crohn's disease: a Scandinavian population-based cohort study. Lancet Gastroenterol Hepatol. 2020;5(5):475–84.
7. Ma Y, Yang W, Song M, Smith-Warner SA, Yang J, Li Y, et al. Type 2 diabetes and risk of colorectal cancer in two large U.S. prospective cohorts. Br J Cancer. 2018;119(11):1436–42.
8. Chan DS, Lau R, Aune D, Vieira R, Greenwood DC, Kampman E, et al. Red and processed meat and colorectal cancer incidence: meta-analysis of prospective studies. PLoS One. 2011;6(6):e20456.
9. Nagtegaal ID, Odze RD, Klimstra D, Paradis V, Rugge M, Schirmacher P, et al. The 2019 WHO classification of tumours of the digestive system. Histopathology. 2020;76(2):182–8.
10. Nguyen LH, Goel A, Chung DC. Pathways of colorectal carcinogenesis. Gastroenterology. 2020;158(2):291–302.
11. Sparks AB, Morin PJ, Vogelstein B, Kinzler KW. Mutational analysis of the APC/beta-catenin/Tcf pathway in colorectal cancer. Cancer Res. 1998;58(6):1130–4.
12. Davies H, Bignell GR, Cox C, Stephens P, Edkins S, Clegg S, et al. Mutations of the BRAF gene in human cancer. Nature. 2002;417(6892):949–54.
13. Spring KJ, Zhao ZZ, Karamatic R, Walsh MD, Whitehall VL, Pike T, et al. High prevalence of sessile serrated adenomas with BRAF mutations: a prospective study of patients undergoing colonoscopy. Gastroenterology. 2006;131(5):1400–7.
14. Guinney J, Dienstmann R, Wang X, de Reynies A, Schlicker A, Soneson C, et al. The consensus molecular subtypes of colorectal cancer. Nat Med. 2015;21(11):1350–6.
15. Jung G, Hernandez-Illan E, Moreira L, Balaguer F, Goel A. Epigenetics of colorectal cancer: biomarker and therapeutic potential. Nat Rev Gastroenterol Hepatol. 2020;17(2):111–30.
16. Cancer Genome Atlas Network. Comprehensive molecular characterization of human colon and rectal cancer. Nature. 2012;487(7407):330–7.
17. Bray F, Ferlay J, Soerjomataram I, Siegel RL, Torre LA, Jemal A. Global cancer statistics 2018: GLOBOCAN estimates of incidence and mortality worldwide for 36 cancers in 185 countries. CA Cancer J Clin. 2018;68(6):394–424.
18. Konyn P, Ahmed A, Kim D. Current epidemiology in hepatocellular carcinoma. Expert Rev Gastroenterol Hepatol. 2021;15(11):1295–307.
19. Villanueva A. Hepatocellular carcinoma. N Engl J Med. 2019;380(15):1450–62.
20. Akinyemiju T, Abera S, Ahmed M, Alam N, Alemayohu MA, Allen C, et al. The burden of primary liver cancer and underlying etiologies from 1990 to 2015 at the global, regional, and national level: results from the global burden of disease study 2015. JAMA Oncol. 2017;3(12):1683–91.
21. Chu YJ, Yang HI, Wu HC, Lee MH, Liu J, Wang LY, et al. Aflatoxin B1 exposure increases the risk of hepatocellular carcinoma associated with hepatitis C virus infection or alcohol consumption. Eur J Cancer. 2018;94:37–46.
22. Han DH, Choi GH, Kim KS, Choi JS, Park YN, Kim SU, et al. Prognostic significance of the worst grade in hepatocellular carcinoma with heterogeneous histologic grades of differentiation. J Gastroenterol Hepatol. 2013;28(8):1384–90.
23. El Jabbour T, Lagana SM, Lee H. Update on hepatocellular carcinoma: pathologists' review. World J Gastroenterol. 2019;25(14):1653–65.
24. Vyas M, Zhang X. Hepatocellular carcinoma: role of pathology in the era of precision medicine. Clin Liver Dis. 2020;24(4):591–610.

25. Llovet JM, Zucman-Rossi J, Pikarsky E, Sangro B, Schwartz M, Sherman M, et al. Hepatocellular carcinoma. Nat Rev Dis Primers. 2016;2:16018.
26. Llovet JM, Montal R, Sia D, Finn RS. Molecular therapies and precision medicine for hepatocellular carcinoma. Nat Rev Clin Oncol. 2018;15(10):599–616.
27. Schulze K, Zucman-Rossi J. Translating the molecular diversity of hepatocellular carcinoma into clinical practice. Mol Cell Oncol. 2016;3(4):e1057316.
28. Schulze K, Imbeaud S, Letouze E, Alexandrov LB, Calderaro J, Rebouissou S, et al. Exome sequencing of hepatocellular carcinomas identifies new mutational signatures and potential therapeutic targets. Nat Genet. 2015;47(5):505–11.
29. Cucarull B, Tutusaus A, Rider P, Hernaez-Alsina T, Cuno C, Garcia de Frutos P, et al. Hepatocellular carcinoma: molecular pathogenesis and therapeutic advances. Cancer. 2022;14(3):621.
30. Ushio J, Kanno A, Ikeda E, Ando K, Nagai H, Miwata T, et al. Pancreatic ductal adenocarcinoma: epidemiology and risk factors. Diagnostics. 2021;11(3):562.
31. Sung H, Ferlay J, Siegel RL, Laversanne M, Soerjomataram I, Jemal A, et al. Global cancer statistics 2020: GLOBOCAN estimates of incidence and mortality worldwide for 36 cancers in 185 countries. CA Cancer J Clin. 2021;71(3):209–49.
32. Rebours V, Boutron-Ruault MC, Schnee M, Ferec C, Maire F, Hammel P, et al. Risk of pancreatic adenocarcinoma in patients with hereditary pancreatitis: a national exhaustive series. Am J Gastroenterol. 2008;103(1):111–9.
33. Golan T, Kanji ZS, Epelbaum R, Devaud N, Dagan E, Holter S, et al. Overall survival and clinical characteristics of pancreatic cancer in BRCA mutation carriers. Br J Cancer. 2014;111(6):1132–8.
34. Leoz ML, Sanchez A, Carballal S, Ruano L, Ocana T, Pellise M, et al. Hereditary gastric and pancreatic cancer predisposition syndromes. Gastroenterol Hepatol. 2016;39(7):481–93.
35. Raimondi S, Lowenfels AB, Morselli-Labate AM, Maisonneuve P, Pezzilli R. Pancreatic cancer in chronic pancreatitis; aetiology, incidence, and early detection. Best Pract Res Clin Gastroenterol. 2010;24(3):349–58.
36. Tramacere I, Scotti L, Jenab M, Bagnardi V, Bellocco R, Rota M, et al. Alcohol drinking and pancreatic cancer risk: a meta-analysis of the dose-risk relation. Int J Cancer. 2010;126(6):1474–86.
37. Waddell N, Pajic M, Patch AM, Chang DK, Kassahn KS, Bailey P, et al. Whole genomes redefine the mutational landscape of pancreatic cancer. Nature. 2015;518(7540):495–501.
38. Bailey P, Chang DK, Nones K, Johns AL, Patch AM, Gingras MC, et al. Genomic analyses identify molecular subtypes of pancreatic cancer. Nature. 2016;531(7592):47–52.
39. Collisson EA, Bailey P, Chang DK, Biankin AV. Molecular subtypes of pancreatic cancer. Nat Rev Gastroenterol Hepatol. 2019;16(4):207–20.
40. Hosoda W, Chianchiano P, Griffin JF, Pittman ME, Brosens LA, Noe M, et al. Genetic analyses of isolated high-grade pancreatic intraepithelial neoplasia (HG-PanIN) reveal paucity of alterations in TP53 and SMAD4. J Pathol. 2017;242(1):16–23.
41. Tang B, Li Y, Qi G, Yuan S, Wang Z, Yu S, et al. Clinicopathological significance of CDKN2A promoter hypermethylation frequency with pancreatic cancer. Sci Rep. 2015;5:13563.
42. Moffitt RA, Marayati R, Flate EL, Volmar KE, Loeza SG, Hoadley KA, et al. Virtual microdissection identifies distinct tumor- and stroma-specific subtypes of pancreatic ductal adenocarcinoma. Nat Genet. 2015;47(10):1168–78.
43. Tiriac H, Belleau P, Engle DD, Plenker D, Deschenes A, Somerville TDD, et al. Organoid profiling identifies common responders to chemotherapy in pancreatic cancer. Cancer Discov. 2018;8(9):1112–29.
44. O'Kane GM, Grunwald BT, Jang GH, Masoomian M, Picardo S, Grant RC, et al. GATA6 expression distinguishes classical and basal-like subtypes in advanced pancreatic cancer. Clin Cancer Res. 2020;26(18):4901–10.

45. Chan-Seng-Yue M, Kim JC, Wilson GW, Ng K, Figueroa EF, O'Kane GM, et al. Transcription phenotypes of pancreatic cancer are driven by genomic events during tumor evolution. Nat Genet. 2020;52(2):231–40.
46. Ho WJ, Jaffee EM. Macrophage-targeting by CSF1/1R blockade in pancreatic cancers. Cancer Res. 2021;81(24):6071–3.
47. Murphy SJ, Hart SN, Lima JF, Kipp BR, Klebig M, Winters JL, et al. Genetic alterations associated with progression from pancreatic intraepithelial neoplasia to invasive pancreatic tumor. Gastroenterology. 2013;145(5):1098–109.
48. Amato E, Molin MD, Mafficini A, Yu J, Malleo G, Rusev B, et al. Targeted next-generation sequencing of cancer genes dissects the molecular profiles of intraductal papillary neoplasms of the pancreas. J Pathol. 2014;233(3):217–27.
49. Wu J, Jiao Y, Dal Molin M, Maitra A, de Wilde RF, Wood LD, et al. Whole-exome sequencing of neoplastic cysts of the pancreas reveals recurrent mutations in components of ubiquitin-dependent pathways. Proc Natl Acad Sci U S A. 2011;108(52):21188–93.

Chapter 19
Current Methods for Intraoperative Application

Francesco Frattini, Michail Mitsis, and Georgios D. Lianos

19.1 Introduction

Recognition of tumor margins is crucial for surgical oncology to ensure therapeutic resection and accurate prognosis and to maintain healthy tissues as well. The last factor is particularly important, for example, in neurosurgery, where the removal of cubic millimeters of brain tissue from eloquent areas could lead to a complete loss of psychomotor functions. Up to date, tumor borders are defined by preoperative imaging [1–3] and tumors are removed with a predetermined "excision margin" defined by the anatomical location of the primary tumor. Despite this approach, it has to be highlighted, for example, that approximately 30% of breast cancers have precarious resection margins. In other cases, where the tumor is approaching important anatomical organs, such as large blood vessels or nerves, more borderline safety zones are used.

It should be reported here that imaging techniques such as CT or MRI scans can "underestimate" the stage of the tumor and inadequately define the anatomy [4]. For this reason, laparoscopy has become very common in gastric [5] and esophageal surgery, and cytology is commonly used to diagnose peritoneal metastasis [6]. What is more, preoperative biopsy data are often not available to the operating surgeon. Finally, according to the principles of surgical oncology, the tumor should not be "cut" to minimize the risk of metastasis. In the case of in situ cancer resection (e.g., anal intraepithelial neoplasm), the surgeon completely ignores the margins of the tumor and will actually perform a "blind" oncological resection.

F. Frattini
Department of Surgery, Istituto Auxologico Italiano IRCCS Ospedale Capitanio, Milano, Italy

M. Mitsis · G. D. Lianos (✉)
Department of Surgery, University Hospital of Ioannina, Ioannina, Greece
e-mail: mmitsis@uoi.gr

G. Alexiou, G. Vartholomatos (eds.), *Intraoperative Flow Cytometry*,
https://doi.org/10.1007/978-3-031-33517-4_19

275

Because of these limitations, more and more intraoperative imaging techniques are being under investigation and several techniques are currently used, including magnetic resonance imaging (MRI), computed tomography (CT), PET, and ultrasound (US). The orientation of the image is facilitated nowadays with the help of modern computer assisting techniques, especially in the case of brain surgery, where it is called "neuronavigation" [7, 8]. Another modern intraoperative technique already used in specialized centers dealing with advanced surgical oncology, is the so-called fluorescence-guided assisted surgery.

19.2 Frozen-Section Histology: The Gold Standard

Since imaging methods do not provide histological identification [9], alternative methods are needed to determine whether the tumor resection is complete or not.

The gold standard for this problem is traditionally frozen-section histology, which provides biological data for the operating surgeon [10]. This technique involves sending various tissue samples to the pathology laboratory in flash-frozen format. The samples are examined with an optical microscope and the results are reported, usually by telephone, back to the operating room in 25–30 min. Often the removed tumor is sent for a rapid biopsy to check the entire surface for the presence of cancer cells, while in other cases, the sentinel lymph nodes are removed and sent for histopathological evaluation [11].

The most important point is the nature of the analysis, including sampling, transfer of the sample to a histopathology laboratory, laboratory sensitivity, and researcher-dependent analysis. This process, which includes rapid freezing, cutting, staining, is time-consuming, laborious, with high economic costs and lacks specialization. In addition, the diagnosis may be affected by artefacts introduced during sample preparation. In addition, the collection and transport of specimens increases the limitations as the complexity of the procedure (average completion time 30 min) significantly prolongs the patient's exposure to general anesthesia and surgical risk. Finally, this approach depends on the detailed verbal description of the samples, making the accurate localization of histological findings in the surgical area a challenge. Histological diagnosis is usually based on the morphological characteristics of cancer cells and tissues that differ from patient to patient and even differ in the same nodule of a liver (the so-called nodule in nodule) [12]. Various techniques have been applied such as conventional morphological examination with hematoxylin and eosin (H&E) staining, immunohistochemistry, and molecular biology [13]. However, these procedures take approximately 30 min. For this reason, a more reliable, time efficient, and less operator dependent-technique is required.

19.3   Mass Spectrometry Techniques

While conventional tumor diagnosis is based on morphological changes in cells and tissues, the chemical composition of the tissue is also important in understanding the full profile of a particular tissue cell type. Therefore, there is an obvious need to identify tissue characteristics in real-time during surgery. Potential intraoperative solutions have been given up to date mainly in the field of neurosurgery. A powerful, innovative solution is represented by tissue fluorescence, which is widely used in high-grade astrocytomas, especially in polymorphic glioblastoma [14]. The labeling is performed by administering the substance to the patient before the interventions, which results in the accumulation of fluorescent dye in the tumors.

Recently, chemical characterization of tissues by spectroscopic techniques has been proposed as an innovative solution. In this way, several decades ago, it was recognized that the chemical composition of tissues follows their histological categorization with astonishing accuracy [15, 16]. Unfortunately, nuclear magnetic resonance (NMR) spectroscopic methods did not reach the feasible level of use due to the low sensitivity of the method and the cost of NMR instruments. Although the information was common, it was not used until a completely different analytical approach emerged in the late 1990s. Matrix-assisted laser desorption ionization (MALDI) was developed in the late 1980s as an advanced ionization method for spectrometric investigation [17].

The MALDI technique was first used as advanced tissue analysis in the late 1990s and it was immediately recognized that spectroscopic information follows histology in a manner similar to spectroscopic NMR. It is reported that MALDI imaging provides tissue information that is consistent with histological analysis of samples. In addition, the most important issue is that the underlying mass spectrometric information is fully independent of the staff performing the analysis [18]. However, it is not superior to "rapid biopsy" and is significantly behind in terms of time required [19]. Several studies show mass spectrometric methods can be used to clearly identify tissues. Until now, however, no mass spectrometric ionization technique has been able to provide the required data in order to present a valid and reliable alternative to histopathology.

It has to be highlighted that mass spectrometry (MS) was introduced to the clinical field 50 years ago and is commonly used to identify and quantify exogenous or endogenous molecules, such as drugs, metabolites, or proteins in tissue and blood samples by measuring the mass-to-load ratio (m/z) of molecular ions or their charged fragments [20, 21]. It has been used as a powerful tool in screening for congenital metabolic diseases in neonates [22]. MS can also be used to classify tissues and provide valuable prognostic information, such as subtype and grade of tumor. In addition, MS technologies for tissue analysis have yielded encouraging results in intraoperative evaluation of surgical margins in common cancers, such as breast and pancreatic cancer, glioma, lung cancer, brain tumors, and HCC [23–30]. These molecular approaches are mainly based on the detection of MS signals, specific to cancer cells against non-cancerous tissue, or against a specific cancer subtype. The lesions that are detected are usually attributed to the modification of the cellular metabolism or the microenvironment of the tumor.

MS techniques that have been used successfully to determine tumor resection limits are currently grouped into two main categories: MS imaging (MSI) of tissue slices, and direct tissue sampling under ambient conditions [31–33]. The first may be very useful for tissue classification based on the distribution of specific molecules, but its use in a clinical and surgical routine is complex and requires time-consuming preparation. Since the introduction of MS in surgery over a decade, 25 different techniques have been used and have been classified into two main groups: online direct intraoperative MS and offline sampling probe-based methods. Two of the most commonly used online approaches are Rapid Evaporative Ionization Mass Spectrometry (REIMS) [26, 34, 35] and the MasSpec Pen [30, 36].

Rapid evaporative ionization mass spectrometry (REIMS) was developed exclusively for intraoperative tissue research in vivo [34, 37, 38]. The technique is based on the discovery that surgical techniques, such as electrosurgery or laser surgery, also function as a method of ionization, such as the molecular conversion of vital biological tissue components into ions by direct mass spectrometric analysis. Since then, while the concept of the smart knife was initially developed for electrosurgery [34], alternative surgical techniques (e.g., laser and ultrasound surgery [36, 39]) have also been successfully associated with mass spectrometric analysis. The "intelligent knife" has the potential to revolutionize the recognition of tumor borders in two fundamental ways: first, it can develop a "warning function" for the surgeon when resecting the tumor and when working close to it. Whenever the tumor is approached, the device "alerts" the surgeon to lead the resection line further. Mass spectrometric chemical profiling also allows the detection of the tumor without cutting the tumor, hence the risk of metastasis does not increase significantly with this approach. Second, the smart knife can be used in the so-called microprobe mode where a tiny catheter (not necessarily a surgical tool) is used to pump small amounts of tissue. Rapid evaporative ionization mass spectrometry technology allows the identification of only 50 µg of tissue material, so sampling is minimally invasive. In this case, the surgeon, endoscope or radiologist can sample any suspicious tissue in the surgical site and receive histological identification in just one second.

Recently, probe electrospray ionization (PESI) has been used to diagnose human renal cell carcinoma and chemically induced mouse HCC [40, 41]. The major advantage is the ability to produce ions directly from tissues in real time, with minimal sample processing [42]. Functional ease of use and real-time evaluation of tissue molecular information make MS extremely attractive, potentially meeting the requirements for clinical use as a routine examination. Kiritani et al. in 2021 emphasize that the combination of PESI-MS and a machine learning distinguish colorectal liver metastasis (CRLM) from non-cancerous tissue with high accuracy. Phospholipids categorized as monounsaturated fatty acids contributed to the difference between CRLM and the normal parenchyma and may also be a useful diagnostic biomarker and therapeutic target for CRLM [12].

In terms of the usefulness of Raman spectroscopy, it has been widely demonstrated for tissue characterization and disease differentiation, however current implementations with either 785 or 830 nm near-infrared (NIR) excitation have been ineffective in highly autofluorescent tissues such as the liver. Pence et al. in 2015 report the use of a Raman 1064 nm dispersion system using a low-noise Indium-Gallium-Arsenide (InGaAs) array for a high distinction between adenocarcinoma and hepatocellular carcinoma of a healthy liver. The resulting spectra have been combined with an algorithm, sparse multinomial logistic regression (SMLR), to predict healthy and diseased tissues [43].

Complete surgical resection with negative margins is one of the pillars in the treatment of liver tumors. However, current techniques for intraoperative evaluation of tumor resection thresholds are time-consuming and empirical. MS in combination with artificial intelligence (AI) is useful for tissue classification and provides valuable prognostic information. Giordano et al. in 2020 [12] attempted to develop an MS-based system for the rapid and objective identification and classification of liver cancer in 222 patients with hepatocellular carcinoma and in 96 patients with cholangiocarcinoma. The authors conclude that the MS-based system, in combination with AI, allows the detection of liver cancer with exceptional accuracy. Minimal sample preparation and short working time are the main advantages. From diagnosis to treatment, it has the potential to influence the decision-making process in real time with the ultimate goal of improving the treatment of cancer patients [44].

19.4 Fluorescence-Guided Surgery

Recently, the use of fluorescence-guided surgery (FGS) to treat visceral, hepatobiliary, and pancreatic neoplasms (benign and malignant) has significantly increased [45]. FGS deals with the fluorescence signal emitted by injected substances (fluorophores) after being illuminated by ad hoc laser sources to help guide the surgical procedure and provide the surgeon with real-time visualization of the fluorescent structures of interest [45].

The imaging of fluorescence emitted by indocyanine green (ICG) is a simple, fast, relatively inexpensive, and harmless tool with numerous different applications in surgical oncology field especially in visceral and hepatobiliary neoplasms. It can also be used in benign pathologiew. ICG, being a small-diameter hydrodynamic molecule, negotiates quickly through the lymphatics, lymph nodes, and blood vessels. It emits fluorescence that can be detected by fluorescent imaging and enables the evaluation of tissue perfusion, uptake, distribution, and clearance of dye-marked fluid [45]. Following submucosal or intradermal injection, ICG disperses in lymph, binds to lipoproteins, and is drained via lymphatic pathways and nodes. The resulting ICG fluorescence lymphography can be used to visualize the lymphatic vessels allowing surgeons to locate a functional lymphatic vessel, identify lymphatic and chyle leaks, assist in lymphaticovenous anastomoses (LVA), and map the sentinel lymph nodes [45].

Following intravenous (iv) injection, ICG binds to plasma proteins making the agent confined within the intravascular compartment. This property has been used for the assessment of flap vascularity, evaluation of organ and anastomotic perfusion. The liver excretes the ICG protein complexes in bile. The presence of ICG fluorescence in the bile has been used for real-time visualization of the extra hepatic bile ducts during fluorescence cholangiography (FC) [46]. Intraluminal injection of ICG in the bronchus, ureters, and bowel can be used to identify pulmonary subsegments, enable ureteric visualization during complicated pelvic procedures, and accurately localize enterocutaneous fistulas. ICG-enhanced laparoscopic surgery can be applied during different procedures offering to the surgeon additional information on anatomy, perfusion, or lymphatic drainage [47].

19.5 Conclusions

In conclusion, there has been a significant technical progress in recognizing tumor margins in recent decades. As histopathology gradually moves toward the detection of genetic markers and expression markers for individualized medical treatment and stratification of patient groups, in vivo tissue identification is increasingly becoming the task of medical imaging, combined with spectroscopic methods.

References

1. Risholm P, Golby AJ, Wells W. Multimodal image registration for preoperative planning and image-guided neurosurgical procedures. Neurosurg Clin N Am. 2011;22:197–206.
2. McSweeney SE, O'Donoghue PM, Jhaveri K. Current and emerging techniques in gastrointestinal imaging. J Postgrad Med. 2010;56:52–9.
3. Plana MN, Carreira C, Muriel A, et al. Magnetic resonance imaging in the preoperative assessment of patients with primary breast cancer: systematic review of diagnostic accuracy and meta-analysis. Eur Radiol. 2012;22:26–38.
4. Leufkens AM, van den Bosch M, van Leeuwen MS, Siersema PD. Diagnostic accuracy of computed tomography for colon cancer staging: a systematic review. Scand J Gastroenterol. 2011;46:887–94.
5. El Abiad R, Gerke H. Gastric cancer: endoscopic diagnosis and staging. Surg Oncol Clin N Am. 2012;21:1–19.
6. La Torre M, Ferri M, Giovagnoli MR, et al. Peritoneal wash cytology in gastric carcinoma. Prognostic significance and therapeutic consequences. Eur J Surg Oncol. 2010;36:982–6.
7. Kubben PL, ter Meulen KJ, Schijns O, et al. Intraoperative MRI-guided resection of glioblastoma multiforme: a systematic review. Lancet Oncol. 2011;12:1062–70.
8. Vranic A. New developments in surgery of malignant gliomas. Radiol Oncol. 2011;45:159–65.
9. Dent OF, Chapuis PH, Haboubi N, Bokey L. Magnetic resonance imaging cannot predict histological tumour involvement of a circumferential surgical margin in rectal cancer. Color Dis. 2011;13:974–81.
10. Winther C, Graem N. Accuracy of frozen section diagnosis: a retrospective analysis of 4785 cases. APMIS. 2011;119:259–62.
11. Nakhleh RE. Quality in surgical pathology communication and reporting. Arch Pathol Lab Med. 2011;135:1394–7.

12. Giordano S, Takeda S, Donadon M, et al. Rapid automated diagnosis of primary hepatic tumour by mass spectrometry and artificial intelligence. Liver Int. 2020;40:3117–24.
13. Schlageter M, Terracciano LM, D'Angelo S, Sorrentino P. Histopathology of hepatocellular carcinoma. World J Gastroenterol. 2014;20:15955–64.
14. Sherman JH, Hoes K, Marcus J, et al. Neurosurgery for brain tumors: update on recent technical advances. Curr Neurol Neurosci. 2011;11:313–9.
15. Herfkens R, Davis P, Crooks L, et al. Nuclear magnetic resonance imaging of the abnormal live rat and correlations with tissue characteristics. Radiology. 1981;141:211–8.
16. Postle AD. Phospholipid lipidomics in health and disease. Eur J Lipid Sci Technol. 2009;111:2–13.
17. Karas M, Bachmann D, Bahr U, Hillenkamp F. Matrix-assisted ultraviolet laser desorption of non-volatile compounds. Int J Mass Spectrom. 1987;78:53–68.
18. Gemoll T, Roblick UJ, Habermann JK. MALDI mass spectrometry imaging in oncology (review). Mol Med Rep. 2011;4:1045–51.
19. Chughtai K, Heeren RM. Mass spectrometric imaging for biomedical tissue analysis. Chem Rev. 2010;110:3237–77.
20. Dalgliesh CE, Horning EC, Horning MG, Knox KL, Yarger K. A gas-liquid-chromatographic procedure for separating a wide range of metabolites occurring in urine or tissue extracts. Biochem J. 1966;101:792–810.
21. Fowler KT, Hugh-Jones P. Mass spectrometry applied to clinical practice and research. Br Med J. 1957;1:1205–11.
22. Wagner M, Tonoli D, Varesio E, Hopfgartner G. The use of mass spectrometry to analyze dried blood spots. Mass Spectrom Rev. 2016;35:361–438.
23. Eberlin LS, Margulis K, Planell-Mendez I, et al. Pancreatic cancer surgical resection margins: molecular assessment by mass spectrometry imaging. PLoS Med. 2016;13:e1002108.
24. Calligaris D, Norton I, Feldman DR, et al. Mass spectrometry imaging as a tool for surgical decision-making. J Mass Spectrom. 2013;48:1178–87.
25. Santagata S, Eberlin LS, Norton I, et al. Intraoperative mass spectrometry mapping of an onco-metabolite to guide brain tumor surgery. Proc Natl Acad Sci U S A. 2014;111:11121–6.
26. Balog J, Sasi-Szabo L, Kinross J, et al. Intraoperative tissue identification using rapid evaporative ionization mass spectrometry. Sci Transl Med. 2013;5:194ra93.
27. Pirro V, Alfaro CM, Jarmusch AK, Hattab EM, Cohen-Gadol AA, Cooks RG. Intraoperative assessment of tumor margins during glioma resection by desorption electrospray ionization-mass spectrometry. Proc Natl Acad Sci U S A. 2017;114:6700–5.
28. Jarmusch AK, Alfaro CM, Pirro V, Hattab EM, Cohen-Gadol AA, Cooks RG. Differential lipid profiles of normal human brain matter and gliomas by positive and negative mode desorption electrospray ionization – mass spectrometry imaging. PLoS ONE. 2016;11:e0163180.
29. Alexander J, Gildea L, Balog J, et al. A novel methodology for in vivo endoscopic phenotyping of colorectal cancer based on real-time analysis of the mucosal lipidome: a prospective observational study of the iKnife. Surg Endosc. 2017;31:1361–70.
30. Sans M, Zhang J, Lin JQ, et al. Performance of the MasSpec pen for rapid diagnosis of ovarian cancer. Clin Chem. 2019;65:674–83.
31. Seeley EH, Caprioli RM. MALDI imaging mass spectrometry of human tissue: method challenges and clinical perspectives. Trends Biotechnol. 2011;29:136–43.
32. Amstalden van Hove ER, Smith DF, Heeren RMA. A concise review of mass spectrometry imaging. J Chromatogr A. 2010;1217:3946–54.
33. Giordano S, Zucchetti M, Decio A, et al. Heterogeneity of paclitaxel distribution in different tumor models assessed by MALDI mass spectrometry imaging. Sci Rep. 2016;6:39284.
34. Schäfer K-C, Dénes J, Albrecht K, et al. In vivo, in situ tissue analysis using rapid evaporative ionization mass spectrometry. Angew Chem Int Ed Engl. 2009;48:8240–2.
35. St John ER, Balog J, McKenzie JS, et al. Rapid evaporative ionization mass spectrometry of electrosurgical vapours for the identification of breast pathology: towards an intelligent knife for breast cancer surgery. Breast Cancer Res. 2017;19:59.

36. Zhang J, Rector J, Lin JQ, et al. Nondestructive tissue analysis for ex vivo and in vivo cancer diagnosis using a handheld mass spectrometry system. Sci Transl Med. 2017;9(406):3968.
37. Balog J, Szaniszlo T, Schaefer KC, et al. Identification of biological tissues by rapid evaporative ionization mass spectrometry. Anal Chem. 2010;82:7343–50.
38. Schafer KC, Szaniszlo T, Gunther S, et al. In situ, real-time identification of biological tissues by ultraviolet and infrared laser desorption ionization mass spectrometry. Anal Chem. 2011;83:1632–40.
39. Schafer KC, Balog J, Szaniszlo T, et al. Real time analysis of brain tissue by direct combination of ultrasonic surgical aspiration and sonic spray mass spectrometry. Anal Chem. 2011;83:7729–35.
40. Yoshimura K, Chen LC, Mandal MK, et al. Analysis of renal cell carcinoma as a first step for developing mass spectrometry-based diagnostics. J Am Soc Mass Spectrom. 2012;23:1741–9.
41. Yoshimura K, Mandal MK, Hara M, et al. Real-time diagnosis of chemically induced hepatocellular carcinoma using a novel mass spectrometry-based technique. Anal Biochem. 2013;441:32–7.
42. Monge ME, Harris GA, Dwivedi P, Fernández FM. Mass spectrometry: recent advances in direct open air surface sampling/ionization. Chem Rev. 2013;113:2269–308.
43. Pence IJ, Patil CA, Lieber CA, Mahadevan-Jansen A. Discrimination of liver malignancies with 1064nm dispersive Raman spectroscopy. Biomed Opt Express. 2015;6:2724–37.
44. Takats Z, Denes J, Kinross J. Identifying the margin: a new method to distinguish between cancerous and noncancerous tissue during surgery. Future Oncol. 2012;8:113–6.
45. Baiocchi GL, Diana M, Boni L. Indocyanine green-based fluorescence imaging in visceral and hepatobiliary and pancreatic surgery: state of the art and future directions. World J Gastroenterol. 2018;24(27):2921–30.
46. Ietto G, Amico F, Soldini G, et al. Real-time intraoperative fluorescent lymphography: a new technique for lymphatic sparing surgery. Transplant Proc. 2016;48(9):3073–8.
47. Boni L, David G, Mangano A, et al. Clinical applications of indocyanine green (ICG) enhanced fluorescence in laparoscopic surgery. Surg Endosc. 2015;29(7):2046–55.

Chapter 20
IFC in Primary and Metastatic Liver Tumours

Anastasia D. Karampa, Evangelos G. Baltagiannis, Georgios D. Lianos, and Georgios K. Glantzounis

20.1   Introduction

The main primary liver tumours are hepatocellular carcinoma (HCC), intrahepatic cholangiocarcinoma, and combined hepatocellular cholangiocarcinoma. HCC represents about 90% of primary liver cancers and constitutes a major global health problem.

HCC is the fifth most common cancer and the second most common cause of mortality worldwide for men [1]. Its incidence has increased over the years, representing a significant health issue, and HCC ranks among the most aggressive types of neoplasms [1]. The incidence of HCC increases progressively with advancing age in all populations, reaching a peak at 70 years. Experts in the field in the USA estimate that, in 2030, liver cancer will be the third leading cause of cancer-related deaths in both sexes, surpassing breast, colorectal, and prostate cancers [2]. The primary treatment that offers long-term survival (5 years survival >50%) with the potential for cure is liver resection and liver transplantation [3]. The principle aim of surgical Oncology is to achieve complete removal of the tumour (R0 resection), along with a functional future liver remnant [4].

The liver is also a high metastasis-permissive organ for the most prevalent malignancies, such as colorectal cancer, followed by pancreatic, breast, lung cancer and melanomas [5]. Moreover, liver metastases are much more common than primary hepatic tumours. It is reported that the organotropism of different carcinomas in the liver is influenced by several factors, such as blood flow pattern, tumour stage, and histological subtype of the tumour. There has been a significant progress in

A. D. Karampa · E. G. Baltagiannis · G. D. Lianos · G. K. Glantzounis (✉)
HPB Unit, Department of Surgery, University Hospital of Ioannina, Ioannina, Greece

Faculty of Medicine, School of Health Sciences, University of Ioannina, Ioannina, Greece
e-mail: gglantzounis@uoi.gr

G. Alexiou, G. Vartholomatos (eds.), *Intraoperative Flow Cytometry*,
https://doi.org/10.1007/978-3-031-33517-4_20

managing liver metastases over the last 20 years. The combination of liver resection, chemotherapy, targeted therapy, and immunotherapy has produced satisfactorily long-term survival. Especially for liver metastases from colorectal cancer, neuroendocrine tumours, and genitourinary tumours, the 5-year survival is over 50% [6, 7].

Liver resection has a central role in managing primary and metastatic liver tumours. The present chapter aims to examine the role of intraoperative flow cytometry (IFC) in achieving an R0 resection and assessing tumour biology.

20.2　Primary Liver Tumours

Barcelona clinic liver cancer (BCLC) staging system is the most commonly used system in the Western world for tumour classification, treatment allocation, prognosis, and study comparisons of HCC. It has been adopted and approved for guidance for HCC management by the European Association for the Study of Liver (EASL) and the American Association for the study of Liver Disease (AASLD) [8]. According to the recent BCLC criteria, patients with HCC are classified into five stages: very early-stage disease, early-stage disease, intermediate stage, advanced stage, and terminal stage [1]. Recent data have shown that patients with the very early disease have 80–90% 5-year survival, while the median survival of patients with early HCC reaches 50–70% at 5 years after hepatic resection, liver transplantation or local ablation in selected candidates [1, 8]. Regarding the intermediate stage, 23 studies with 2412 patients undergoing liver resection have shown that the median survival was 37 months and the 5-year survival 35%. Regarding the advanced stage, 29 studies with 3659 patients with HCC undergoing hepatectomy refer that the three and 5-year survival was 33% and 20%, respectively [9].

Cholangiocarcinoma (CCA) comprises a heterogeneous group of malignancies that can arise anywhere in the bile ducts. Despite being a rare disease, over the past 15 years, incidence and mortality rates have increased globally. Many patients have no apparent cause at diagnosis, limiting the ability of early detection by surveillance programmes, while at the same time, the 'asymptomatic' nature of CCA in its early stages and its aggressiveness strongly compromise patient outcomes and survival [10]. Similar to hepatocellular cancer, the main treatment that ensures long-term survival with curative intent is liver resection with complete removal of the tumour (R0 resection) and, in selected cases, liver transplantation.

It also has to be highlighted that in these neoplasms, the role of tumour biology is very significant since it affects diseases' prognosis. According to essential studies, three groups of genes are related to risk factors. (1) CTNNB1 with alcoholic liver disease, (2) TP53 with hepatitis B virus (HBV) induced cirrhosis; and (3) others that do not have a distinct pattern, mainly in patients with hepatitis C virus (HCV) infection, metabolic syndrome, and hemochromatosis [11]. Research in tumour stage demonstrated that TERT promoter mutation was seen more frequently in early-stage tumours. On the other hand, TP53 and CDKN2A alterations and amplification of the chromosome 11 amplicon that encodes FGF3, FGF4, FGF19, and CCND1 were observed more commonly in advanced stages [12]. The advent of functional genetic screening has contributed to the advancement of liver cancer biology, uncovering many novel genes involved in tumorigenesis and cancer progression. Through in vivo and in vitro screens, many novel oncogenes and tumour suppressor genes have been elucidated, deepening our understanding of the tumorigenesis and progression of liver cancer. Regarding biology of cholangiocarcinoma, two different categories of cholangiocarcinomas have been described using an integrative genomic analysis: the inflammation class and the proliferation class. Each class has specific activated oncogenic pathways associated with different clinical outcomes. Shorter survival and earlier recurrence have been observed in patients with proliferation class cholangiocarcinomas [13].

Histopathologic examination is the gold standard diagnostic method to evaluate the surgical margins microscopically and to guide the extent of resection. Detailed histopathologic analysis of liver cancer specimens is crucial for definite diagnosis and patient prognosis. Tumour characteristics such as size, histologic subtype, histologic grade, vascular invasion, pathologic staging, and immunohistochemical characteristics are significant features that predict patient prognosis, recurrence, and metastatic potential.

20.3 Flow Cytometry in Primary Liver Tumours

Flow cytometry is a powerful technique with applications such as phenotypic analysis and quantification of DNA content. Intraoperative flow cytometry is an emerging technique for applying flow cytometry for DNA content/ploidy and cell cycle distribution analysis during surgery for tumour cell analysis and margin evaluation. It has been used for cell analysis of intracranial tumours, head and neck carcinomas, and breast carcinomas, as well as for tumour margin evaluation [14, 15]. The quantification of the state/phenotype of a cell population is among the main advantages of FC to other methods, such as microscopy. DNA analysis is among the first widely used applications of flow cytometry. In contrast, intraoperative flow cytometry (IFC) was based on flow cytometric quantification of DNA content/ploidy and cell cycle distribution during surgery for cancer cell analysis and margin evaluation [16]. IFC offers the ability for intraoperative diagnosis, an alternative to pathology evaluation of tissue sections obtained during surgery. The utility of this powerful emerging technique (IFC) is currently being widely expanded beyond central nervous system tumours into the analysis of tumour margins in several cancer types, including liver cancers [17]. It may represent in the future a very useful tool in the surgical oncology field (Fig. 20.1).

Flow cytometry is a fast technique that allows the analysis of whole-cell populations. Thus, clonal expansion of cancer may be monitored as subpopulations with distinct genetic characteristics. The intraoperative use of flow cytometry contributes to the precise characterization of tumour margins and the potential for complete tumour removal, which is the main goal in surgical oncology. Regarding liver

A. D. Karampa et al.

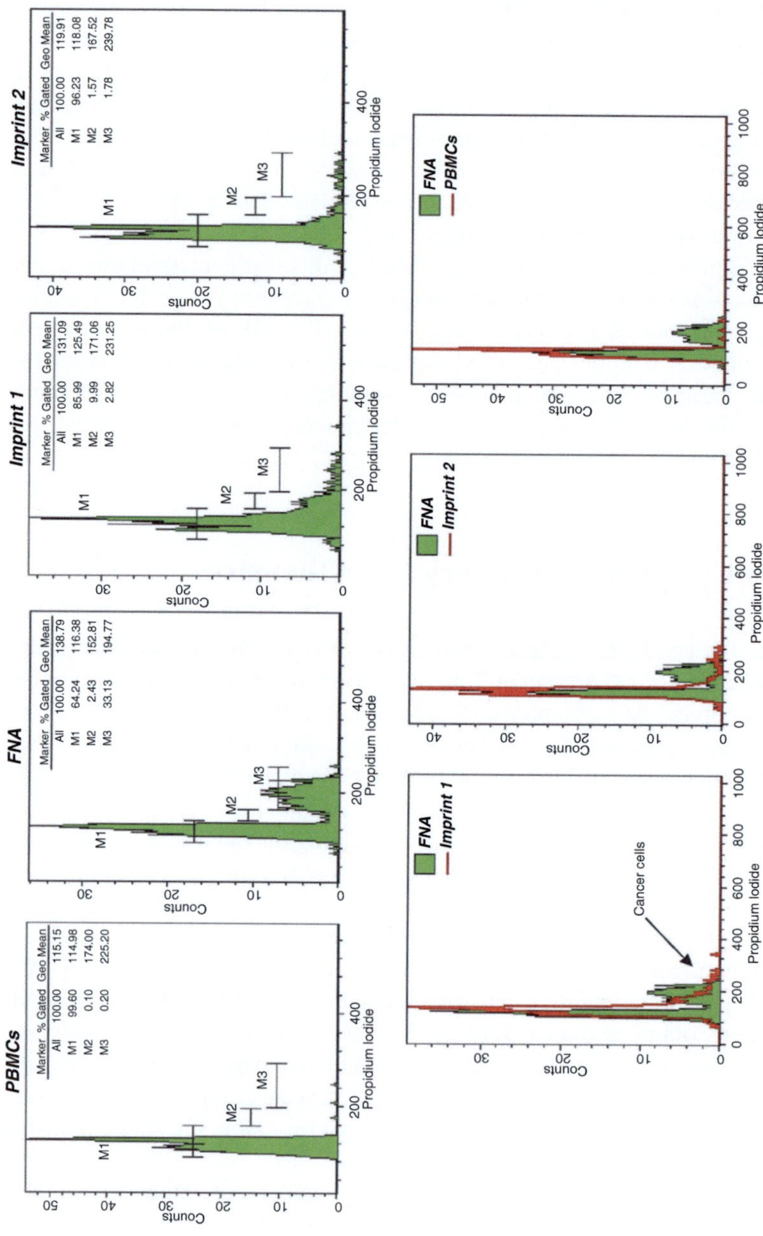

Fig. 20.1 DNA analysis in touch imprint IFC in primary liver tumour (hepatocellular carcinoma). Peripheral blood mononuclear cells (PBMCs) are used as a control for DNA content evaluation. FNA samples are used to characterize malignant cells (in this case cells with a tumour index of 35.5%). Imprint 1 represents a positive margin containing cancer cells, while imprint 2 represents a negative margin. (From Markopoulos et al., Methods Protocol 2021;4(3):66, after permission)

surgery, the information provided from flow cytometry could change the intraoperative strategy with the performance of further liver resection if the future liver remnant is adequate. Furthermore, IFC could also identify those patients who are at high risk for local recurrence, and this is a vital tool because, in this way, adjuvant treatment could be offered in a few weeks postoperatively in patients that are at high risk for recurrence, while at the same time a very close follow-up should be planned as well. Touch imprints have been extensively used in the cytological evaluation of tumour cells in several types of cancer, including hepatic malignancies. Touch imprint IFC offers several advantages to assist clinical management. DNA analysis can be performed within 5–6 min from sample collection, providing information to the surgeon, while flow cytometry analysis can characterize cancer cells taken from fine-needle aspirates (FNAs). The touch imprint covers the surface of the resected liver, allowing analysis of cancer cells for the whole resected area [17] (Fig. 20.2).

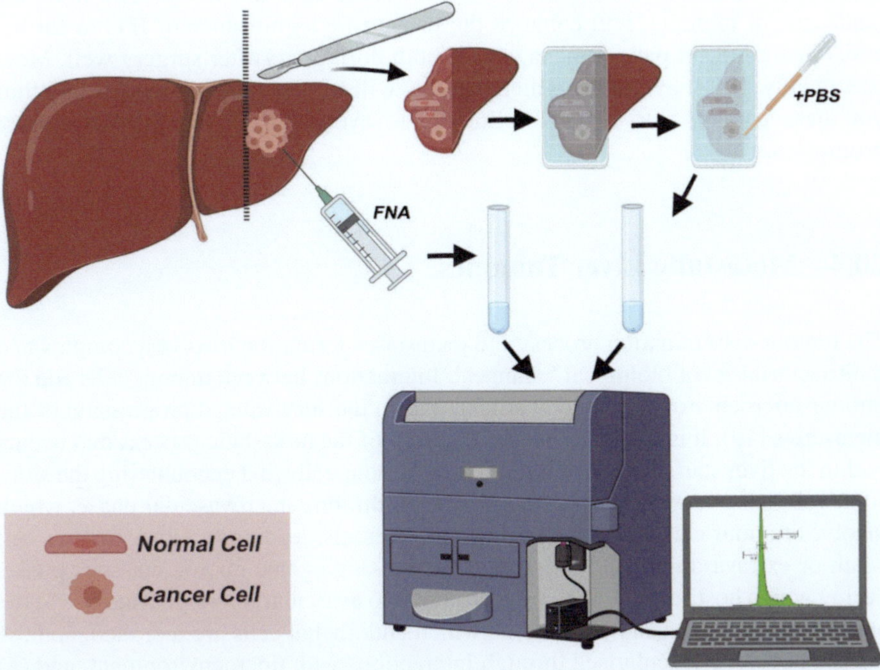

Fig. 20.2 Protocol overview. Immediately after tumour excision, tumour samples are used for the creation of touch imprints into a nylon membrane. The obtained cells are rinsed in phosphate buffered saline into a cell suspension that is further passed through a sterile filter. Cells are counted and are immediately stained with propidium iodide (125 mM). Following 3 min staining, The DNA content of samples is analysed according to 'Ioannina protocol' [18]. Fine-needle aspirates (FNA) taken from the tumour are used as positive control to characterize the DNA content of cancer cells. In parallel, histopathologic examination of the respective tissue samples on permanent tissue sections are performed according to established diagnostic protocols. Evaluation of tumour grade is also performed according to the proposed grading systems. (From Markopoulos et al., Methods Protocol 2021;4(3):66, after permission)

At the same time, histopathologic analysis is the gold standard for malignant cells' characterization. The ability to find cancer cells in the margin area may offer the possibility for further molecular analysis and more intensive follow-up for those patients. The use of intraoperative flow cytometry is currently under investigation. The results presented in a recently published study from the Ioannina IFC group [17] are preliminary and have to be further elucidated in large clinical trials in long-term patient follow-up.

The molecular profile of cancer, including individual driver mutations, has diagnostic, prognostic, and therapeutic value. It has been described that liver cell dysplasias exhibit aneuploid cell populations. Since DNA index is used to characterize cellular malignancy with intraoperative flow cytometry, the possibility of characterizing liver cell dysplasia as a malignant tumour may be a limitation that must be considered. The molecular identification of tumours is now a critical factor for patients' therapeutic and clinical management. In the future, intraoperative flow cytometry, combined with immunohistochemical data and the genetic mutation landscape of tumours, will enhance the prognostic significance of IFC to further assist in significant patient management both during and after surgery well. More specifically, IFC may predict which patients will have a worse prognosis and thus put these patients into a strict follow-up to avoid early recurrence or disease progression.

20.4   Metastatic Liver Tumours

The tumour dissemination process and metastases formation involve a complex and multifactorial set of biological 'changes'. Interactions between tumour cells and the tumour microenvironment play a crucial part in the survival and progression of the metastases [19]. It is reported that the first step of the metastatic process that occurs within the liver starts with the disseminated tumour cells first encountering the sinusoids following four phases: (1) the tumour-infiltrating microvascular phase, which involves tumour cell arrest in the sinusoidal vessels, leading to either tumour cell death or extravasation, (2) the interlobular pre-angiogenic micrometastasis phase, during which host stromal cells are recruited into avascular micrometastases; (3) the angiogenic micrometastasis phase, in which endothelial cells are recruited, and the tumours become vascularised through interactions with microenvironment, and (4) the growth phase that leads to clinically manifested metastases [6].

The major health issue today is, without a doubt, that the incidence of cancer keeps rising dramatically. Specifically, among 2.4 million cancer patients in the Surveillance, Epidemiology, and End Results (SEER) database from 2010 to 2015, 5.14% of patients with cancer are diagnosed with liver metastasis at the time of primary cancer diagnosis [7]. For women ages 20–50, breast cancer is the most common cancer with liver metastases. For men ages 20–50, colon cancer is the most common diagnosis with liver metastases, followed by the primary diagnoses of rectal, lung, and pancreatic cancers. As patients get older, a more heterogeneous population of the top cancers with liver metastases emerges and includes the oesophageal, stomach, small intestine, melanoma, and bladder cancer, in addition to the large proportion of lung, pancreatic, and colorectal cancers [20].

For this reason, management and therapeutic decisions for patients with liver metastases should be discussed at multi-disciplinary team meetings to determine an optimal personalized approach. In this way, management strategies should consider resection as part of a multimodal treatment algorithm, given that surgery, chemotherapy, targeted therapy or immunotherapy represents the best chance of long-term survival.

It is already known that hepatic resection is the gold standard of treatment in patients with resectable liver metastases, while liver transplantation is performed in only a tiny minority of patients [21]. In this way, systemic chemotherapy, as well as surgical treatment for metastatic disease, has enhanced in a significant way the prognosis of patients with liver metastases. It should be noted that the reported 5-year survival rates after surgical treatment are reported to be approximately 71% for patients with solitary colorectal liver metastasis [6].

There is robust evidence that a clear surgical margin is an independent prognostic factor in many types of tumours. Four years ago, a meta-analysis reported that a >1 mm margin (usually defined as R0) is associated with improved survival compared to a submillimetre margin (<1 mm, R1) [22]. In addition, Wang et al. demonstrated recently that an involved margin (0 mm, R1-contact) is associated with poorer survival [7]. In cases of colorectal liver metastases, a systemic disease, the oncological impact of resection margins is still under discussion. Several authors emphasized the importance of achieving >1 mm margin clearance. However, R1 margin may be a surrogate of biological behaviour rather than the result of surgical technique [6].

20.5 Flow Cytometry in Metastatic Liver Tumours

The significance of R0 resection in liver metastases is clear [23], but the method to intra-operationally confirm it is only through a rapid histopathological report. This method harbours many issues as it concerns a small segment, not the whole margin line, but remains the gold standard. In this background, flow cytometry (FC) [24] came to give a potential intraoperative tool to the operating surgeon. As mentioned above, this method was developed in the University Hospital of Ioannina [15, 18], firstly used for central nervous tumours and is currently being expanded to cancer cell characterization and margin detection during the excision of primary and metastatic liver neoplasms [17].

Flow cytometry analysis offers several advantages for tumour diagnosis [25]. The intraoperative use of flow cytometry contributes towards the precise characterization of tumour margins and the potential for complete tumour removal (R0 resection), which is the main goal in surgical oncology. In the field of liver surgery, the information provided by FC on the presence of cancer cells in the hepatic transection surface could change the intraoperative management with the performance of further liver resection if the future liver remnant is adequate (for primary and for metastatic liver tumours). Furthermore, the presence of cancer cells in the resection area will offer us important information regarding tumour biology. This will help the postoperative management either with early onset of effective chemotherapy or close follow-up for early recurrence.

Touch imprint IFC offers several advantages to assist clinical management [17]. DNA content analysis based on the 'Ioannina protocol' can be performed rapidly, providing information to the surgeon, while flow cytometry analysis can accurately characterize cancer cells taken from fine-needle aspirates (FNAs). The new methodology presented in 'Ioannina protocol' undoubtedly provides a 'roadmap' on the use of touch imprint IFC during hepatectomies. However, as this is the first clinical trial on this new implementation of FC, the results are preliminary and must be further investigated in large clinical trials. Furthermore, the clinical significance of our findings needs to be explored in long-term patient follow-up. A key solution to these issues may be the integration of next-generation sequencing as the molecular characterization of tumours becomes the new standard and is now a critical factor for the therapeutic and clinical management of patients in the new era of Cancer Precision Medicine [26].

In conclusion, the current literature does not offer comprehensive and robust scientific information about the role of IFC in the effective management of liver neoplasms. However, there are significant indications that IFC has the potential to offer important information which will guide the intraoperative and postoperative management of primary and metastatic liver tumours. After the preliminary encouraging results above, our group prospectively continues this challenging research project. It has to be highlighted that IFC in liver tumours can potentially be a very useful intraoperative and postoperative tool that can help surgeons and oncologists to increase survival rates of patients with primary and metastatic liver tumours.

References

1. Galle PR, Forner A, Llovet JM, Mazzaferro V, Piscaglia F, Raoul J-L, et al. EASL clinical practice guidelines: management of hepatocellular carcinoma. J Hepatol. 2018;69(1):182–236.
2. Sung H, Ferlay J, Siegel RL, Laversanne M, Soerjomataram I, Jemal A, et al. Global cancer statistics 2020. GLOBOCAN estimates of incidence and mortality worldwide for 36 cancers in 185 countries. CA Cancer J Clin. 2021, 71:209–49.
3. Glantzounis GK, Karampa A, Peristeri DV, Pappas-Gogos TK, Tzimas P, et al. Recent advances in the surgical management of hepatocellular carcinoma. Ann Gastroenterol. 2021;34(4):453. https://doi.org/10.20524/aog.2021.0632.
4. Anastasopoulos N-A, Lianos GD, Tatsi V, Karampa A, Goussia A, Glantzounis GK. Clinical heterogeneity in patients with non-alcoholic fatty liver disease associated with hepatocellular carcinoma. Expert Rev Gastroenterol Hepatol. 2020;14:1025–33.
5. Siegel RL, Miller KD, Jemal A. Cancer statistics, 2020. CA Cancer J Clin. 2020;70:7–30.
6. Tsilimigras DI, Brodt P, Clavien PA, Muschel RJ, D'Angelica MI, Endo I, et al. Liver metastases. Nat Rev Dis Primers. 2021;7(1):27.

7. Wang S, Feng Y, Swinnen J, Oyen R, li Y, Ni Y. Incidence and prognosis of liver metastasis at diagnosis: a pan-cancer population-based study. Am J Cancer Res. 2020;10:1477–517.
8. Heimbach JK, Kulik LM, Finn RS, Sirlin CB, Abecassis MM, Roberts LR, et al. AASLD guidelines for the treatment of hepatocellular carcinoma. Hepatology. 2018;67:358–80.
9. Glantzounis GK, Paliouras A, Stylianidi MC, Milionis H, Tzimas P, Roukos D, et al. The role of liver resection in the management of intermediate and advanced stage hepatocellular carcinoma. A systematic review. Eur J Surg Oncol. 2018;44(2):195–208.
10. Izquierdo-Sanchez L, Lamarca A, Casta AL, Buettner S, Utpatel K, Klumpen HJ, et al. Cholangiocarcinoma landscape in Europe: diagnostic, prognostic and therapeutic insights from the ENSCCA registry. J Hepatol. 2022;76:1109–21.
11. Khemlina G, Ikeda S, Kurzrock R. The biology of hepatocellular carcinoma: implications for genomic and immune therapies. Mol Cancer. 2017;16(1):149.
12. Castelli G, Pelosi E, Testa U. Liver cancer: molecular characterization, clonal evolution and cancer stem cells. Cancer. 2017;9:127.
13. Banales JM, Marin JJ, Lamarca A, Rodrigues PM, Khan SA, Roberts LR, et al. Cholangiocarcinoma 2020: the next horizon in mechanisms and management. Nat Rev Gastroenterol Hepatol. 2020, 17:557–88.
14. Andreou M, Vartholomatos E, Harissis H, Markopoulos GS, Alexiou GA. Past, present and future of flow cytometry in breast cancer-a systematic review. EJIFCC. 2019;30:423–37.
15. Vartholomatos G, Basiari L, Exarchakos G, Katsanioudakis I, Komnos I, Michali M, et al. Intraoperative flow cytometry for head and neck lesions. Assessment of malignancy and tumour-free resection margins. Oral Oncol. 2019;99:104344.
16. Horan PK, Wheeless J. Quantitative single cell analysis and sorting. Science. 1977;198:149–57.
17. Markopoulos GS, Glantzounis GK, Goussia AC, Lianos GD, Karampa A, Alexiou GA, et al. Touch imprint intraoperative flow cytometry as a complementary tool for detailed assessment of resection margins and tumor biology in liver surgery for primary and metastatic liver neoplasms. Methods Protoc. 2021;4:66.
18. Vartholomatos E, Vartholomatos G, Alexiou GA, Markopoulos GS. The past, present and future of flow cytometry in central nervous system malignancies. Methods Protoc. 2021;4(1):11.
19. Li X, Ramadori P, Pfister D, Seehawer M, Zender L, Heikenwalder M. The immunological and metabolic landscape in primary and metastatic liver cancer. Nat Rev Cancer. 2021;21:541–57.
20. Horn SR, Stolzfus KC, Lehrer EJ, Dawson LA, Tchelebi L, Gusani NJ, et al., et al. Epidemiology of liver metastases. Cancer Epidemiol. 2020;67:101760.
21. Kambakamba P, Hotie, Cremen S, Braun F, Becker T, Lineker M. The evolution of surgery for colorectal liver metastases: a persistent challenge to improve survival. Surgery. 2021;170:1732–40.
22. Margonis GA, Sergentanis TN, Ntanasis-Stathopoulos I, Andreatos N, Tzanninis I-G, Sasaki K, et al. Impact of surgical margin width on recurrence and overall survival following R0 hepatic resection of colorectal metastases: a systematic review and meta-analysis. Ann Surg. 2018;267:1047–55.
23. Ausania F, Landi F, Mertinez-Perez A, Sandomenico R, Cuatrecasas M, Pages M, et al. Impact of microscopic incomplete resection for colorectal liver metastases on surgical margin recurrence: R1-contact vs R1 < 1 mm margin width. J Hepatobiliary Pancreat Sci. 2022;29:449–59.
24. McKinnon KM. Flow cytometry: an overview. Curr Protoc Immunol. 2018;120:5.1.1–5.1.11.
25. Suo Y, Gu Z, Wei X. Advances of in vivo flow cytometry on cancer studies. Cytometry A. 2020;97:15–23.
26. Priestley P, Baber J, Lolkema MP, Steeghs N, Bruijn ED, Shale C, et al. Pan-cancer whole-genome analyses of metastatic solid tumours. Nature. 2019;575:210–6.

Chapter 21
Intraoperative Flow Cytometry in Colorectal Cancer

Christina Bali and Vaia K. Georvasili

21.1 Colorectal Cancer

21.1.1 Epidemiology

Colorectal cancer (CRC) constitutes the third most common human malignancy and 10% of all cancer diagnoses. According to the GLOBOCAN 2020 data, 1.9 million new colorectal cancers were estimated to occur in 2020. Regarding sex, men are more often diagnosed with CRC than women. The risk of developing CRC increases with age, and over 90% of sporadic CRCs occur in individuals over the age of 50. Worldwide, CRC is a disease that affects more the developing countries. The highest colon cancer incidence rates are found in Eastern Europe, Australia/New Zealand, North America, and Eastern Asia. All regions of Africa, as well as Southern Asia, have the lowest incidence rates of CRC. Predisposing factors in Western societies are the increased intake of animal-source foods (especially red meat), the lower intake of fibers, the decreased physical activity and increased body weight, smoking habits and alcohol consumption.

CRC has a major impact in human life, as it constitutes the second leading cause of cancer-related mortality, responsible for approximately 935,000 deaths in 2020 [1, 2].

C. Bali (✉) · V. K. Georvasili
Department of Surgery, Medical School, University Hospital of Ioannina, Ioannina, Greece
e-mail: cbali@uoi.gr

21.1.2   Pathogenesis

Most colorectal cancers (90%) arise from the cells of the inner layer of the large bowel called epithelium. The colon epithelium forms crypts and consists mostly of mucous-secreting (goblet) cells, columnar absorptive cells, enteroendocrine cells, Paneth cells and stem cells located at its base [3]. The cell of origin for most colorectal cancers is currently assumed to be a stem cell or a stem-cell-like cell of the epithelium crypt base. The cancerous transformation of these stem cells is believed to be a consequence of genetic and epigenetic alterations that inactivate tumor-suppressor genes and/or activate oncogenes [3]. Cancer stem cells have lost control of replication and differentiation, which leads to tumorigenesis.

CRC usually begins with the non-cancerous proliferation of mucosal epithelial cells called polyps. The polyps derived from the glandular cells are called adenomas. The traditional adenoma–carcinoma pathway is considered responsible for the development of 70–90% of colorectal cancers. This transformation usually takes 10–15 years, which allow early diagnosis and removal of these premalignant or early malignant lesions. Depending on the origin of the mutation, colorectal carcinomas can be classified as sporadic (70%), inherited (5%), and familial (25%). Currently, three molecular pathways have been recognized. These are the chromosomal instability (CIN) pathway, microsatellite instability (MSI) pathway, and the CpG island methylator phenotype (CIMP) pathway [4]. One or more pathways may coexist in some tumors.

21.1.2.1   Chromosomal Instability (CIN) Pathway

Chromosomal instability is the most common cause of genomic instability in CRC. It is responsible for 65–70% of sporadic CRC. In molecular basis, there is an accelerated rate of gains or losses of whole or large portions of chromosomes that results in karyotypic variability from cell to cell. The consequence of CIN is an imbalance in chromosome number (aneuploidy), sub-chromosomal genomic amplifications, and a high frequency of loss of heterozygosity (LOH). Chromosomal instability phenotypes typically develop following genomic events initiated by an APC mutation, followed by RAS activation or function loss of TP53 [4].

21.1.2.2   Microsatellite Instability (MSI) Pathway

Microsatellites are small (1–6 base pairs) repeating segments of DNA scattered throughout the entire genome and account for approximately 3% of the human genome. Due to their repetitive nature, they are prone to mutations. Instability of microsatellites results from the inability to correct DNA duplication errors by the mismatched repair system (MMR). The latter consist of different proteins coded by MSH2, MLH1, MSH6, PMS2, MLH3, MSH3, PMS1, and Exo1 genes. Germline mutation in MMR genes results in Hereditary Non-Polyposis Colorectal Cancer (HNPCC), while somatic mutation or hypermethylation silencing of MMR genes accounts for about 15% of sporadic CRC [4, 5]. MSI-high tumors usually are diploid with less LOH and have fewer mutations in KRAS and p53. Sporadic MSI-high CRC are more common in older women, and mostly located proximal to the splenic flexure. The histology pattern shows increased lymphocytic infiltration, mucinous histology, and poor differentiation [4].

21.1.2.3 CpG Island Methylator Phenotype (CIMP) Pathway

DNA methylation occurs commonly at the 5′-CG-3′ (CpG) dinucleotide and causes epigenetic changes in gene expression/function. Methylation of a gene promoter region may interfere with gene expression and halter its function. In colorectal carcinogenesis silenced genes by DNA hypermethylation are APC, MCC, and MLH1. Hypermethylation of MSH1 is found in MSI-high sporadic CRC. The presence of such hypermethylation in several genes creates the CpG Island Methylator Phenotype (CIMP). CIMP is found in 15–20% of sporadic CRC [4].

21.1.3 CRC Dissemination

CRC like every neoplasm tends to grow locally and disseminate throughout the body. CRC dissemination begins with the invasion of the submucosa, the layer outside epithelium, which is rich in blood/lymph vessels and nerves and predisposing to spread via the blood stream to distant organs (liver, lung, etc.), or along the regional or distal lymph nodes (Fig. 21.1). Other ways of recognized CRC spread are through invasion of serosa and tumor seeding across the peritoneal cavity and through viable tumor cells, which exfoliate intraluminaly, and grow distally to the tumor, especially on the colonic anastomosis.

Cancer spread is the main factor for treatment failure and survival compromise in CRC patients and the research has been focused on the comprehension of the pathways that lead to metastasis. Cancer metastasis constitutes a complicated process, which involves several modifications in, primary or metastasis site, cancer cells (seed), and microenviroment (soil). The activation of invasion and metastasis is triggered by epigenetic factors that are regulated by environmental stimuli, adhesive signals from extracellular matrix (ECM) components and mechanical pressures, cell–cell interactions, soluble signals, immune response, and the intratumoral microbiota. Secondary sites do not receive invading cancer cells passively. In fact, the host microenvironment is selectively primed by the primary tumor even before the initiation of metastasis. Metastatic cancer encompasses a diverse collection of cells that possess different genetic and phenotypic characteristics. Studies have been shown that this intratumoral cell heterogenity could predispose to cancer recurrence and resistance to treatment [5].

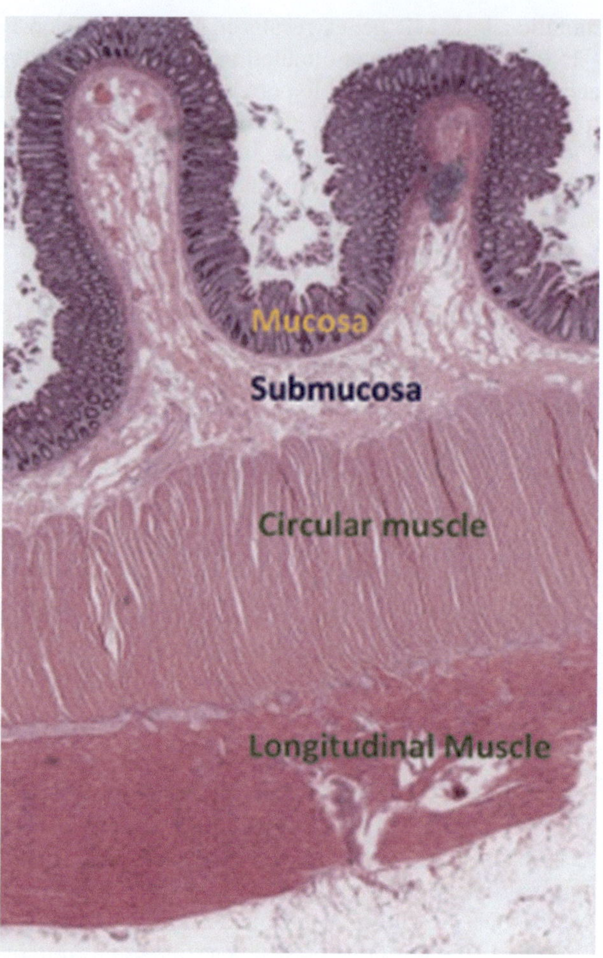

Fig. 21.1 Microscopic anatomy of colon wall

21.1.4 CRC Staging

The identification of the CRC spreading sites is called staging. The American Joint Committee on Cancer (AJCC) TNM staging system is the most widely used prognostic staging system for CRC (Table 21.1). This system estimates three parameters: the tumor invasion through the bowel wall (T), the status of the regional lymph nodes (N), and the presence of distant metastasis (M). The current 8th edition (2017) of the TNM staging classification recognize additional factors implicating in the appropriate treatment, including preoperative CEA levels, the tumor regression score, lymphovascular and perineural invasion, MSI, and KRAS/NRAS/BRAF mutation status [6].

Table 21.1 TMN staging system in CRC

TNM staging
Primary tumor staging (T)
Tx: primary tumor cannot be assessed
T0: no evidence of primary tumor
Tis: carcinoma in situ
T1: invasion into submucosa
T2: invasion into muscularis propria
T3: invasion of the subserosa or non-peritonealized pericolic tissues
T4 a: penetration of the visceral peritoneal layer
b: penetration or adhesion to adjacent organs
Nodal status (N)
Nx: nodes cannot be assessed
N0: no evidence of nodal involvement
N1 a: involvement of one regional node
b: involvement of 2–3 regional nodes
c: deposits involving serosa or non-peritonealized pericolic/perirectal tissues without regional nodal metastasis
N2 a: involvement of 4–6 nodes
b: involvement of $\geq$7 nodes
Metastases (M)
Mx: presence of metastases cannot be assessed
M0: no evidence of metastases
M1 a: distant metastases confined to one organ (e.g., liver, lung, ovary, non-regional node)
b: distant metastases confined to more than one organ or to the peritoneum

Table 21.2 Classification of CRC stages according to TNM, and patient prognosis by stage

Stage	TNM	5-year survival (%)
0, I	Tis-T1, N0, M0	>90
I	T2, N0, M0	80–85
II	T3-4, N0, M0	70–75
III	T2, N1-3, M0	70–75
III	T3, N1-3, M0	50–65
III	T4, N1-2, M0	25–45
IV	M1	<10

Preoperative staging is based on physical examination, but most decisively in imaging methods as computed or/magnetic tomography of the abdomen, pelvis, and chest. The definite and most accurate TNM staging is based on postoperative microscopy findings of pathology report, and according to this, patients are classified in four stages (Table 21.2). Stage constitutes the most important factor in the choice of the optimal treatment, but also remains the most significant prognostic factor for the patient's survival (Table 21.2) [7].

21.1.5 CRC Treatment

The major regulator of CRC treatment is preoperative stage. Surgery remains the cornerstone of the available treatment modalities, and the only one that can provide the prospective of cure for localized colon cancer. For stages I–III, standard colectomies according to the location of tumor are performed. Principles of surgical resection in colon cancer include resection of bowel lumen in adequate margins (10 cm in either direction from tumor) along with the regional lymph nodes [8]. The long colon length permits these wide excisions without any functional implications to the patient.

The rectal cancer treatment strategy is currently focused on organ (rectum) sparing methods, which do not compromise the oncological outcome, but preserve the defecation function per anus. In rectal tumors, a 10 cm distal margin in most patients is synonym to abdominoperineal resection and permanent stoma due to the proximity to anal sphincters. Another difference in rectal tumors is related to higher local recurrence rate comparing to colon. The role of mesorectum and the necessity of its complete resection, along the plane of mesorectal fascia, has been highlighted in the 80s and has become the revolution in the field of rectal cancer treatment [9]. The negative circumferential resection margin (non-cancerous invasion of mesorectal fascia) has been also found to be a significant prognostic factor [8]. Accurate preoperative staging provides the selection of rectal cancer patients to be treated by either local resection or neoadjuvant chemoradiation (CRT) plus resection. In both cases, the required distal resection margin of rectum is 1cm, which enables preservation of anal canal [10].

Stage V patients do not benefit by surgery due to spread of cancer outside the operation field. These patients are offered only chemotherapy [ChT] (±radiation in rectal cancer) and the prognosis in most of them is dismal (Table 21.2). Resection of primary tumor is performed only in cases of complicated cancers (bleeding, perforation, obstruction) and in cases where the metastatic sites are considered surgically resectable (liver, lungs) [8, 11].

Following a proper oncological resection, in colon and preoperatively irradiated rectal cancer, adjuvant ChT has an established role for patients with "high-risk" stage II and stage III (N+) disease to prevent tumor recurrence, metastasis and death [12, 13]. High -risk criteria for stage II patients that will benefit from adjuvant ChT are lymph nodes sampling <12, pT4 stage including perforation, poorly differentiated tumor, lymphovascular and perineural invasion, obstructing tumor, high preoperative CEA levels, and MSI stable tumors [13].

21.2 Flow Cytometry (FC)

Flow cytometry is a technology that rapidly analyzes single cells or particles and has been utilized in multiple scientific areas such as immunology, virology, molecular biology, cancer biology, and infectious disease monitoring. FC is a useful for the quantification of cellular phenotype and analysis of cellular processes, such as cell

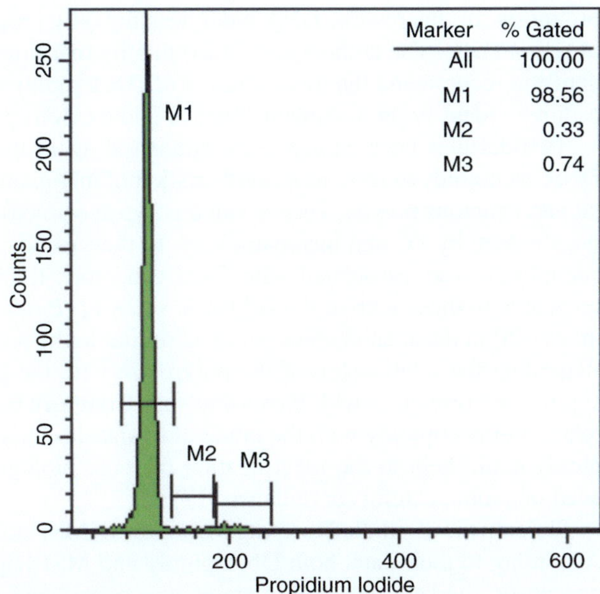

Fig. 21.2 DNA content histogram by flow cytometry. The M1 area corresponds to G0/G1, the M2 area to S, and the M3 area to the G2/M cell cycle phase of a diploid cell population

proliferation and death. DNA analysis has been established among the first applications of FC. Cell cycle analysis assays consist of staining DNA with a saturating amount of DNA binding dye. Samples are analyzed using ploidy modeling software to determine the cell cycle phases [14].

DNA cytometry is currently the most widely used method to detect aneuploidy. In normal state, human cells are genetically diploid, consisting of two DNA content units (one chromosome from each parent) (Fig. 21.2). Aneuploidy represents an abnormal quantity of DNA. In 2004, the "aneuploidy theory of carcinogenesis" was proposed, suggesting that aneuploidy is the primary cause of genomic instability and carcinogenesis. The CIN pathway that was mentioned previously reflects the role of aneuploidy in tumorigenesis in CRC [15].

21.2.1 Flow Cytometry (FC) in CRC

21.2.1.1 Ploidy Status

Since 1982, several studies have implicating FC in detecting ploidy status in either paraffin embedded or fresh/fresh frozen tumor specimens and elucidating its role in CRC diagnosis and prognosis.

Grabsch et al. reviewing the existing data tried to answer the question of the clinical value of routine DNA ploidy measurement in several gastrointestinal pathologies, including CRC. Regarding CRC, they found that DNA aneuploidy incidence was ranging from 38 to 93%. DNA aneuploidy was also variable (up to 38%) in different sites of primary tumor and lymph node metastasis and did not consistently correlate with histological tumor type or grade of differentiation or prognosis. In this review, DNA index was the only prognostic marker independent of tumor stage. The authors concluded that by that time there was not enough evidence to recommend the measurement of DNA ploidy as a routine diagnostic procedure to identify premalignant changes in the colon epithelium [16].

Two decades later, Stoian et al. addressed again the question of the ability of DNA aneuploidy to serve as an early marker of malignant transformation of colorectal adenomatous polyps. They divided polyp specimens in two and examined each one of them by FC and histopathology. In their results, adenomas presenting with aneuploidy were associated with focal cancerous lesions in a greater proportion compared to those with diploidy [100% vs 28%] ($P < 0.01$). Additionally, the DNA index (DI) in the adenomatous part was similar to the one of the carcinomatous part. Regarding the relationship of the polyp size with the ploidy status, they reported significant correlation with increasing size. Contrariwise, they did not find any correlation of aneuploidy with the grade of dysplasia. They conclude that polyp aneuploidy could help to the identification of more biologically aggressive lesions in need of a more careful surveillance [17].

Sinicrope et al. studied the prognostic role of MSI along with DNA ploidy status. According to their data, both DNA ploidy and MSI-High status were independent prognostic markers, but ploidy status was considered more significant. Diploidy tumors were associated with better survival in both MSI-High and in MSS/MSI-Low patients [18]. The same conclusion was reported by Walther et al. in their meta-analysis of CIN and prognosis in colorectal cancer [19].

Araujo et al., in a meta-analysis of non-randomized studies, showed reduction in 5-year overall mortality from 43.2% for patients with aneuploid tumors to 29.2% for patients with diploid tumors. The same percentage of overall mortality reduction was noticed in stage II colon cancer with diploid tumors. This observation highlighted the possibility of aneuploidy status as a new criterion for high-risk characterization of stage II patients [20]. In VICTOR trial, Muradov et al. studied prognostic factors regarding survival in CRC stage II and III patients. In their results, MSI and CIN were independent predictors of disease-free survival [DFS] (for MSI, hazard ratio (HR) = 0.58, 95% confidence interval (CI) 0.36–0.93, and p = 0.021; for CIN, HR = 1.54, 95% CI 1.14–2.08, and p = 0.005). Higher levels of CIN were associated with poorer DFS. Also, the combination of MSI+/CIN+ tumors was rare (2.7%). The authors suggested that identification of MSI and CIN status has the potential to drive the selection of stage II/III CRC patients, who may benefit from more aggressive investigation and therapy [21]. Comparable results showed by Hveem et al. in a 952 CRC patients series. They also confirmed that CIN was an independent predictor of early relapse and death among stage II patients [22]. A meta-analysis published in 2015 focused on the association of the individual tumor stages with the ploidy status. After analysis of 7072 CRC patients by image and flow cytometry, aneuploidy was ranged from 39 to 81%. Overall, aneuploidy was detected significantly more frequently in late-stage (III and IV) than in early-stage (I and II) CRC (p = 0.0001). Almost half of the studies included described a significant prognostic impact of aneuploidy for overall, disease-specific, and recurrence-free survival. The conclusion implied an increased genomic instability with CRC progression, although for the individual tumor stages, only a minority of studies described statistical significances in survival differences for aneuploid versus euploid tumors [23]. The same authors had also reported previously that both elevated CEA level and aneuploidy were independent predictive markers for metachronous metastasis in their series [24].

21.2.1.2 Circulating Tumor Cells Detection

Another application of FC in CRC is the identification of circulating tumor cells (CTC) in peripheral blood samples. Although CTCs were first discovered in 1860, more than a century has passed till it became feasible and affordable to measure them in blood and evaluate its role in CRC patient prognosis. There is increasing evidence that CTCs comprise a heterogeneous pool of cells that includes epithelial tumor cells, tumor cells undergoing EMT, and tumor stem cells. Many believe that the later are responsible for metastatic disease progression because, even though curative resection, CRC patients develop recurrence in 20–30% during follow-up. It is believed that either occult metastatic foci continue to grow postoperatively or that viable tumor cells with proliferative and metastatic potential have been shed into the bloodstream from the primary tumor site during resection [25, 26]. In a systematic review, the presence of CTCs in peripheral blood at least 24 h after resection of CRCs was found to be an independent prognostic marker of recurrence and poor survival [25]. Additionally, studies have shown that the CTC count reflects tumor burden to some extent and increases with increasing tumor stage [26]. The identification of CTCs in metastatic CRC (mCRC) patient samples potentially indicates the reseeding of metastasis from metastatic lesions [27].

Evaluation of CTCs is currently a developing technique which is expected to contribute to better identification of high-risk patients and personalization of treatments.

Several methods have been utilized in the detection and quantification of CTCs including reverse transcriptase-PCR, membrane array, immunocytochemical staining, microfluidics, and FC. Different methodologies regarding the amount of blood taken or sampling time before or after CRC treatment have been utilized to have the best result in CTC isolation. To isolate CTCs from other blood cells several antibody labeling surface markers have been used such as CD326 (epithelial cell adhesion molecule), cytokeratins (CK19, CK20, CK7), 4,6-diamidino-2-phenylindole (DAPI), CD26, CD133, CD44, and CEA [26].

The advantage of flow cytometry is the ability of single-cell analysis which permits to include or exclude from the analysis cell populations of doubtful origin at any time after sample acquisition and to detect as low as one cell in less than 20 mL of blood [28].

Galizia et al. applied FC to detect CTCs (CD326$^+$, CD45$^-$) in CRC patients both prior and post-surgical resection (after 1 month). In 71% of patients ≥3 CTC/7.5 ml of blood were found. The CTC count was significantly related to CRC stage and elevated CEA and noticeably all stage IV patients were CTC positive. Most of the patients had significant decrease in CTC levels postoperatively, but 23% of those continue to have countable CTCs, which questions the effect of radical resection. Many of those who remained CTC high postoperatively developed recurrence. The latter implicates the possible role of postoperative CTC evaluation in different treatment selection or early metastasis detection [28]. In a similar study, Musina et al. evaluated the CTC count before and after CRC specimen resection in blood taken intraoperatively. A threshold of CTC positive patients was set at ≥ 4 CTCs/4mL blood. They found no statistical difference in the CTCs count, which would have been provoked by surgical manipulation of the tumor. In multivariate analysis, only the female sex and the tumor location at the colon were significantly associated with CTC positivity after resection.

The detection of CTCs is a rather time-consuming process and most of the researchers need at least 2 hours. Lopresti et al. reported a new FC methodology that manages to limit the blood sample processing for CTCs in less than 1 h. They studied blood taken from malignant and nonmalignant patients and reported accurate prediction of which samples are derived from cancer donors [29].

21.2.1.3   Intraoperative Flow Cytometry

During the last decade, FC has been utilized in the clinical setting as an adjunct diagnostic tool intraoperatively. In surgical oncology, the major goal is to provide the patient with a complete tumor resection. To accomplish that in most of the tumors is important to define the adequacy of the resection margins. Traditionally, this refers to intraoperative consultation by a pathologist, which includes gross inspection of the integrity of the specimen, frozen section (FS) of the tumor or the resection margins, and cytology evaluation. The pathologist usually gives a report regarding the existence or not of malignancy in frozen sections or cytology in approximately 20 min. This report guides the surgeon to proceed or not to further excision to accomplish the desired tumor free margins. The overall accuracy of FS as a diagnostic test is approximately 95.1% and may vary between tissue types and sampling methods [30].

In CRC every colonic resection specimen has at least three surgical resection margins: the proximal, the distal, and the radial margin. As stated in the previous section, in colon resection the adequate margins are easily succeed due to the adequate length of the bowel. Contrariwise, in rectal cancer, it is of great importance for the patient not only to become tumor free but also to retain the anus. These sphincter-sparing procedures are made possible by neoadjuvant CRT and evolution in surgical technique. Studies have shown that a minimum of 1 cm free distal margin can ensure adequate oncological resection [31]. In surgical practice, although most of the positive margins are located at the circumferential margin, a 30% are still affects the distal resection margin. Therefore, some suggest that the intraoperative pathological assessment should be routinely used in very low rectal cancer with potentially insecure margins [32]. Khoury et al. estimated the distal margins in rectal specimens of CRC by FS and reported that the overall sensitivity, specificity, and accuracy of FS examination were high: 83%, 98%, and 95%, respectively. This accuracy rate did not alter by neoadjuvant CRT [33].

Several reports have highlighted that intraoperative FC (iFC) is a promising method for intracranial tumor surgery, which can identify the tumor's grade, diagnose lymphoma, and define the gliomas boundaries in approximately 6 min, and also have a prognostic role in glioma [34]. Comparable accuracy of iFC to pathology has also been seen in recent publications, regarding the evaluation of excision margins in breast cancer conserving surgery, in liver and head and neck malignancies [35–37].

The role of iFC in CRC is a relatively new prospect that aspires to become the guidance tool of the colorectal surgeon in the acquisition of tumor free margins. Our research team, which introduced the Ioannina Protocol in iFC, having already the knowledge in assessing resection margins, have utilized this method in CRC for the first time [38]. We retrieved tissue samples of 3–5 mm from normal and cancerous mucosa from patients with endoscopic biopsy confirmed CRC. The study group included patients with both colon and rectal cancer and there were also cases which received neoadjuvant CRT. The samples were procured immediately after the completeness of standard colorectal excision according to the current CRC guidelines (Fig. 21.3). The study methodology is summarized in Fig. 21.4. An expert cytometrist, who was blinded to the origin of the tissue, following the Ioannina Protocol, reported in 10 minutes on the sample origin. Additional confirmation was added by subsequently histology examination of the sites that the tissue samples had been procured. The FC method included the estimation of DNA ploidy, which was given by the DNA index, defined as a proportion of the modal DNA values of the tumor G0 and G1 cells (peak channel) to the DNA content of the diploid standard and the tumor index, which was defined as the percentage of cells in S and G2/M cell cycle phase. Representative DNA content histograms of normal and cancerous epithelium in CRC patients with different DNA ploidy tumors are shown in Fig. 21.5a–c.

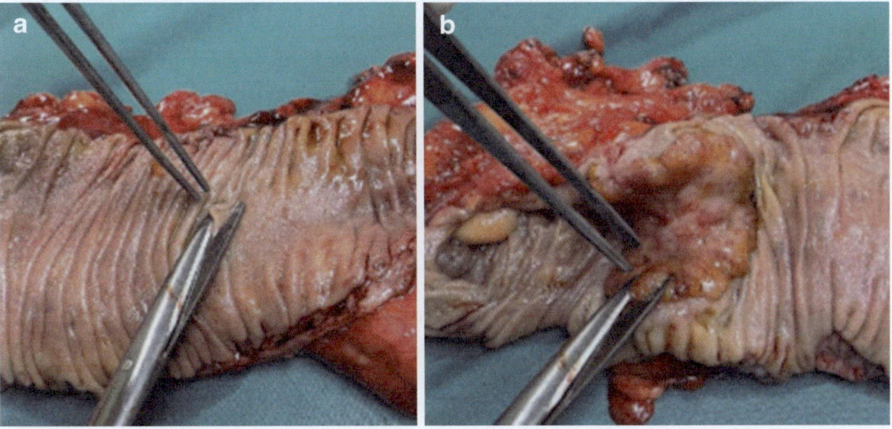

Fig. 21.3 Intraoperative sampling of normal (**a**) and cancerous (**b**) epithelium following colorectal specimen excision

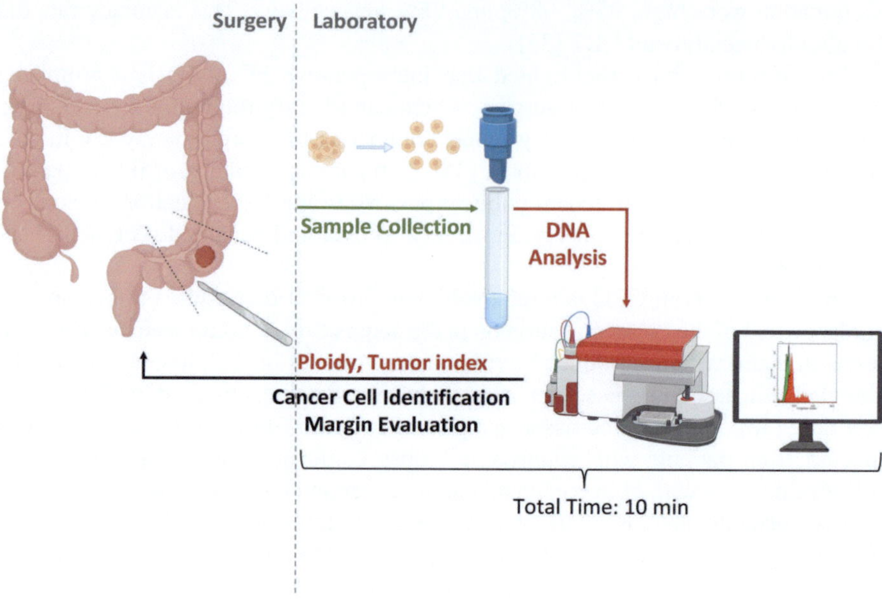

Fig. 21.4 iFC study workflow. Tissue samples were procured following colorectal resection and sent to the molecular biology laboratory. The standard protocol includes tissue homogenization, stain of cells with propidium iodide, and flow cytometry analysis of the DNA content. Tumor index and DNA index are the parameters used to identify and characterize cancer cells and evaluate tumor margin status. (Reproduced from [38] with permission from Elsevier)

In our results, the percentage of G0/G1 cells in cancer cells was significantly lower and additionally the tumor index was significantly higher in all cancer samples, irrespectively of tumor stage. We estimated that a cut-off value of 10.5% for tumor index predicts the presence of tumor cells with approximately 91% accuracy (82.2% sensitivity, 99.9% specificity). The administration of neoadjuvant CRT altered the accuracy of iFC. In the subgroup of rectal cancer, the overall accuracy of iFC in predicting the presence of tumor cells was 85% (88% in no neoadjuvant group and 79% in neoadjuvant group) (Fig. 21.5d). In the interpretation of this difference between neoadjuvant and non-neoadjuvant groups, we identified six rectal cancer patients that received neoadjuvant CRT. In these patients no cancer cells were detected by iFC. In two of them there was complete tumor response to treatment, in one patient the histology confirmed no tumor at the sample site and in the rest of them the histology showed residual cancer or isolated tumor foci in the deeper layers of bowel wall or inside the post treatment fibrosis [38].

Although, this study consists of a preliminary evaluation of iFC in CRC, the results highlight its potential role as an auxiliary tool in the detection of cancer cells and further estimation of distal resection margin in rectal cancer. Further confirmation by larger studies and probably different sampling techniques in cases with neoadjuvant CRT might improve the iFC accuracy and provide a guiding tool for the future surgeon.

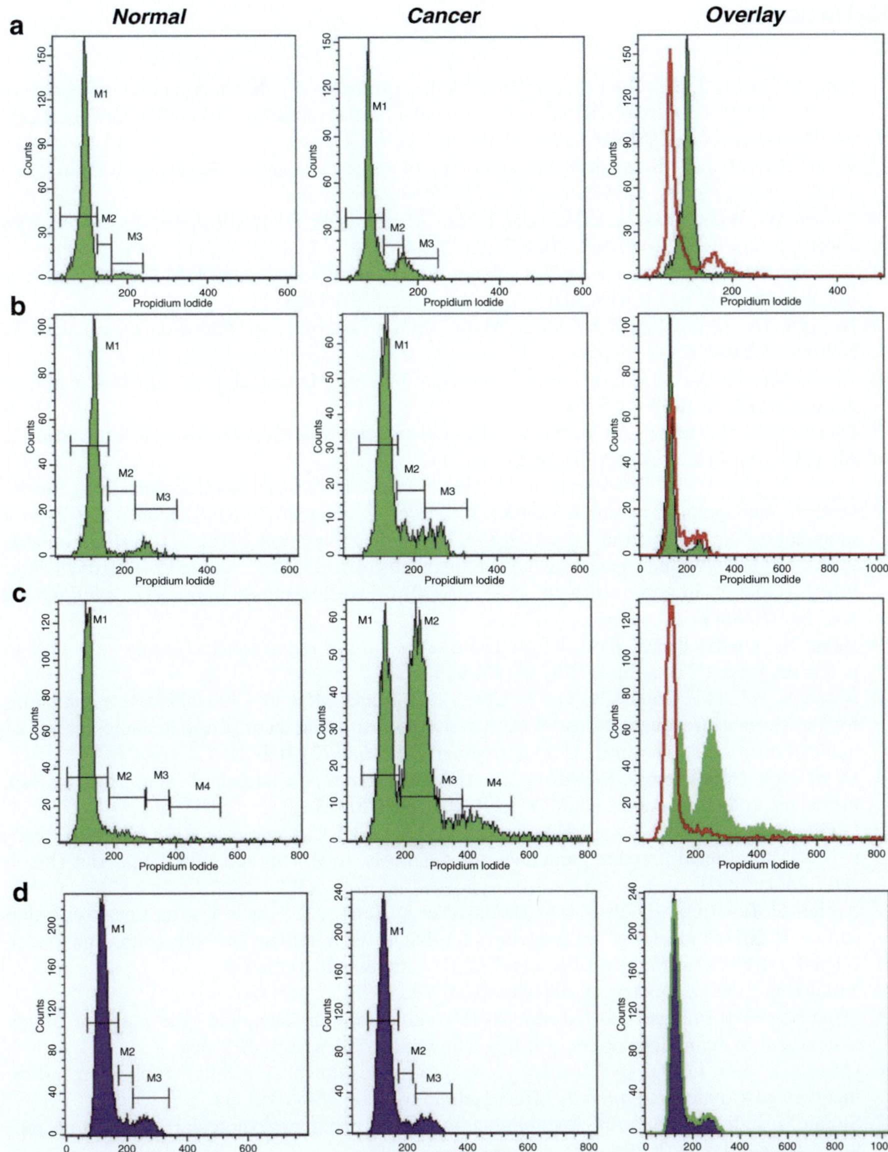

Fig. 21.5 Analysis of representative cases with iFC. In each case, histograms of DNA content are presented. Left column of histograms contains the analysis of normal cells of respective case, middle column of histograms the analysis of cancer cells, and an overlay is depicted in the right. (**a**) A hypoploid tumor (DNA index = 0.9) sample from a 75-years-old male patient with stage IIA (T3N0M0) sigmoid colon cancer, (**b**) a diploid tumor with significantly higher tumor index (22.5%) than that of normal cells (7%)—55-years-old male with stage IIA (T3N0M0) descending colon cancer, (**c**) a hyperploid tumor with high tumor index (DI = 1.5)—75-years-old female patient with stage IIA (T3N0M0) transverse colon cancer, (**d**) Cancer cells with similar tumor index (11.5%) to that of normal cells (10.5%) in a rectal cancer patient, who received neoadjuvant CRT and presented with complete tumor response (TRG = 0). (Courtesy by G. Vartholomatos)

References

1. Sung H, Ferlay J, Siegel RL, Laversanne M, Soerjomataram I, Jemal A, et al. Global cancer statistics 2020: GLOBOCAN estimates of incidence and mortality worldwide for 36 cancers in 185 countries. CA Cancer J Clin. 2021;71(3):209–49.
2. Rawla P, Sunkara T, Barsouk A. Epidemiology of colorectal cancer: incidence, mortality, survival, and risk factors. Prz Gastroenterol. 2019;14(2):89–103.
3. Munro MJ, Wickremesekera SK, Peng L, Tan ST, Itinteang T. Cancer stem cells in colorectal cancer: a review. J Clin Pathol. 2018;71(2):110–6.
4. Al-Sohaily S, Biankin A, Leong R, Kohonen-Corish M, Warusavitarne J. Molecular pathways in colorectal cancer. J Gastroenterol Hepatol. 2012;27(9):1423–31.
5. Nojadeh JN, Sharif SB, Sakhinia E. Microsatellite instability in colorectal cancer. EXCLI J. 2018;17:159–68.
6. Weiser MR. AJCC 8th edition: colorectal cancer. Ann Surg Oncol. 2018;25(6):1454–5. https://doi.org/10.1245/s10434-018-6462-1.
7. Fadaka AO, Pretorius A, Klein A. Biomarkers for stratification in colorectal cancer: MicroRNAs. Cancer Control. 2019;26(1):1–11.
8. Xynos E, Gouvas N, Triantopoulou C, Tekkis P, et al. Clinical practice guidelines for the surgical management of colon cancer: a consensus statement of the hellenic and cypriot olorectal cancer study group by the HeSMO. Ann Gastroenterol. 2016;29(1):3–17. Available from http://www.annalsgastro.gr/index.php/annalsgastro/article/download/2360/1658%5Cn; http://ovidsp.ovid.com/ovidweb.cgi?T=JS&PAGE=reference&D=emed18a&NEWS=N&AN=607690440.
9. Heald RJ, Husband EM, Ryall RDH. The mesorectum in rectal cancer surgery—the clue to pelvic recurrence? Br J Surg. 1982;69(10):613–6.
10. Xynos E, Tekkis P, Gouvas N, Vini L, Chrysou E, Tzardi M, et al. Clinical practice guidelines for the surgical treatment of rectal cancer: a consensus statement of the hellenic society of medical oncologists (hesmo). Ann Gastroenterol. 2016;29(2):103–26.
11. De Falco V, Napolitano S, Roselló S, Huerta M, Cervantes A, Ciardiello F, et al. How we treat metastatic colorectal cancer. ESMO Open. 2020;4:e000813.
12. Glynne-Jones R, Wyrwicz L, Tiret E, Brown G, Rödel C, Cervantes A, et al. Rectal cancer: ESMO clinical practice guidelines for diagnosis, treatment and follow-up. Ann Oncol. 2017;28(4):22–40.
13. Argilés G, Tabernero J, Labianca R, Hochhauser D, Salazar R, Iveson T, et al. Localised colon cancer: ESMO clinical practice guidelines for diagnosis, treatment and follow-up. Ann Oncol. 2020;31(10):1291–305. https://doi.org/10.1016/j.annonc.2020.06.022.
14. Villas BH. Flow cytometry: an overview. Cell Vis. 1998;5(1):56–61.
15. Danielsen HE, Pradhan M, Novelli M. Revisiting tumour aneuploidy-the place of ploidy assessment in the molecular era. Nat Rev Clin Oncol. 2016;13(5):291–304.
16. Grabsch H, Kerr D, Quirke P. Is there a case for routine clinical application of ploidy measurements in gastrointestinal tumours? Histopathology. 2004;45(4):312–34.
17. Stoian M, Indrei L, Stoian B. Aneuploidia: marker of malignant colorectal adenomatous polyps. Clin Res Trials. 2020;6(3):1–6.
18. Sinicrope FA, Rego RL, Halling KC, Foster N, Sargent DJ, La Plant B, et al. Prognostic impact of microsatellite instability and DNA ploidy in human colon carcinoma patients. Gastroenterology. 2006;131(3):729–37.
19. Fichera A. Association between chromosomal instability and prognosis in colorectal cancer: a meta-analysis. Dis Colon Rectum. 2008;51(11):1733–4.
20. Araujo SEA, Bernardo WM, Habr-Gama A, Kiss DR, Cecconello I. DNA ploidy status and prognosis in colorectal cancer: a meta-analysis of published data. Dis Colon Rectum. 2007;50(11):1800–10.

21. Mouradov D, Domingo E, Gibbs P, Jorissen RN, Li S, Soo PY, et al. Survival in stage II/III colorectal cancer is independently predicted by chromosomal and microsatellite instability, but not by specific driver mutations. Am J Gastroenterol. 2013;108(11):1785–93.

22. Hveem TS, Merok MA, Pretorius ME, Novelli M, Bævre MS, Sjo OH, et al. Prognostic impact of genomic instability in colorectal cancer. Br J Cancer. 2014;110(8):2159–64.

23. Laubert T, Freitag-Wolf S, Linnebacher M, König A, Vollmar B, Habermann JK. Stage-specific frequency and prognostic significance of aneuploidy in patients with sporadic colorectal cancer—a meta-analysis and current overview. Int J Color Dis. 2015;30(8):1015–28.

24. Laubert T, Bente V, Freitag-Wolf S, Voulgaris H, Oberländer M, Schillo K, et al. Aneuploidy and elevated CEA indicate an increased risk for metachronous metastasis in colorectal cancer. Int J Color Dis. 2013;28(6):767–75.

25. Peach G, Kim C, Zacharakis E, Purkayastha S, Ziprin P. Prognostic significance of circulating tumour cells following surgical resection of colorectal cancers: a systematic review. Br J Cancer. 2010;102(9):1327–34. https://doi.org/10.1038/sj.bjc.6605651.

26. Hardingham JE, Grover P, Winter M, Hewett PJ, Price TJ, Thierry B. Detection and clinical significance of circulating tumor cells in colorectal cancer—20 years of progress. Mol Med. 2015;21(1):25–31.

27. Nanduri LK, Hissa B, Weitz J, Schölch S, Bork U. The prognostic role of circulating tumor cells in colorectal cancer. Expert Rev Anticancer Ther. 2019;19(12):1077–88. https://doi.org/10.1080/14737140.2019.1699065.

28. Galizia G, Gemei M, Orditura M, Romano C, Zamboli A, Castellano P, et al. Postoperative detection of circulating tumor cells predicts tumor recurrence in colorectal cancer patients. J Gastrointest Surg. 2013;17(10):1809–18.

29. Lopresti A, Malergue F, Bertucci F, Liberatoscioli ML, Garnier S, DaCosta Q, et al. Sensitive and easy screening for circulating tumor cells by flow cytometry. JCI Insight. 2019;4(14):1–14.

30. Winther C, Græm N. Accuracy of frozen section diagnosis: a retrospective analysis of 4785 cases. APMIS. 2011;119(4–5):259–62.

31. Manegold P, Taukert J, Neeff H, Fichtner-Feigl S, Thomusch O. The minimum distal resection margin in rectal cancer surgery and its impact on local recurrence - a retrospective cohort analysis. Int J Surg. 2019;69(April):77–83.

32. Rickenbacher A, Watson J, Horisberger K, Töpfer A, Weber A, Kessler H, et al. Direct intraoperative assessment of total mesorectal excision specimens by expert pathologists in patients with very low rectal cancer prevents unnecessary abdominoperineal resections. Int J Color Dis. 2020;35(4):755–8.

33. Khoury W, Abboud W, Hershkovitz D, Duek SD. Frozen section examination may facilitate reconstructive surgery for mid and low rectal cancer. J Surg Oncol. 2014;110(8):997–1001.

34. Vartholomatos E, Vartholomatos G, Alexiou GA, Markopoulos GS. The past, present and future of flow cytometry in central nervous system malignancies. Methods Protoc. 2021;4(1):1–13.

35. Vartholomatos G, Harissis H, Markopoulos GS, Alexiou GA. The role of intraoperative flow cytometry in breast-conserving surgery. Ann Surg Oncol. 2021;28(s3):785–6. https://doi.org/10.1245/s10434-021-10794-5.

36. Vartholomatos G, Basiari L, Kastanioudakis I, Psichogios G, Alexiou GA. The role of intraoperative flow cytometry in surgical margins of head and neck malignancies. Ear Nose Throat J. 2021;100(10):989S–90S.

37. Markopoulos GS, Glantzounis GK, Goussia AC, Lianos GD, Karampa A, Alexiou GA, et al. Touch imprint intraoperative flow cytometry as a complementary tool for detailed assessment of resection margins and tumor biology in liver surgery for primary and metastatic liver neoplasms. Methods Protoc. 2021;4:3.

38. Georvasili VK, Markopoulos GS, Batistatou A, Mitsis M, Messinis T, Lianos GD, et al. Detection of cancer cells and tumor margins during colorectal cancer surgery by intraoperative flow cytometry. Int J Surg. 2022;104(June):106717. https://doi.org/10.1016/j.ijsu.2022.106717.

Chapter 22
Future Perspectives of iFC

Georgios S. Markopoulos, Georgios Alexiou ⓘ, Evrysthenis Vartholomatos, and Georgios Vartholomatos ⓘ

22.1 Introduction: Revisiting the State of the Art

A foundation stone of treatment of cancer and the first line of treatment is surgical management [1]. Over 4 out of 5 of the ~15 million cases in the year 2015 were candidates for surgery, while by 2030, it has been estimated that >45 million surgical procedures will be carried out, regarding cancer cases [1]. The timely characterization of tumor biology and margin status is essential for clinical management. Positive margins are an indication of local recurrence, require adjuvant chemotherapy, and lead to significant financial and prognostic implications for the patient [2]. The necessity for accurate resection margin evaluation makes the development of next-generation techniques that would detect the presence of cancer cells in a given sample, such as intraoperative flow cytometry (iFC) [3].

A concept revisited throughout this book is that iFC contributes to tumor cell detection and resection margin status evaluation with a considerably high accuracy. The methodology exhibits a high sensitivity and specificity in several types of malignancy, including brain [4], head-and-neck [5], breast [6], liver [7], and colorectal cancer [8]. With a high level of accuracy that in most cases is beyond 90%, iFC

G. S. Markopoulos · E. Vartholomatos
Haematology Laboratory - Unit of Molecular Biology and Translational Flow Cytometry, University Hospital of Ioannina, Ioannina, Greece

Faculty of Medicine, Neurosurgical Institute, School of Health Sciences, University of Ioannina, Ioannina, Greece

G. Alexiou
Department of Neurosurgery, University Hospital of Ioannina, Ioannina, Greece
e-mail: galexiou@uoi.gr

G. Vartholomatos (✉)
Unit of Molecular Biology, University Hospital of Ioannina, Ioannina, Greece

G. Alexiou, G. Vartholomatos (eds.), *Intraoperative Flow Cytometry*, https://doi.org/10.1007/978-3-031-33517-4_22

has developed to now be considered as a reliable diagnostic tool in the operation theater. The main advantage of iFC is based on the high throughput of data acquisition and analysis performed by a flow cytometer, which offers a precise characterization of phenotypic properties at the cellular level [9]. The implementation of a uniquely rapid analysis framework below 8 min, the Ioannina protocol, is another advantage of iFC that allows implementation in a surgical procedure.

In this chapter, the most recent developments and the future perspectives for iFC will be discussed. We envision that further progress and implementation of iFC protocols would prove an irreplaceable ally in our fight against cancer.

22.2   Future Perspectives A: Novel Protocols

Flow cytometry, since its development in the late twentieth century, has been evolved as the science of quantification of cellular phenotype and into a powerful tool assisting both research and diagnosis purposes.

The successful application of iFC in several types of malignancy warrants the further development of iFC protocols, in order to be applied as a universal diagnostic technique during surgery in the characterization of cancer cells and the evaluation of resection margins status. Toward this end, iFC is currently applied in novel protocols that include gynecological and urological malignancies.

Gynecological malignancies affect organs throughout the female reproductive tract, with endometrium, cervix, ovaries, and vulva being the most commonly affected [10, 11]. It has been estimated that gynecological malignancies represent account for more than 1.3 million new cases and approximately almost 650 thousand deaths annually, emerging as an alarming global health issue [12].

An original pilot study from our research group investigated the impact of iFC in samples from 42 women with gynecological malignancies [13]. The study by Anastasiadi et al. accomplished a response time for iFC to obtain results was 5–6 min/sample, which is similar to the most developed iFC assays to date. DNA-index calculation, an index of chromosomal abnormalities, informed that 21 women the samples were aneuploid. The proliferative potential of cancer cells was mirrored in an increase of tumor index, revealed that iFC had 100% sensitivity and 90.5% specificity (an accuracy of ~95%) in detecting cancer cells in a given sample. The analysis of a representative case of endometrial cancer, is presented if Fig. 22.1. The data from iFC were corroborated from the final pathology assessment.

Bladder cancer represent the majority of urological cancers and is the most common malignancy of the male urinary tract, with an elevated frequency in males than females [14]. In 2020 bladder cancer reached almost 450,000 cases and 160,000 deaths in male patients [12]. Transurethral resection is the golden standard methodology that offers both toward diagnosis and therapy of non-invasive bladder cancer [15]. However, a successful operation is based on variables that require an accurate characterization of cancer cells for both diagnostic and therapeutic management [15]. Recently, we enlisted patients for the first application of iFC in bladder cancer and urological malignancies. The preliminary results from our pilot study including

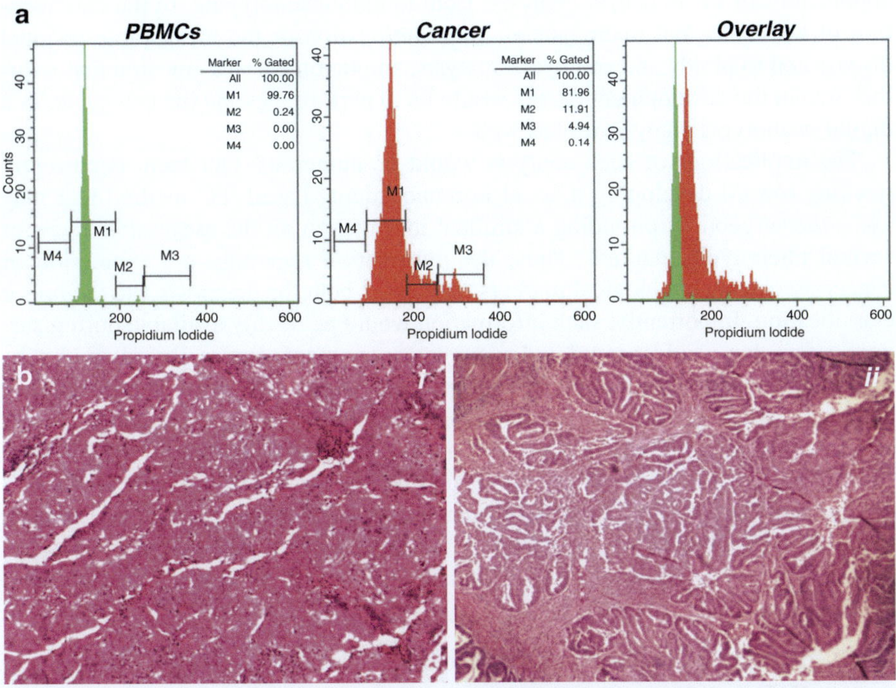

Fig. 22.1 Analysis of endometrial cancer by iFC and pathology assessment. (**a**) DNA content analysis by iFC in normal peripheral blood monocytes (PBMCs, in green color) and cancer cells (red color). The percentage of cells corresponding at different cell cycle phases is presented in the right part, inside each respective histogram. (**b**) Pathology assessment: a moderately differentiated (Grade II) ovary cancer, following hematoxylin/eosin stain at a ×40 (I) and ×200 (II) magnification. The figure was published under an open access Creative Common CC BY license and reproduced from citation [13]

52 individuals indicates a positive predictive value of 96.2%, a negative predictive value of 100% and ultimately an accuracy of 98.1% (unpublished data).

The ongoing results from both the aforementioned studies warrant the development of iFC in the surgical management of additional malignancies. Both studies indicate a highly accurate (>95%) diagnostic potential. Based on the present encouraging results, we project the development of novel iFC in other types of cancer-excision surgery and that iFC might soon recognized as a universal tool in surgical management of cancer.

22.3 Future Perspectives B: Beyond the Cell Cycle

A main reason behind the fact that Flow Cytometry is among the most effective single-cell analysis techniques is the capacity to perform phenotypic analysis, based on specific cellular marker characterization. This dynamic leads to several applications of FC in cancer analysis: from immunophenotyping, to the classification of hematological malignancies, to quantification of the measurable residual disease and to ploidy and cell cycle analysis, among others. We envision that a further step in the development of iFC would be to perform beyond the cell cycle, as a digital phenotypic analysis tool as well.

The implications of such analysis would be numerous. Our team is currently working toward developing a novel immunostaining-based iFC method that may assist the surgeon by providing additional information on the expression levels of several phenotypic markers. Thus, the information regarding the expression of cancer-associated histological markers may assist both the diagnosis and the tumor classification. Importantly, such information would be readily available during surgery, a fact that would a rapid and accurate cancer management. Based on unpublished data, using a cytokeratin phenotypic analysis in orthopedic surgeries as an archetype, we found that our methodology could be applied as an adjunct to the standard histopathological examination of tumor samples. Our preliminary results warrant further investigation in a clinical study in order to develop a novel iFC methodology that would offer a more accurate cancer typification, beyond the standard cell cycle analysis.

22.4 Future Perspectives C: Towards Sarissa, a Real-Time iFC Analyzer

The rapid analysis made possible by iFC, with times for sample preparation and analysis that can fall below 5 minutes, gives a promise for a future real-time analyzer that may be applied directly in the operation theater. Our research team has previously suggested the development of a real-time analyzer for brain tumor analysis, namely Sarissa [16]. The rationale of Sarissa is based on two principles. First, it is known that Cavitron ultrasonic surgical aspirator (CUSA) is a system that assist neurosurgical dissections for the removal of brain malignancies. CUSA dissections result in an aspirate that is an abundant and viable source of cells that can be compatible for flow cytometry analysis [17]. Second, online real-time flow cytometry is now possible, having successfully applied in the analysis of microbial populations [18] and circulating tumor cells [19]. The development of a device that combines CUSA (or analogous aspiration systems for other types of malignancy) and a real-time flow cytometer would make Sarissa a reality.

22.5 Future Perspectives D: Correlation with Imaging Findings

Imaging has a crucial role in patient's management. Magnetic resonance imaging (MRI) is the examination of choice for central nervous system tumor imaging. MRI provides high image resolution, fast image acquisition, and high safety profile for patients. Nuclear medicine techniques namely positron emission tomography (PET) and single photon emission tomography (SPECT) provide information on metabolism, physiology, and functionality of the neoplasms beyond anatomical imaging that MRI offers. Advanced MRI techniques namely diffusion weighted imaging (DWI), perfusion-weighted imaging (PWI), and spectroscopy provide additional important information for the evaluation of a space occupying lesion. Alexiou et al. evaluated whether glioma aggressiveness as assessed by flow cytometry correlated with DWI metric, such as apparent diffusion coefficient (ADC) values that measure water diffusivity, and PWI metrics, such as rCBV that measures the state of the tumor vascular bed. Decreased ACD values and increased rCBV usually correlates with increased malignancy. The study included 30 glioma patients and a significant correlation was found between G2/M and S + G2/M phase fractions with rCBV. A significant negative correlation was demonstrated between ADC and S + G2/M. No correlation was found between MRI metrics and ploidy status [20]. Likewise, in a study that included 14 meningiomas, tumors that exhibited increased perfusion, as assessed by rCBV, had significant lower G0/G1 phase fraction and increased G2/M phase fraction. A significant correlation was also observed between fractional anisotropy ratio and G0/G1 phase fraction. Both studies used the intraoperative "Ioannina protocol" for sample analysis by flow cytometry [21].

Flow cytometry metrics have been also correlated with SPECT findings in brain tumor patients. A prospective pilot study included 10 patients, suspicious of having a glioma, that underwent metabolic imaging by 99mTc-Tetrofosmin SPECT a week prior to tumor removal. Radiotracer accumulation in tumors was first assessed visually. Then semiquantitative analysis was performed to the reconstructed SPECT images, by measuring the lesion-to-normal (L/N) uptake ratio. High-grade tumors usually exhibit increased L/N ratio compared to low-grade tumors. Post-surgery samples were analyzed for DNA content distributions. The results of the study demonstrated a significant positive linear correlation between radiotracer uptake and S-phase fraction. Thus, tumors that exhibited increased radiotracer uptake had high S-phase phase fraction [22]. Furthermore, radiotracer uptake also correlated with S-phase fraction in a study that included meningioma patients. This study also found a significant correlation between a SPECT radiotracer uptake and level of aneuploidy and tumor grade [23].

References

1. Sullivan R, Alatise OI, Anderson BO, Audisio R, Autier P, Aggarwal A, Balch C, Brennan MF, Dare A, D'Cruz A. Global cancer surgery: delivering safe, affordable, and timely cancer surgery. Lancet Oncol. 2015;16:1193–224.
2. Orosco RK, Tapia VJ, Califano JA, Clary B, Cohen EE, Kane C, Lippman SM, Messer K, Molinolo A, Murphy JD. Positive surgical margins in the 10 most common solid cancers. Sci Rep. 2018;8:1–9.
3. Vartholomatos G, Alexiou GA, Tatsi V, Harissis H, Markopoulos GS. Next-generation margin evaluation techniques in breast conserving surgery: a memorandum on intraoperative flow cytometry. Eur J Surg Oncol. 2022;48:1439.

4. Alexiou GA, Vartholomatos G, Goussia A, Batistatou A, Tsamis K, Voulgaris S, Kyritsis AP. Fast cell cycle analysis for intraoperative characterization of brain tumor margins and malignancy. J Clin Neurosci. 2015;22:129–32.

5. Vartholomatos G, Basiari L, Exarchakos G, Kastanioudakis I, Komnos I, Michali M, Markopoulos GS, Batistatou A, Papoudou-Bai A, Alexiou GA. Intraoperative flow cytometry for head and neck lesions. Assessment of malignancy and tumour-free resection margins. Oral Oncol. 2019;99:104344. https://doi.org/10.1016/j.oraloncology.2019.06.025.

6. Vartholomatos G, Harissis H, Andreou M, Tatsi V, Pappa L, Kamina S, Batistatou A, Markopoulos GS, Alexiou GA. Rapid assessment of resection margins during breast conserving surgery using intraoperative flow cytometry. Clin Breast Cancer. 2021;21:e602–10.

7. Markopoulos GS, Glantzounis GK, Goussia AC, Lianos GD, Karampa A, Alexiou GA, Vartholomatos G. Touch imprint intraoperative flow cytometry as a complementary tool for detailed assessment of resection margins and tumor biology in liver surgery for primary and metastatic liver neoplasms. Methods Protocols. 2021;4:66.

8. Georvasili VK, Markopoulos GS, Batistatou A, Mitsis M, Messinis T, Lianos GD, Alexiou G, Vartholomatos G, Bali CD. Detection of cancer cells and tumor margins during colorectal cancer surgery by intraoperative flow cytometry. Int J Surg. 2022;104:106717.

9. Shapiro HM. Practical flow cytometry. Hoboken: Wiley; 2005.

10. Stepanian M, Cohn DE. Gynecologic malignancies in adolescents. Adolesc Med Clin. 2004;15:549.

11. Lõhmussaar K, Boretto M, Clevers H. Human-derived model systems in gynecological cancer research. Trends Cancer. 2020;6:1031–43.

12. Sung H, Ferlay J, Siegel RL, Laversanne M, Soerjomataram I, Jemal A, Bray F. Global cancer statistics 2020: GLOBOCAN estimates of incidence and mortality worldwide for 36 cancers in 185 countries. CA Cancer J Clin. 2021;71:209–49.

13. Anastasiadi Z, Mantziou S, Akrivis C, Paschopoulos M, Balasi E, Lianos GD, Alexiou GA, Mitsis M, Vartholomatos G, Markopoulos GS. Intraoperative flow cytometry for the characterization of gynecological malignancies. Biology. 2022;11:1339. https://doi.org/10.3390/biology11091339.

14. Zhu S, Yu W, Yang X, Wu C, Cheng F. Traditional classification and novel subtyping systems for bladder cancer. Front Oncol. 2020;10:102. https://doi.org/10.3389/fonc.2020.00102.

15. Richterstetter M, Wullich B, Amann K, Haeberle L, Engehausen DG, Goebell PJ, Krause FS. The value of extended transurethral resection of bladder tumour (TURBT) in the treatment of bladder cancer. BJU Int. 2012;110:E76–9. https://doi.org/10.1111/j.1464-410X.2011.10904.x.

16. Vartholomatos G, Alexiou GA, Batistatou A, Lykoudis E, Voulgaris S, Kyritsis AP. GV/GA sarissa-Lancet: a proposed real-time flow cytometer for intraoperative identification of glioma margins. Surg Innov. 2016;23:104–5. https://doi.org/10.1177/1553350615589860.

17. Day BW, Stringer BW, Wilson J, Jeffree RL, Jamieson PR, Ensbey KS, Bruce ZC, Inglis P, Allan S, Winter C. Glioma surgical aspirate: a viable source of tumor tissue for experimental research. Cancer. 2013;5:357–71.

18. McEvoy B, Lynch M, Rowan NJ. Opportunities for the application of real-time bacterial cell analysis using flow cytometry for the advancement of sterilization microbiology. J Appl Microbiol. 2021;130:1794–812.

19. Juratli MA, Sarimollaoglu M, Siegel ER, Nedosekin DA, Galanzha EI, Suen JY, Zharov VP. Real-time monitoring of circulating tumor cell release during tumor manipulation using in vivo photoacoustic and fluorescent flow cytometry. Head Neck. 2014;36:1207–15.

20. Zikou AK, Alexiou GA, Vartholomatos G, et al. Correlation of diffusion tensor and dynamic susceptibility contrastMRI with DNA ploidy and cell cycle analysis of gliomas. Clin Neurol Neurosurg. 2015;139:119–24.

21. Alexiou AG, Zikou KA, Vartholomatos G, Goussia A, Voulgaris S, Kyritsis AP, Argyropoulou MI. Correlation of DNA ploidy and cell cycle analysis with diffusion tensor and dynamic susceptibility contrast MRI metrics in meningiomas. Hell J Radiol. 2018;3(3):1–6.
22. Alexiou GA, Tsiouris S, Vartholomatos G, et al. Correlation of glioma proliferation assessed by flow cytometry with 99mTc-Tetrofosmin SPECT uptake. Clin Neurol Neurosurg. 2009;111:808–11.
23. Alexiou GA, Vartholomatos G, Tsiouris S, et al. Evaluation of meningioma aggressiveness by 99mTc-Tetrofosmin SPECT. Clin Neurol Neurosurg. 2008;110:645–8.